AN ATLAS OF CLOSED NAILING OF THE TIBIA AND FEMUR

AN ATLAS OF CLOSED NAILING OF THE TIBIA AND FEMUR

Charles M Court-Brown

MD FRCS Ed (Orth)

Senior Lecturer
Department of Orthopaedic Surgery
University of Edinburgh

Consultant Orthopaedic Surgeon
Royal Infirmary of Edinburgh

Springer-Verlag
New York Berlin Heidelberg
London Paris Tokyo
Hong Kong Barcelona

MARTIN DUNITZ

First published in the United States in 1991
by Springer-Verlag New York Inc.,
175 Fifth Avenue, New York NY10010

First published in the United Kingdom in 1991
by Martin Dunitz Ltd, 7–9 Pratt Street
London NW1 0AE

ISBN 0-387-91396-3 Springer-Verlag
New York Berlin Heidelberg

Phototypeset by Scribe Design, Gillingham, Kent

Origination, printed and bound in Singapore by
Toppan Printing Company (S) Pte Ltd

CONTENTS

FOREWORD

Care of major fractures has changed dramatically in the past three decades. Although internal fixation of these fractures was pioneered in the early years of this century, the masters of non-operative care, such as Laurence Bohler, `Sir Reginald Watson-Jones, and others, dominated. Fractures of the femur were treated with traction, in itself a major advance. During World War I, many lives were saved by this technique, as advocated by Sir Robert Jones. Fractures of the tibia were treated with plaster cast immobilization and occasional external skeletal fixation. The natural history of that particular treatment was clearly outlined by Nichol and Evans, who indicated that those tibial fractures with a poor personality, that is, with major comminution, displacement and an open wound, generally had poor outcomes. It was not until the era of modern anaesthesia, advances in critical care management and surgical asepsis, allowing internal fixation to be performed with a minimal risk of infection, that internal fixation of major fractures could advance. The AO group placed the fixation of fractures on firm biomechanical principles. However, many controversies still remain concerning the role of plates, external fixators and intramedullary nails. The indications for each of these techniques are finding their place in our armamentarium through carefully documented prospective studies.

Although some questions remain unanswered, there can no longer be any doubt that closed intramedullary nailing of the tibia and the femur is a safer and a more effective technique than open nailing: the indications for its use can be expanded to include the polytraumatized patient, on account of reduced intraoperative bleeding, and the more distal and proximal fractures on account of locking techniques. Also, in severe comminuted fractures the soft tissue attachments to the bony fragments remain intact, allowing healing to occur more rapidly. Therefore, the closed technique is more physiological, and has become the treatment of choice for the indications so comprehensively covered in this book.

There is certainly a need for *An Atlas of Closed Nailing of the Tibia and Femur:* it has been clearly and concisely written and is well illustrated with drawings and radiographs. Although titled an 'atlas', Charles Court-Brown has enhanced the book with chapters on the history of intramedullary nailing, the indications for the technique, and in particular the complications. The author's interest and experience in the management of major trauma has led him to produce many scientific studies on intramedullary nailing. It is this expertise that allows him to write with such authority on the technical details included in this book. His considerable personal experience with this particular technique makes this book even more valuable, since it is full of 'pearls'. This book will become required reading for all surgeons, registrars, residents and house officers managing major fractures of the femur and tibia. It should be kept not only in one's library, but also in every operating theatre for ready reference.

MARVIN TILE
Professor of Surgery
Sunnybrook Health Science Center
University of Toronto, Ontario, Canada

PREFACE

It is inevitable that this book will be regarded as advocating the use of locking intramedullary nails for virtually all femoral and tibial fractures. There is obviously some justification for this view but the purpose of writing the book is to describe the techniques of intramedullary nailing that the surgeon might employ once the decision has been made to use an intramedullary nail.

The book has a marked clinical bias and does not include chapters dealing with biomechanics or fracture healing. This information is available in other texts. It is hoped that this book will be used by those surgeons who are taking up the technique of intramedullary nailing. Few references are included in the text but a list of useful references is included at the end of the book.

I am indebted to my colleagues Margaret McQueen and James Christie for their help and to Genevieve Stewart-Smith for typing the manuscript. Inevitably, in Edinburgh, much of the photographic work was undertaken by Mike Devlin and Sonia Miller. My thanks to them.

C M C-B

CHAPTER 1
INTRAMEDULLARY NAILING

Intramedullary devices in various forms have been used to stabilize long bone fractures for many years. It is recorded that the Aztecs used wooden intramedullary nails 500 years ago (Hæger, 1988). Early orthopaedic surgeons such as Senn, Lambotte and Hey Groves investigated the use of ivory, bone and metal nails. It is interesting to note that in the first 20 years of this century, Lambotte and Hey Groves investigated the role of both external fixation and intramedullary nailing in the management of diaphyseal fractures. However, the debate regarding the merits of these two procedures still continues.

Although all current intramedullary techniques, like other surgical procedures, have evolved from earlier surgical operations, the intramedullary techniques that are in common use today derive mainly from the work of Gerhard Küntscher in Germany and the Rush family in the USA. Küntscher is unquestionably the father of reamed intramedullary nailing. Together with Pohl, an instrument maker and metallurgist, he produced a series of nails with a V-shaped profile made of corrosion-resistant steel. Subsequently he invented a number of nails of different shapes culminating in his design of a slotted nail with a clover-leaf cross-section (Figure 1.1a and b). This nail gained world-wide acceptance and is the basis for the design of many modern intramedullary nails. The only bone in which he used a nail of a different shape was the tibia. Initially he developed a nail with a double-V cross-section, but the results were poor. Herzog, however, used Küntscher's femoral nail design and designed a nail with a clover-leaf cross-section of an overall shape suitable for the tibia (Figure 1.2).

Küntscher believed that the enlargement of the medullary canal was of the greatest importance in the practice of intramedullary nailing. He felt that reaming the endosteal surface of the cortex was important for three reasons:

- It permitted the insertion of a nail of sufficient thickness to take over the function of the bone.
- It increased the area of endosteal contact made by the nail.
- It allowed an accurate fit between the nail and the reamed part of the endosteal cortex.

He also believed that the technique provided favourable conditions for callus formation and was not only simple to undertake but applicable to many common fractures.

Küntscher considered that for successful fracture fixation, the incision should be as far from the fracture as possible. He thus also pioneered the concept of closed reamed intramedullary nailing. To achieve this and to adhere to his philosophy of accurate reaming, he invented flexible guided reamers. His reamer design has been adapted over the years but closed reaming has become an essential part of closed intramedullary nailing of both the femur and the tibia. Successful closed nailing also requires the use of image intensification to allow immediate imaging of the fracture at all times during surgery. These techniques were also largely pioneered by Küntscher.

At about the time that Küntscher was developing the reamed intramedullary nail, the Rush family were pursuing the concept of the unreamed nail. They initially used a Steinmann pin and cerclage wiring to immobilize a Monteggia fracture dislocation, and following the success of this procedure they developed the Rush pin. This is a smooth, solid, thin stainless-steel pin with a proximal bend (Figure 1.3). The pins are supplied in different diameters and lengths and are used singly or in pairs to achieve fracture stability.

Following the invention of both reamed and unreamed nails, opinions among orthopaedic surgeons became polarized according to which nailing philosophy was favoured. Such polarization is regrettable as all good trauma surgeons should be familiar with both philosophies and be able to use nails of both types in treating fractures.

Since Küntscher's time, the evolution of the reamed nail has followed two main paths. First the femoral nail shape was altered to correspond with the natural anterior bow of the femur although the overall shape of the tibial nail remained essentially unchanged (Figure 1.4). The second modification involved perforation of the nail to allow the introduction of cross-screws capable of transfixing both bone and nail. This type of 'locking' or 'interlocking' nail was initially introduced by Küntscher but the design has been modified by Huckstep, Klemm, Grosse and Kempf and others. Most current designs permit two cross-screws distal to the fracture with either one, two or three proximal cross-screws. Commonly used examples of this type of nail are the Grosse-Kempf nail (Figure 1.5) and the AO nail (Figure 1.6).

The evolution of unreamed nails has also progressed over the years. Ender produced shaped nails suitable for metaphyseal and diaphyseal fractures (Figure 1.7), these being somewhat more flexible than the Rush nail. Russell and Taylor combined the concept of the unreamed intramedullary nail in the design of larger diameter nails and produced an unreamed, unslotted nail used for virtually the same indications as the reamed locking nail (Figure 1.8).

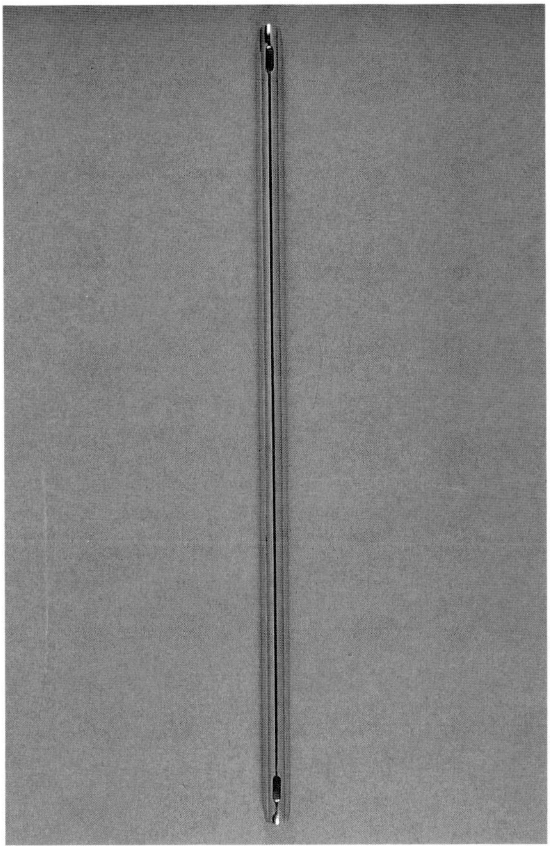

Figure 1.1

a The Küntscher nail: a straight, stainless-steel intramedullary nail designed for use in the femur and humerus. There is a slot at each end of the nail to facilitate nail extraction.

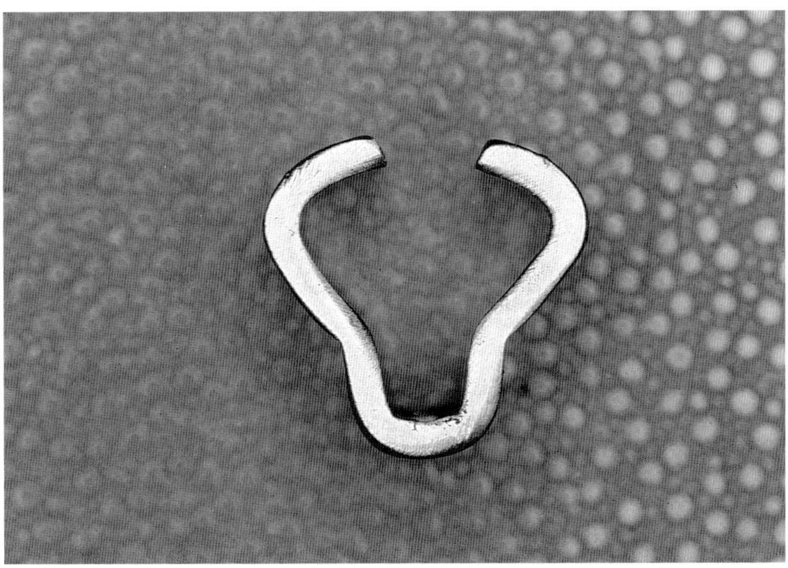

b A combination of the clover-leaf cross-section with the posteriorly located slot allows for compression of the nail during insertion. This facilitates endosteal contact, thereby increasing fracture stability.

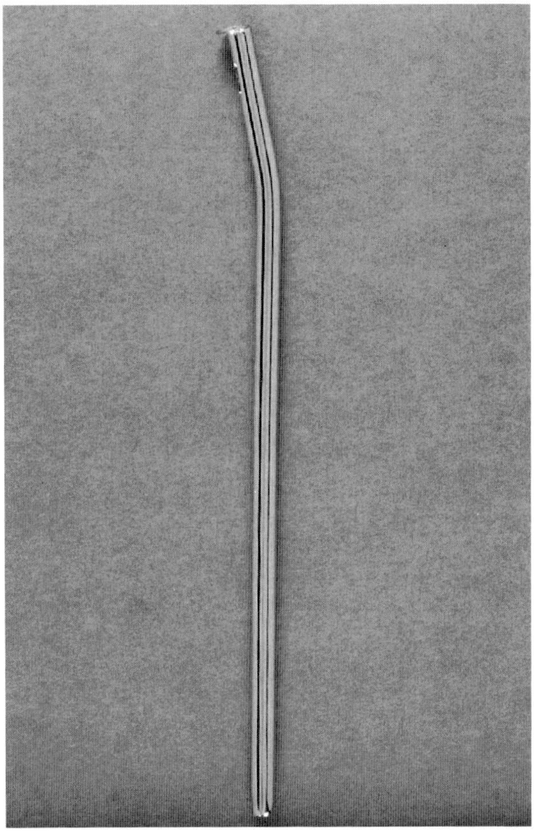

Figure 1.2

The Küntscher-Herzog tibial nail has a clover-leaf cross-section and a posteriorly located slot to aid endosteal contact. The proximal end of the nail is curved to facilitate placement within the tibia.

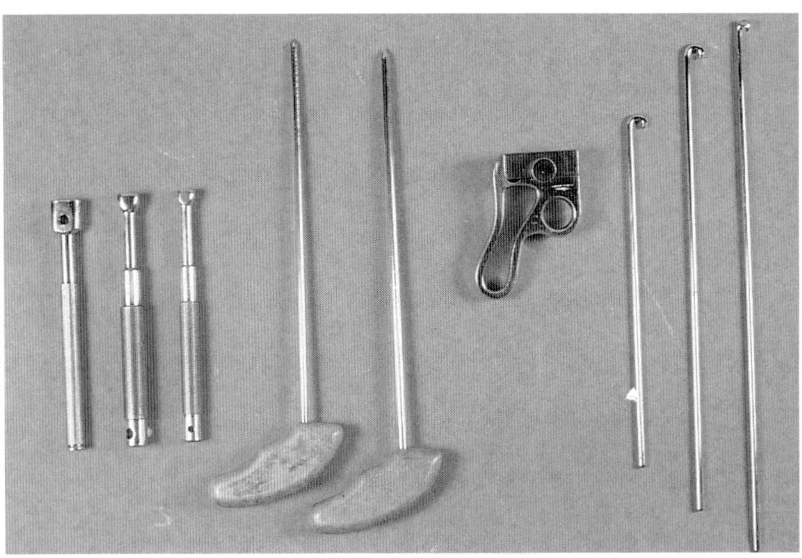

Figure 1.3

Rush pins and equipment necessary for their insertion. From left to right, the photograph shows Rush pin introducers, reamers, handle for gripping the proximal end of the pins and the Rush pins themselves.

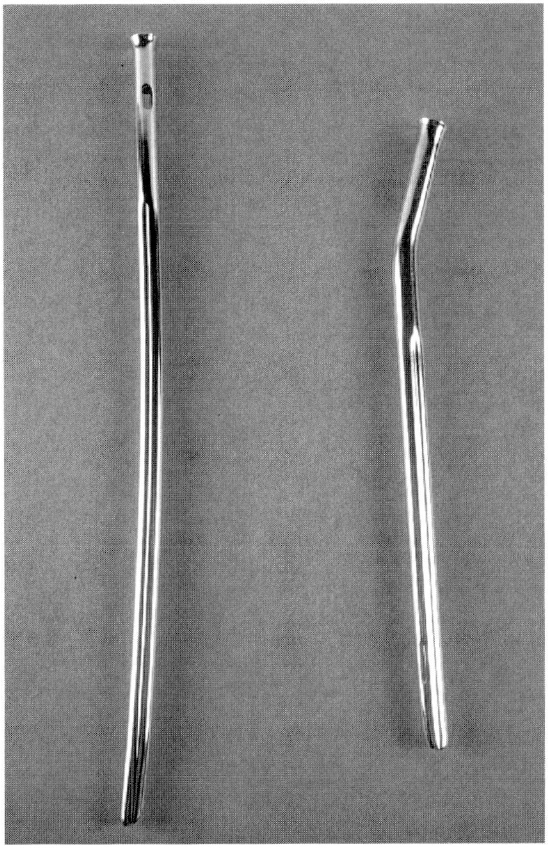

Figure 1.4

The original AO femoral and tibial nails. The femoral nail was curved to correspond to the normal femoral shape. The tibial nail was of a conventional shape but had distal slots cut bilaterally to allow for the insertion of anti-rotation wires.

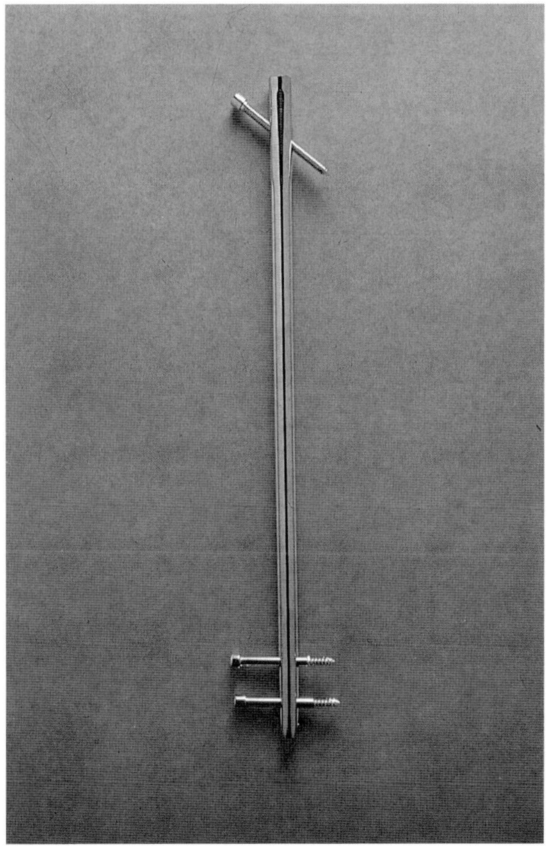

Figure 1.5

The Grosse-Kempf locking femoral nail: a stainless-steel nail with an anterior bow and a posteriorly located slot. The proximal part of the nail is unslotted to allow for insertion of the nail introducer and the proximal cross-screw. The design permits the use of one oblique proximal cross-screw and two transverse distal cross-screws. The obliquity of the proximal screw means that there are right- and left-sided nails.

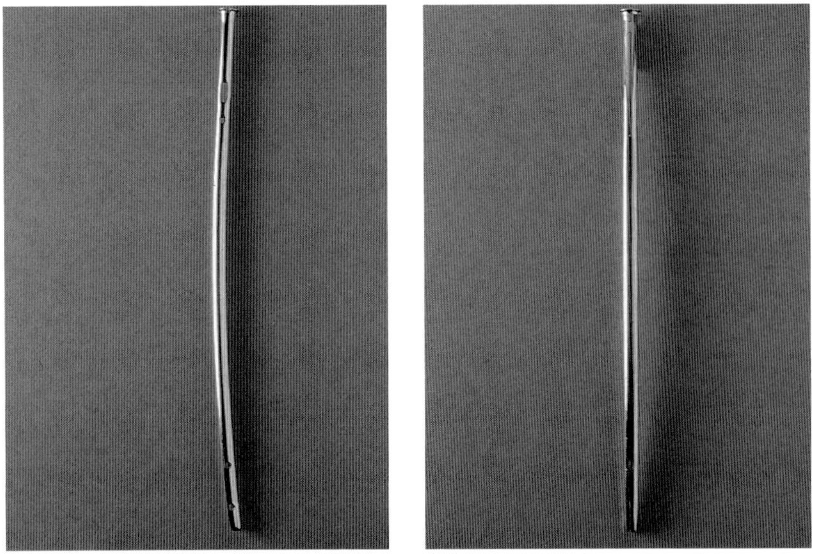

Figure 1.6

The AO femoral locking nail. This nail also has an anterior bow but the slot is placed anteriorly over most of its length. The proximal part of the nail is also slotted, although proximally the slot is narrow. One transverse proximal screw and two transverse distal screws can be used. The transverse nature of the proximal screw means that the nails are interchangeable between right and left femora.

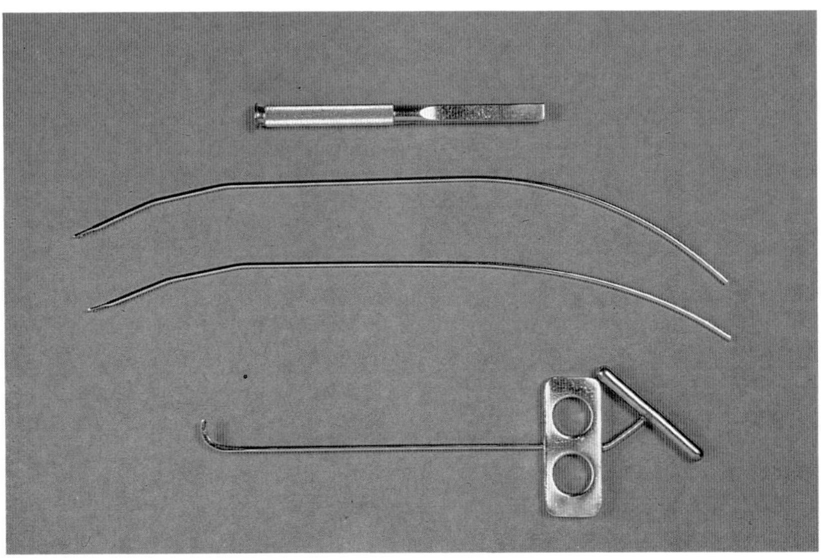

Figure 1.7

Ender nails and the equipment required for their use. From top to bottom is shown an introducer, two flexible Ender nails and an extractor.

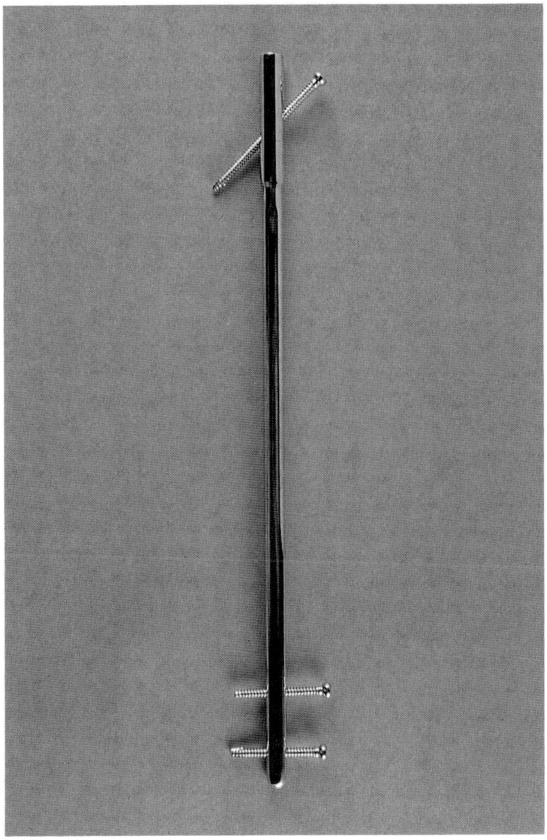

Figure 1.8

a The Russell-Taylor locking femoral nail. This nail is unslotted and mechanically stiffer than the equivalent sizes of unslotted nails. The proximal screw is oblique but the nail is drilled so that left or right screws can be inserted. The nail can therefore be used for either femur. There are two distal cross-screws.

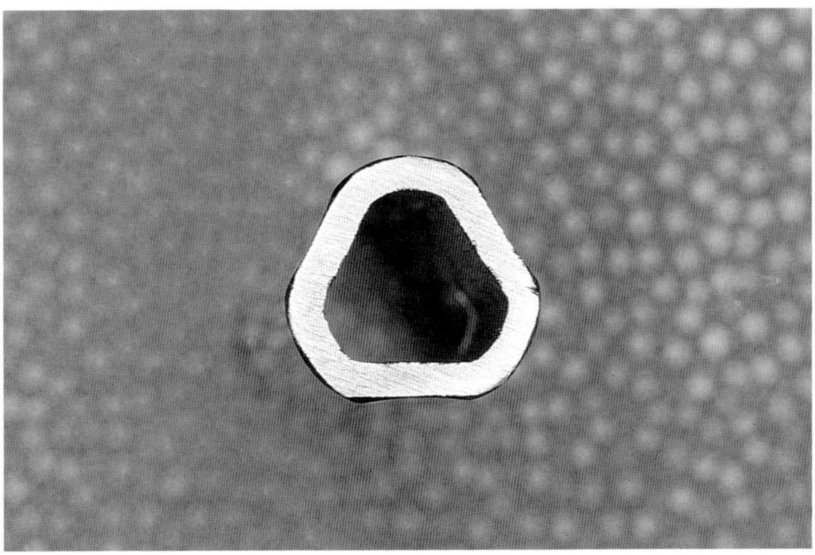

b The cross-section of the nail shows that Küntscher's clover-leaf shape has been retained although the nail is unslotted. The combination of the continuous wall with increased wall thickness stiffens the nail, allowing smaller nails to be inserted.

CHAPTER 2 TYPES OF INTRAMEDULLARY NAIL

A knowledge of the evolution of intramedullary nailing allows the surgeon to appreciate why there are a number of different nail designs on the market. All the available nails can be placed in four groups depending on the requirement for reaming and the potential to insert cross-screws.

Unreamed unlocked nails

The two main examples of this type of nail are the Rush pin (Figure 1.3) and the Ender nail (Figure 1.7). Neither nail requires reaming for its insertion. The Rush pin can be used in two principal ways. A single Rush pin can be used to stabilize fractures in one of the smaller long bones, such as the fibula, radius or ulna. This technique is often used to stabilize lateral malleolar fractures in elderly patients where the bone is osteoporotic (Figure 2.1). In this situation, the close apposition between the nail and the endosteal surface of the cortex maintains fracture reduction, although this is also helped by the hooked end of the nail.

Another way of using Rush pins is to employ two of them to gain stability in a wider medullary canal, as is encountered in the femur (Figure 2.2) or the tibia (Figure 2.3). In this technique thicker, stiffer Rush pins are bent into a curve and used to provide three-point fixation within the medullary canal. The opposing forces produced by insertion of the two appropriately bent nails provide stability. It is obvious that adequate stability can only exist when the fracture is stable after reduction and fixation. In the case of spiral or comminuted fractures Rush pins will not provide the same stability as a locked, reamed or unreamed nail. Surgeons who prefer the use of unreamed, unlocked nails in these situations may have to supplement the fixation with a postoperative functional brace to help maintain fracture reduction.

The Ender nail can be used in a similar manner to the Rush pin, but its inherent flexibility lends itself to stacking. Stacking of these nails involves inserting a number of them into the medullary canal. Under these circumstances, diaphyseal stability can be conferred by contact between the stacked nails and the endosteal surface of the cortex. Metaphyseal stability is conferred by fanning out the ends of the nails. This principle can be used in the management of proximal femoral fractures (Figure 2.4) or in the treatment of distal diaphyseal or metaphyseal femoral fractures (Figure 2.5). The usual portals of insertion of Ender nails or Rush pins in the femur and tibia are shown in Figures 2.6 and 2.7. When used for proximal femoral fractures, a medial portal of entry in the lower femur is employed although, if a diaphyseal or lower metaphyseal fracture is to be stabilized, both medial and lateral portals are used in a similar manner to the insertion of Rush pins. A trochanteric portal of entry has also been described for the treatment of femoral diaphyseal fractures (Walters et al, 1990).

Unreamed locked nails

Some surgeons attempt to 'lock' Ender nails by inserting bone cement into the entry portal of the bone or by cross-wiring the ends of the Ender nails by passing stainless-steel wire through the eyes that are located at the proximal end of each nail. Alternatively, a small bone screw can be placed through the eye into the bone. Increased stability with unreamed nails has been gained by the use of hollow nails of larger diameter and the insertion of cross-screws as in reamed locked nails. An example of this type of nail is the Russell-Taylor femoral nail (Figure 1.8). This is an unslotted nail which has retained the traditional clover-leaf pattern. The absence of a slot in the nail makes these nails stiffer than the locked reamed nails. They are, however, inserted in a similar way to locked reamed nails and thus their mode of insertion will not be separately discussed.

The indications for the use of unreamed locked nails are basically the same as for reamed locked nails. Surgical preference is largely based on the theoretical advantage of one type of nail over the other. Unfortunately good comparative prospective documentation does not yet exist to indicate which type of nail is of advantage in a particular situation. The main theoretical advantage of using unreamed nails is that the medullary blood supply is less traumatized than if it is reamed out prior to nail insertion. This theory may be correct but the success of reamed locked nails in healing both femoral and tibial fractures suggests that the intramedullary blood supply may be only one parameter that affects bone union. Rhinelander (1968) demonstrated a rapid regeneration of the nutrient system in fractures stabilized with loosely fitting nails and Rand et al (1977) showed a greater overall blood flow in nailed dog ulnar osteotomies than occurred after plating.

Recent work by Strachan et al (1990), using radioactive labelled microspheres, suggests that the importance of the medullary blood supply and the nutrient arterial supply in long bone diaphyses has been exaggerated. They have shown that it is the periosteal blood supply that is important – and they argue that the periosteal blood supply reserve is so great that it will more than compensate for any damage to the medullary supply.

Reamed unlocked nails

Reamed unlocked nails such as the Küntscher, Samson or early AO femoral nails or the Küntscher-Herzog, Lottes or early AO tibial nails have been superseded by the reamed locked nails. The only indication to use reamed unlocked nails nowadays is the unavailability of locked nails. However, many surgeons will come into contact with nails such as the Küntscher and therefore a brief description of their use will be given. If a locked nail is available its use is preferred.

The use of reamed unlocked nails is similar in both tibia and femur, although the relative scarcity of tibial fractures at or near to the isthmus means that fewer tibial than femoral fractures are suitable for stabilization with such a nail. The Küntscher femoral nail will be used to illustrate the technique.

The standard Küntscher nail can be successfully used to stabilize a number of long bone fractures. The ideal fracture for the use of this straight unlocked nail is situated at or close to the isthmus where good apposition between the endosteal cortex and the nail on both sides of the fracture can be achieved. Figure 2.8a illustrates an oblique femoral fracture situated just below the isthmus.

The shape of the fracture is important when nailing is considered. Oblique and transverse fractures that are situated close to the isthmus can often be stabilized with an unlocked nail. Figure 2.8b shows that good reduction has been achieved by the use of a closed technique and Figure 2.8c shows that the position has been maintained until union occurred. Characteristically a considerable amount of callus has been formed.

Transverse fractures (Figure 2.9a) usually have an irregular surface and, if accurate reduction is obtained, then the interdigitation of the bone ends will aid stability. Figure 2.9b shows that good reduction has been obtained and Figure 2.9c indicates that the position has been maintained until union has commenced. Figures 2.8 and 2.9 both illustrate the slight straightening of the femoral shaft which occurs when a straight nail is used to stabilize a mid-diaphyseal fracture.

Unlocked intramedullary nails may be used to treat fractures which occur at a greater distance from the isthmus. Figure 2.10a shows a fracture distal to the isthmus where there is minor comminution. Despite the comminution the transverse nature of the fracture has ensured sufficient stability to maintain fracture position until union (Figure 2.10b). The position has been maintained despite the failure of the surgeon to place the nail fully into the metaphyseal bone in the distal femur. In low diaphyseal fractures, maximum stability is maintained by placing the nail as far distally as possible, as insertion into the harder subchondral bone improves stability.

Fractures proximal to the isthmus can be treated with an unlocked nail but, as proximal stability depends solely on the contact between the nail and the proximal femoral cortex, the reduction may not be maintained and a coxa vara may result. Figure 2.11 shows a proximal fracture which is united but there is a degree of coxa vara present. This can be avoided by the use of a locking nail with a proximal cross-screw.

In fractures associated with comminution, the closed insertion of an unlocked Küntscher nail is not the correct treatment. Where comminution is recognized pre-operatively, an open procedure can be performed and the fragments wired back into position if possible. However, if the surgeon fails to realize that the fracture is inherently unstable, problems may ensue. Figure 2.12a shows such a fracture. The lateral view shows slight splaying of the upper fragment demonstrating the presence of a longitudinal fracture. Despite this, a closed Küntscher nail was inserted and the postoperative X-ray scan (Figure 2.12b) shows that the longitudinal fracture line has opened further. Three months later, the fracture is healing but there is considerable shortening secondary to the initially unrecognized comminution (Figure 2.12c).

Spiral fractures of the femur usually occur below the isthmus and are impossible to stabilize adequately using a Küntscher nail. An example of this is seen in Figure 2.13 where an open Küntscher nailing procedure was undertaken on a multiply injured patient. The initial position as seen on the antero-posterior X-ray scan is satisfactory (Figure 2.13a) but, shortly after surgery, the leg became externally rotated and a further antero-posterior X-ray scan showed that the fracture had undergone rotatory displacement (Figure 2.13b). The solution for this problem is to use a locking intramedullary nail such as the Grosse-Kempf nail shown in Figure 2.13c. The distal cross-screw maintained the stability of the distal fragment. It was removed after 6 weeks to dynamize the fracture and Figure 2.13d shows that the fracture reduction was maintained until bone union.

The use of the unlocked reamed intramedullary nail can be extended if the technique is combined with other methods of fracture treatment. However, to do this, the fracture site must often be opened. Figure 2.14a shows a segmental fracture with longitudinal fractures within the segment. The surgeon has used cerclage wiring to stabilize the segment and a Küntscher nail has been used to stabilize the transverse fracture sites (Figure 2.14b). Three months after surgery, union is proceeding well and the position of the fracture is maintained (Figure 2.14c).

In addition to cerclage stainless-steel wiring, plastic banding techniques can be used to stabilize the bone fragments or a bone plate may be applied across the fractures with the screws placed only through one cortex. Alternatively, cast bracing may be used to maintain rotation following the use of an unlocked nail to maintain axial alignment. It is important to realize that open surgical techniques combined with intramedullary nailing merely serve to increase the amount of soft-tissue damage at the fracture site and, therefore, are detrimental to fracture union and cannot be advocated.

A better solution than a combination of different techniques in the treatment of difficult femoral or tibial fractures is to use a locking nail such as the Grosse-Kempf nail. Figure 2.15a shows a tibial fracture which could not easily be stabilized by conventional operative techniques. The use of a locking nail with proximal and distal locking screws confers stability (Figure 2.15b). Three months after the fracture was treated, healing is proceeding and length and alignment have been maintained (Figure 2.15c).

Reamed locked nails

The invention of reamed locked nails has revolutionized intramedullary nailing by extending the technique to include all diaphyseal and many metaphyseal fractures. It has therefore become possible to stabilize closed comminuted fractures of the tibia and femur without opening the fracture site or without using casting methods or traction (Figure 2.15). Most reamed locked nails consist of a slotted tube of appropriate shape for the femur or tibia perforated by a number of proximal and distal holes. Examples of this type of nail are the Grosse-Kempf and AO femoral and tibial nails. The differences between the two femoral nails (Figures 1.5 and 1.6) are fairly minor and relate mainly to the transverse location of the AO proximal screw compared with the obliquity of the Grosse-Kempf proximal screw. This obliquity extends the scope of the Grosse-Kempf nail very slightly.

The Grosse-Kempf and AO tibial nails (Figures 2.16 and 2.17) are somewhat different with the curve in the AO nail being distal to the curve on the Grosse-Kempf nail. In addition, all proximal screws in the AO nail are in the coronal plane while there is one coronal and one sagittal proximal cross-screw in the Grosse-Kempf nail. These differences are not major and it is unlikely that one nail is superior to the other to a significant extent.

Most reamed and unreamed locked nails can be inserted in dynamic or static modes. Dynamic locking refers to the practice of placing cross-screws at one end of the nail only while in the static mode there are cross-screws at both ends. Dynamic locking can be proximal or distal, depending on the position and type of fracture. The theoretical advantage of dynamic locking is that it permits axial movement at the fracture site. This mode is used when there is a fracture above or below the isthmus of a type that is stable after nailing; examples are shown in Figures 2.18a and b.

If there is any comminution, or if the fracture is segmental, a static lock should be used (Figure 2.19). This gives stability to the fracture, allowing for the maintenance of length and correct alignment. However, axial loading of the fracture is minimized. Dynamization is the practice of converting the static mode to either a proximal or a distal dynamic mode. This is usually carried out between 6 and 8 weeks after the fracture has occurred.

Most surgeons perceive that the hardest part of inserting a locked intramedullary nail is the insertion of the distal cross-screws. This belief has led to a number of ingenious devices designed to aid distal cross-screw insertion. These will be discussed in Chapter 6, but the problem of distal screw insertion has led to a radical new design of reamed locked nail – the flanged nail. This modification has been introduced in the Brooker-Wills, Derby and Medinov® nails. The Brooker-Wills nail is shown in Figure 2.20a. It is a curved nail of clover-leaf cross-section with a metal insert carrying two sharp flanges (Figure 2.20b). After nail introduction, the flanges are advanced and a proximal screw is used to maintain the flange extension by pressing down on the central metal rod that lies between the proximal screw and the distal flanges. This nail abolishes the problems of distal screw insertion, although occasionally the flanges may be difficult to retract prior to nail extraction. Its main theoretical disadvantage is that it can only be used with a proximal dynamic lock or with a static lock. Thus, the distal dynamic locked mode that might be used with the Grosse-Kempf or AO nails in the treatment of fractures below the isthmus cannot be used. The Medinov® nail has solved this problem by the use of a small proximal plastic plug.

The theoretical advantages of reamed over unreamed large diameter hollow locked nails are that larger stronger nails can be used, although the abolition of the slot in the unreamed Russell-Taylor nail strengthens it. A number of surgeons also believe that the reamings from the endosteal surface of the cortex have a bone graft effect and thereby enhance bone union. Figure 2.21 shows the extent to which medullary bone reamings can be extruded during reaming. It is probable that this material is osteogenic. The last possible advantage of reamed nails is that the creation of an endosteal tube of comparable size to the nail will allow the use of more dynamic rather than static fixation. If an unreamed nail is to be used, the contact between nail and endosteum will probably be less and static fixation will be necessary to ensure stability. Good prospective trials are required to investigate the advantages and disadvantages of both nail types.

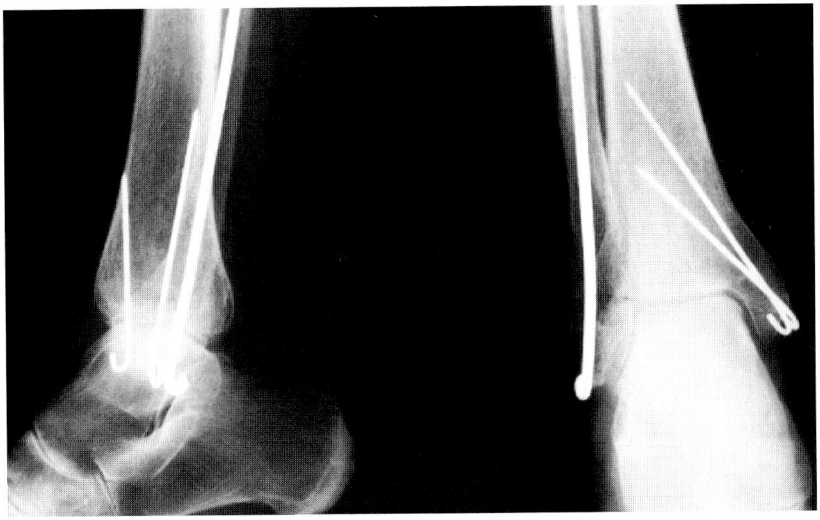

Figure 2.1

Internal fixation of a bimalleolar ankle fracture in an elderly patient with osteoporotic bone. The combination of Kirschner wires for the medial malleolus and a Rush pin for the fibula fracture is appropriate for this type of bone.

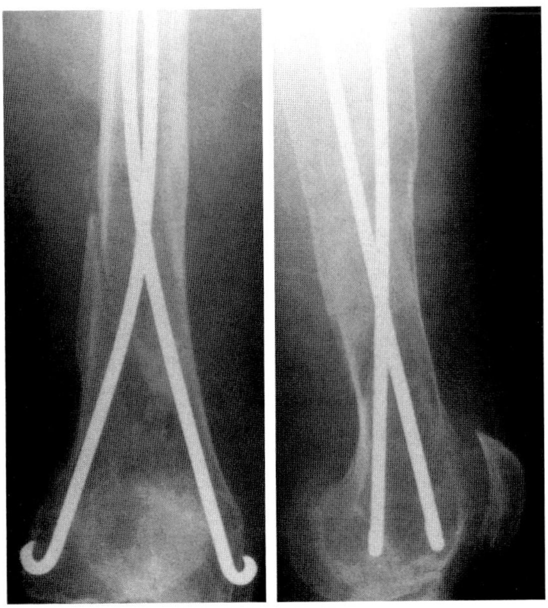

Figure 2.2

Two pre-bent Rush pins can be used to gain stability in diaphyseal or metaphyseal long bone fractures. In this case, two Rush pins have been used to stabilize a femoral fracture in an elderly lady who had sustained a previous femoral fracture which had been conservatively managed. It was felt that the resulting mal-union mitigated against the use of a locking femoral nail.

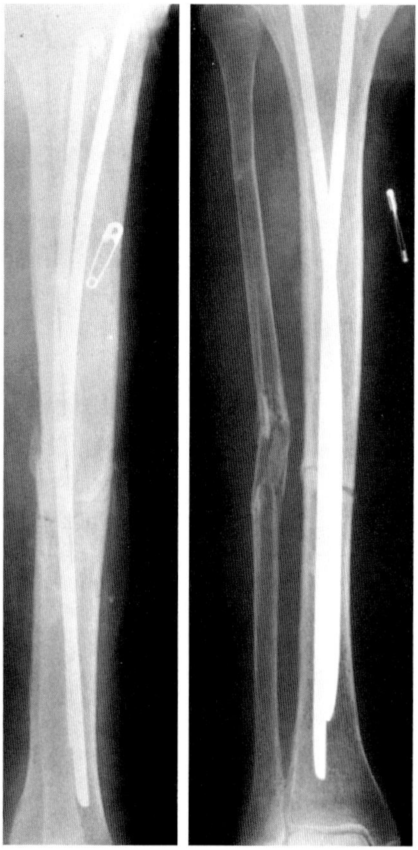

Figure 2.3

Two Rush pins used to stabilize a mid-diaphyseal tibial fracture in a multiply injured patient. In this case the method was chosen because of the relative speed with which the two nails can be inserted.

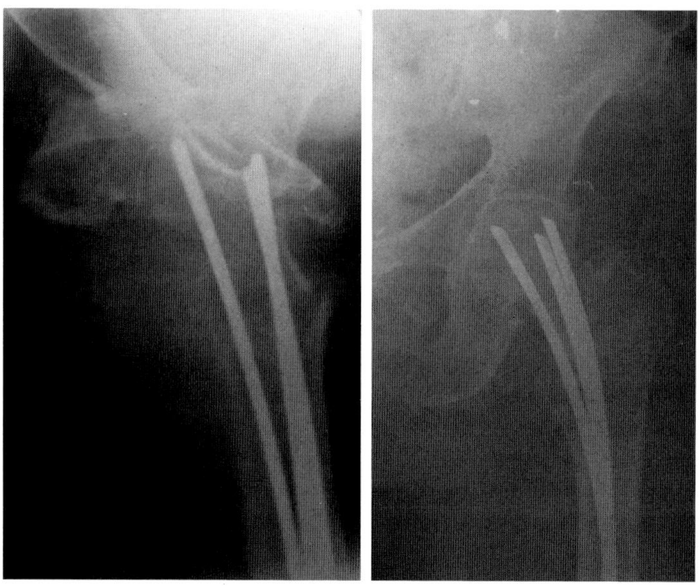

Figure 2.4

A proximal femoral fracture stabilized by the use of three Ender nails. The nails should always be fanned out to provide maximum stability.

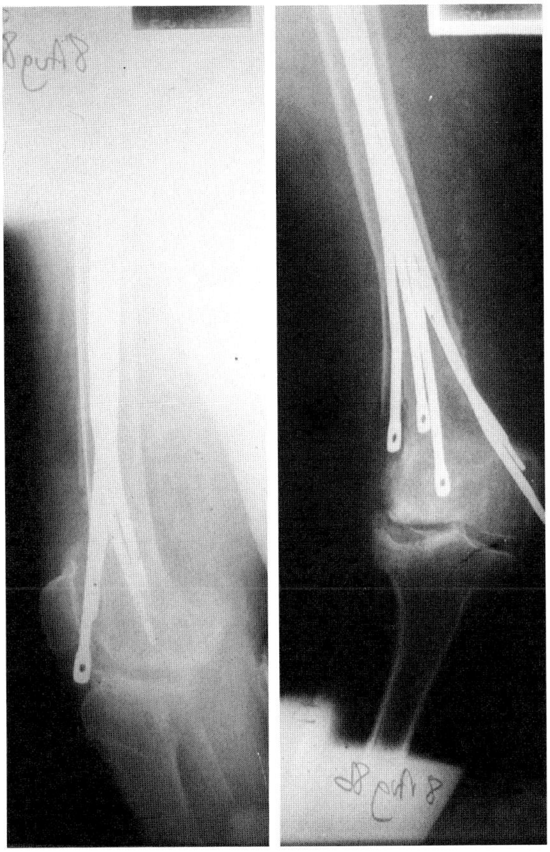

Figure 2.5

In this case, five Ender nails have been used to provide stability to a lower femoral fracture in an 84-year-old woman. The bone was markedly osteoporotic. The Ender nails held the fracture well and union was achieved, although subsequently the nails were removed because of impingement of the soft tissues around the knee.

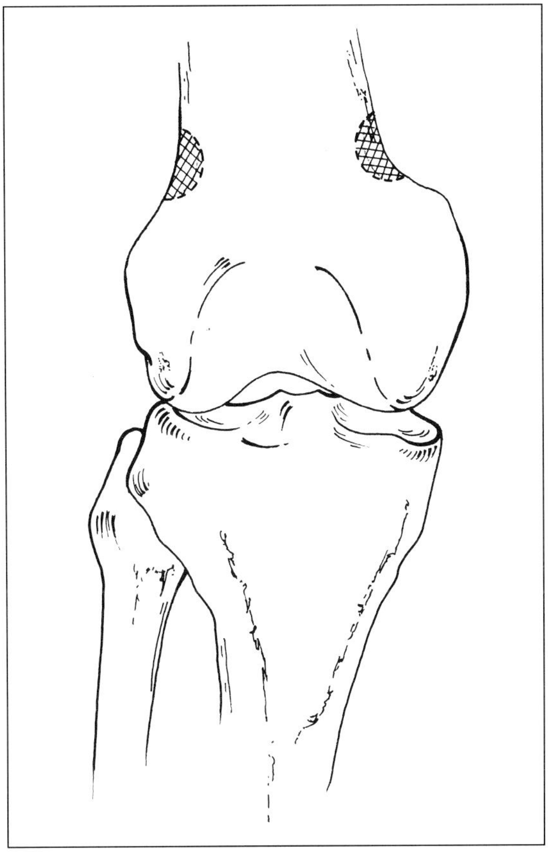

Figure 2.6

Rush pins and Ender nails are usually inserted distally and passed proximally up the femur. The usual sites of insertion are on the lowest part of the medial and lateral supracondylar ridges, as demonstrated in this diagram.

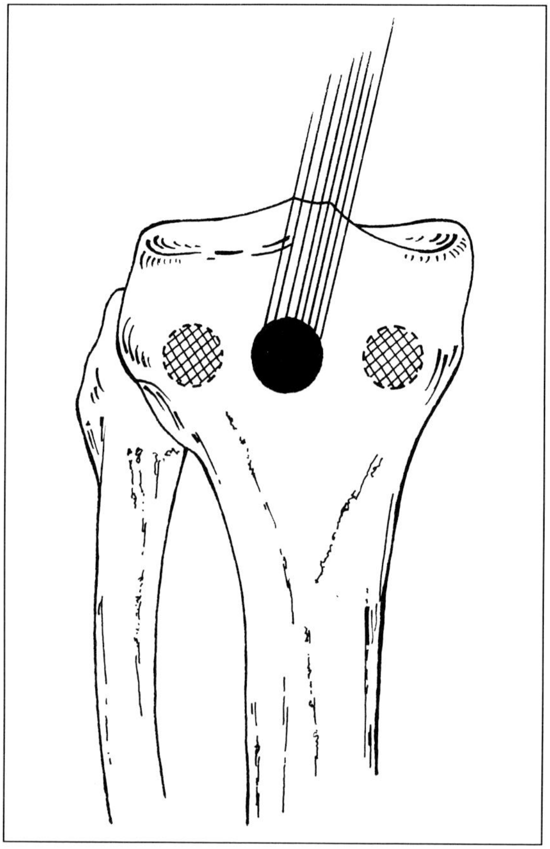

Figure 2.7

It is usual to introduce Rush pins or Ender nails into the tibia through medial and lateral approaches at the level of the tibial tuberosity.

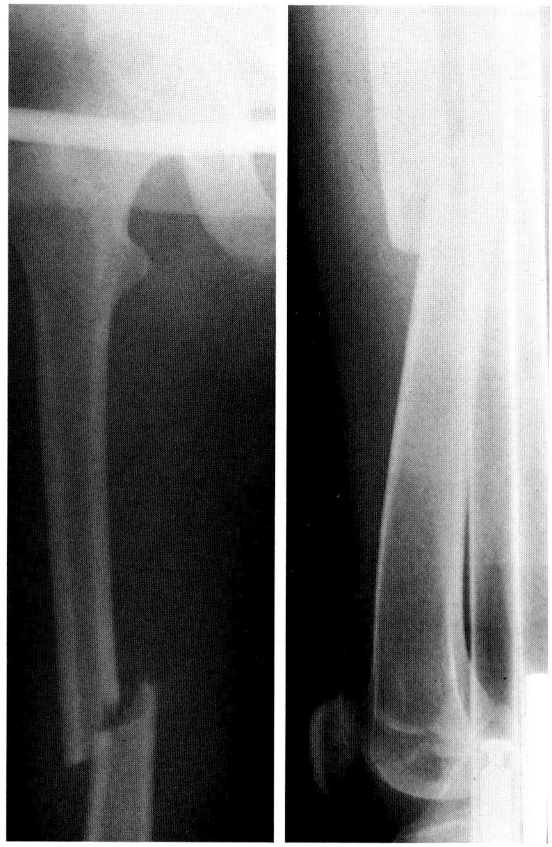

Figure 2.8

a A closed oblique femoral fracture which has been treated with a Küntscher nail. As the fracture is below the isthmus, it would be technically correct to use a distally locked nail.

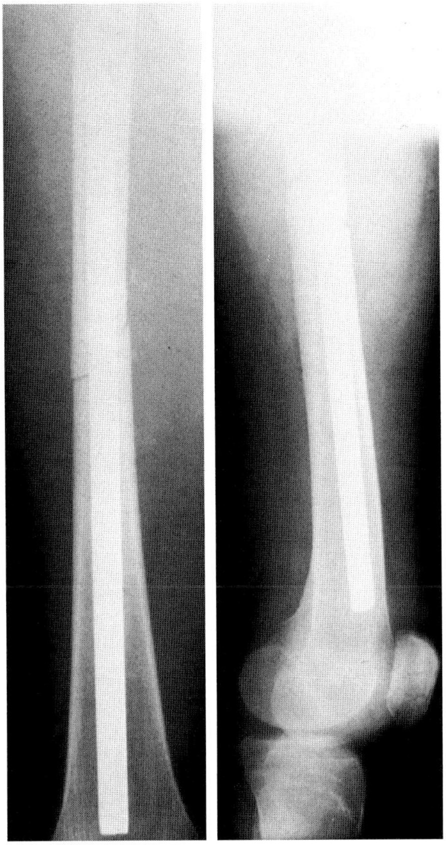

b In this case, the obliquity of the fracture has ensured stability after nailing. The slight straightening of the femur following the use of a straight nail is demonstrated.

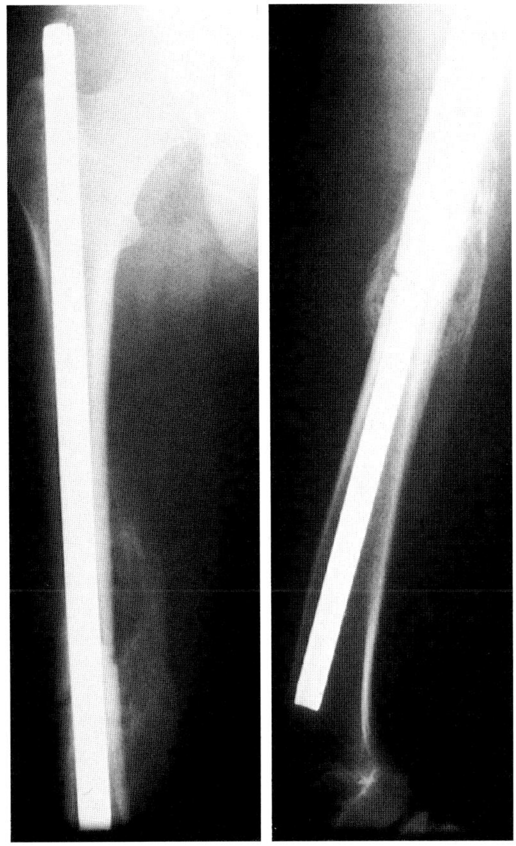

c The fracture has healed without loss of position. Characteristically a considerable amount of callus has formed. The X-ray scan also shows calcification related to the proximal end of the nail.

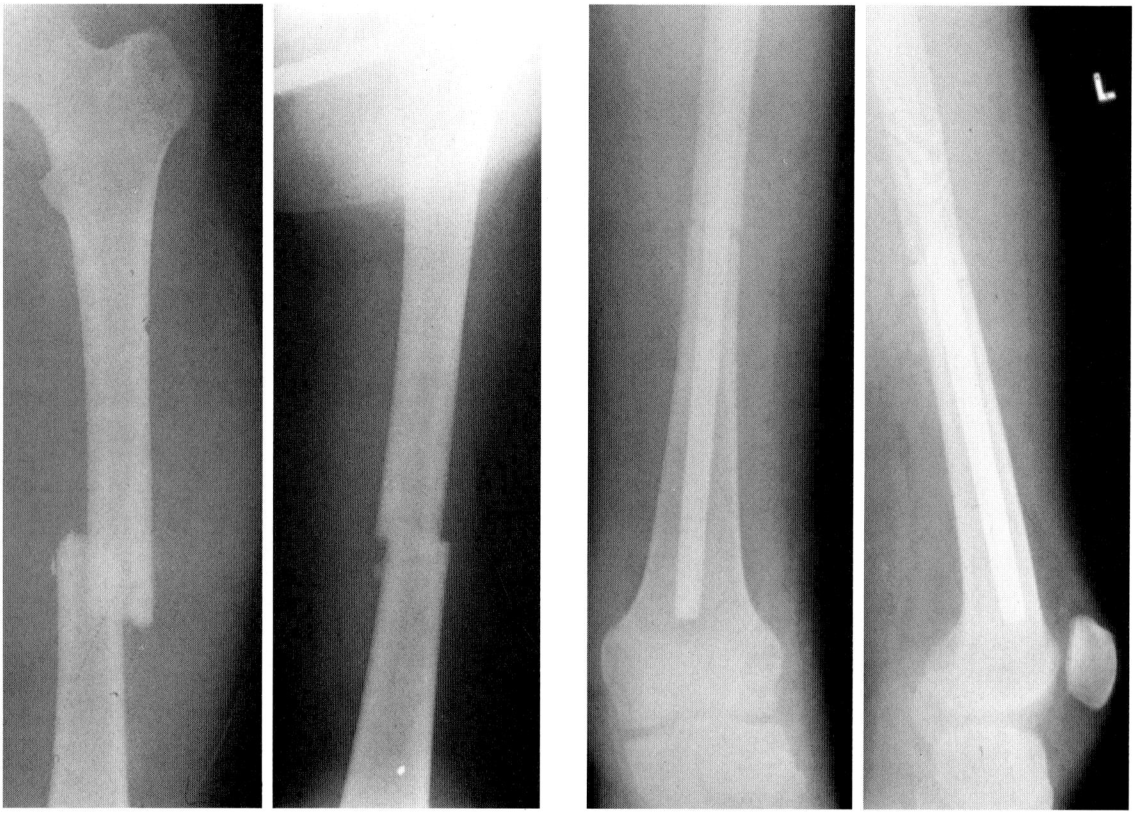

Figure 2.9

a A transverse femoral fracture situated just below the isthmus.

b Oblique or transverse fractures just below or above the isthmus can be stabilized with an unlocked nail. Again there has been slight straightening of the femoral shaft following the use of a straight nail.

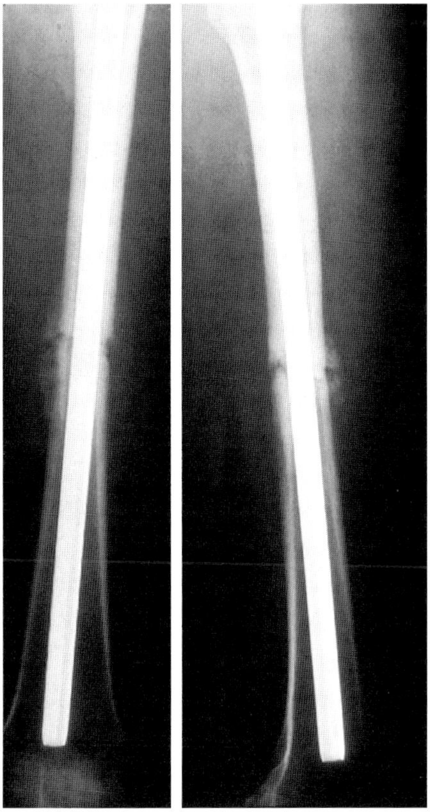

c Reduction has been maintained until union.

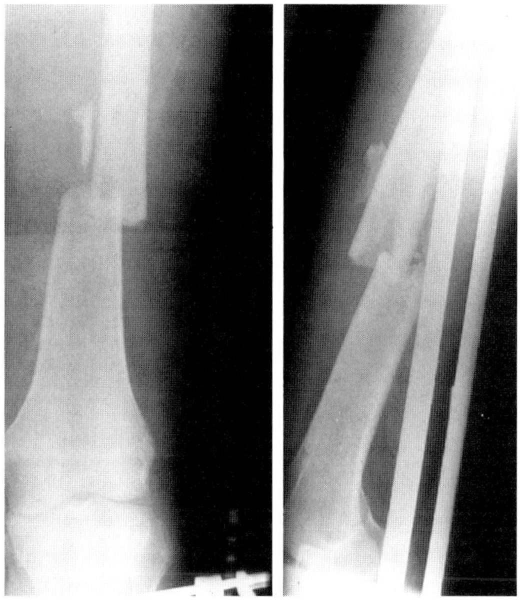

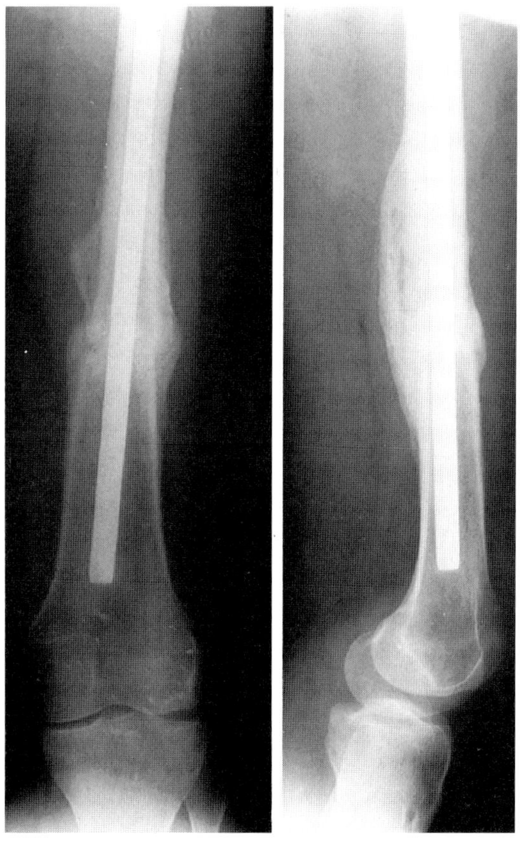

Figure 2.10

a Few surgeons nowadays would use an unlocked nail to stabilize this fracture. A distally locked nail should be used. This fracture was treated before the use of locked nails became popular at the author's centre.

b If an unlocked nail is to be used for a fracture in the distal third of the femur or tibia, the nail should be hammered into the lower metaphysis. If this is not done, there is a risk of the fracture displacing. In this case, the surgeon was fortunate that the fracture position was maintained.

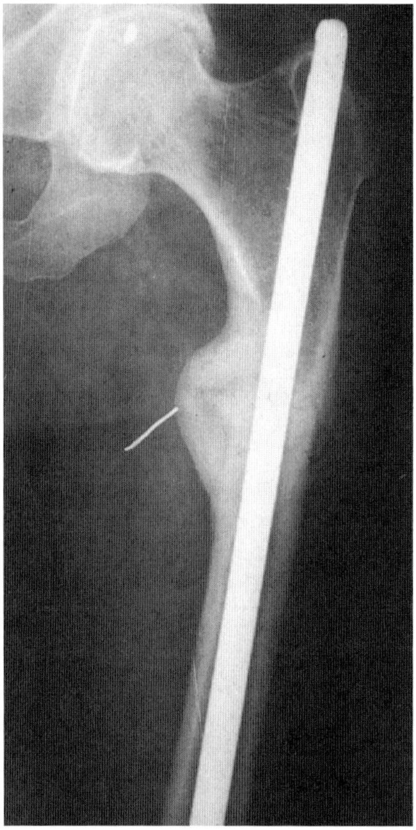

Figure 2.11

Nowadays this fracture would be treated with a proximally locked nail. If an unlocked nail is used, the surgeon relies on contact between the greater trochanter and the nail for stability. As the stability is inadequate, a coxa vara has resulted.

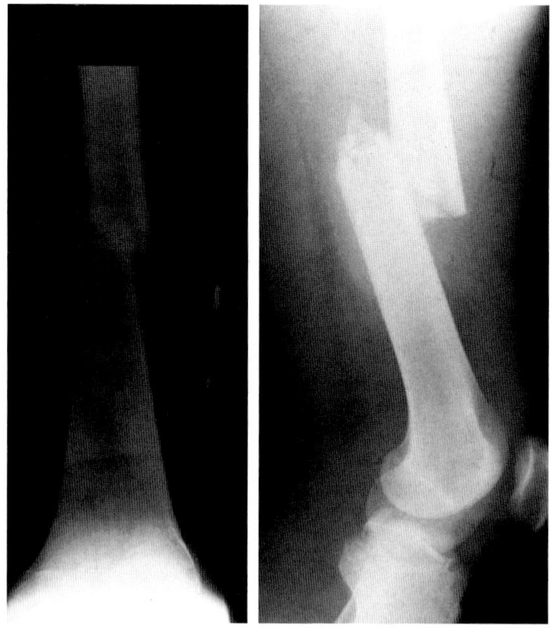

Figure 2.12

a A distal femoral fracture. It is obvious that there is comminution of the proximal femoral fragment and a statically locked nail should be used.

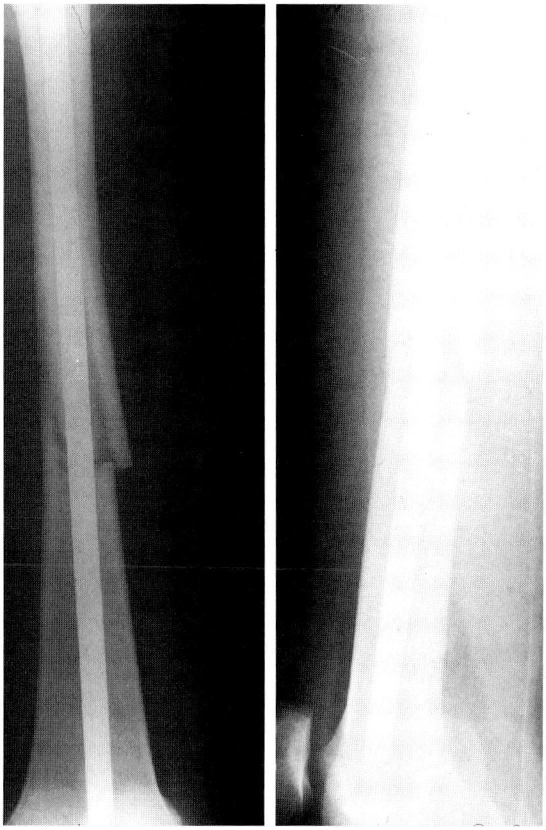

b At first sight, it would seem that a reasonable reduction has been achieved, but there has been displacement of a piece of bone proximal to the fracture. It could be predicted that this fracture would not be adequately held by an unlocked nail.

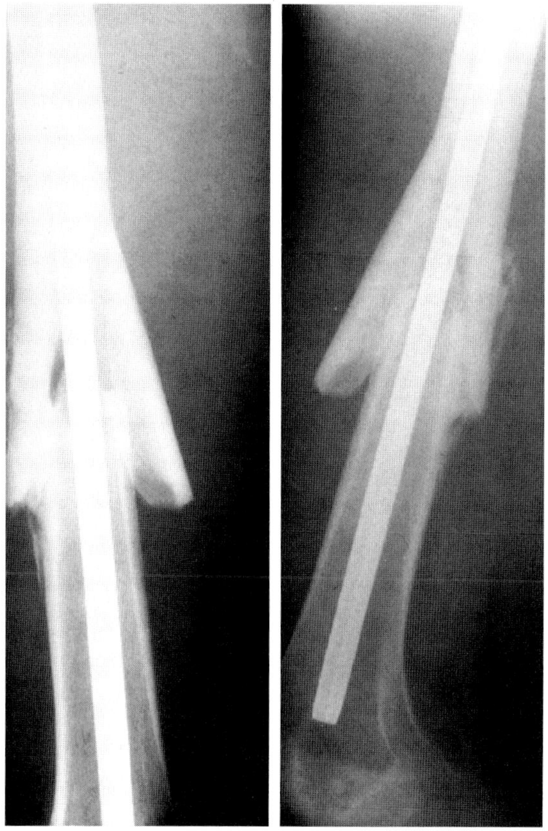

c The nail has failed to hold this femoral fracture. There has been displacement of the comminuted bone fragments proximal to the fracture and shortening of the femur. This would have been avoided with a statically locked nail.

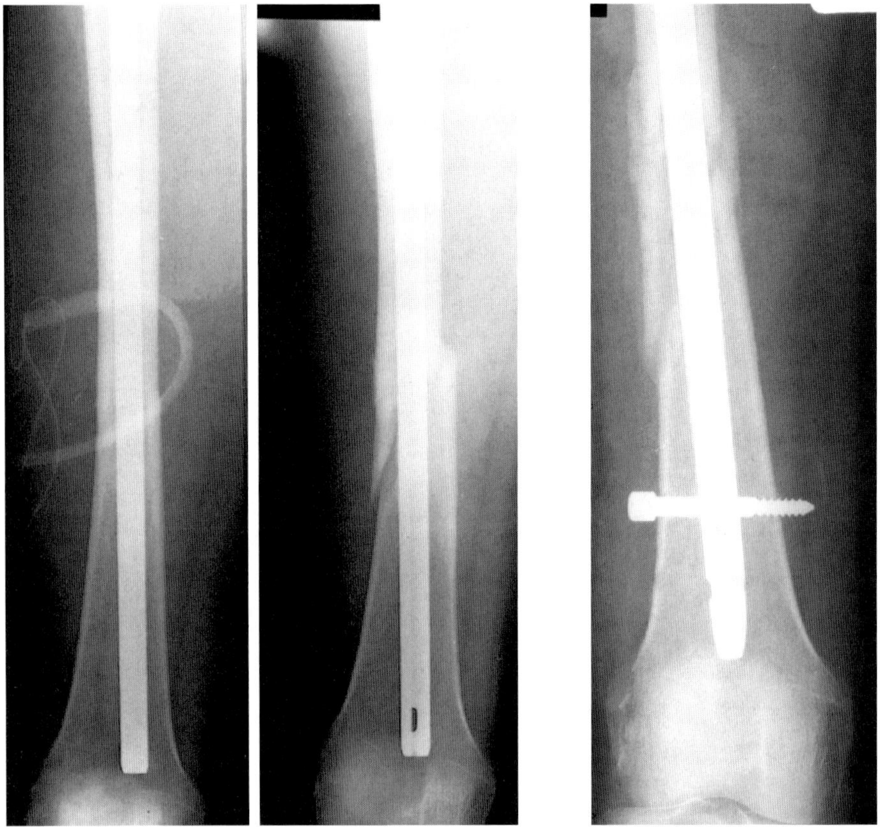

Figure 2.13

a A spiral fracture situated below the isthmus in a 45-year-old female with multiple injuries. A locking nail was not available to the surgeon and a Küntscher nail was used.

b (right) After 3 days, it became clear that the spiral fracture had opened and the distal femoral fragment rotated externally.

c The patient was returned to theatre and a distally locked nail was inserted.

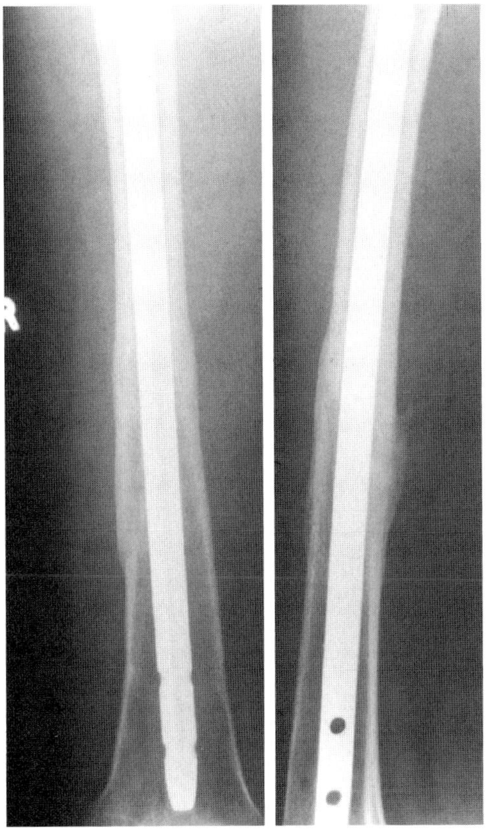

d The distal cross-screw was removed to facilitate dynamization and the fracture healed without any further complications.

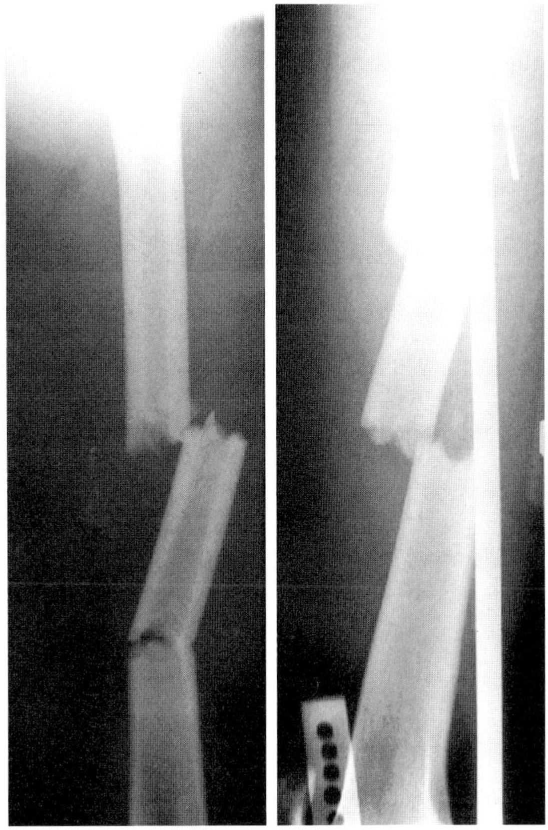

Figure 2.14

a A segmental femoral fracture with two transverse fractures. The segment is also fractured longitudinally.

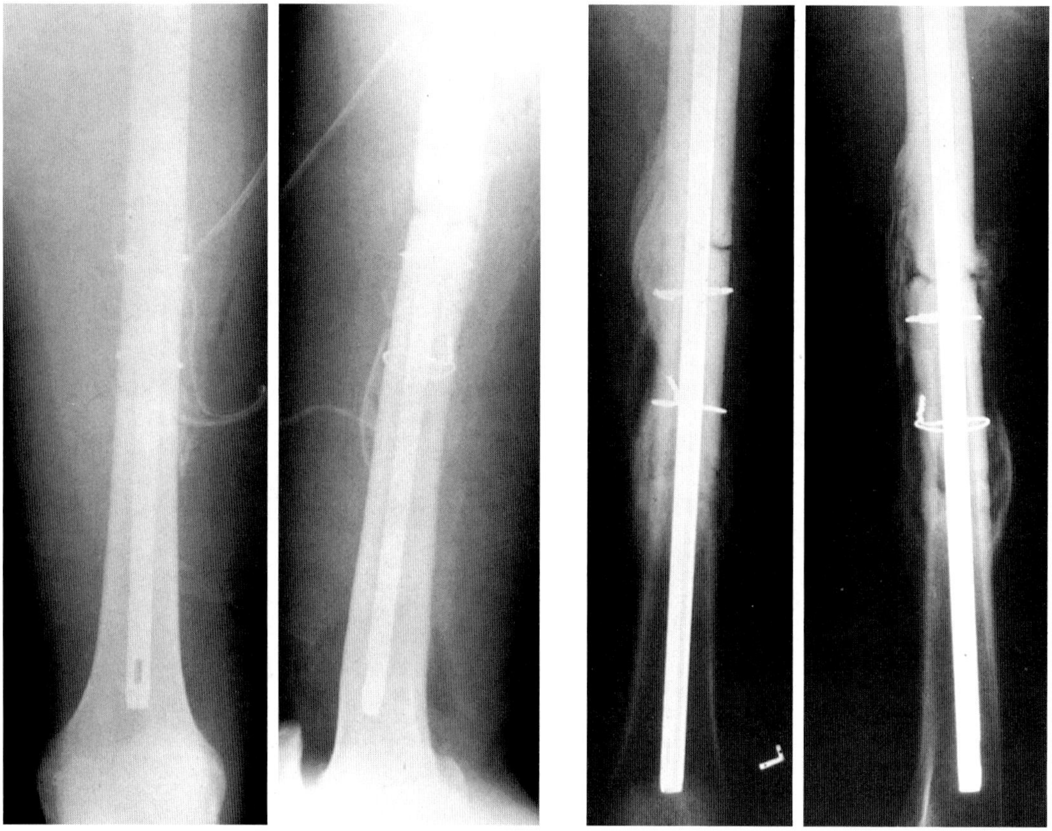

Figure 2.14 *continued*

b A combination of treatment methods has been used to stabilize this fracture. The fractures within the segment have been stabilized with cerclage wiring. The segment has been repositioned and the fracture nailed at an open operation.

c The transverse nature of both fractures has ensured stability and, despite the soft-tissue stripping required to perform an open operation, abundant callus has formed. Nowadays a closed statically locked nail would be used to treat this fracture.

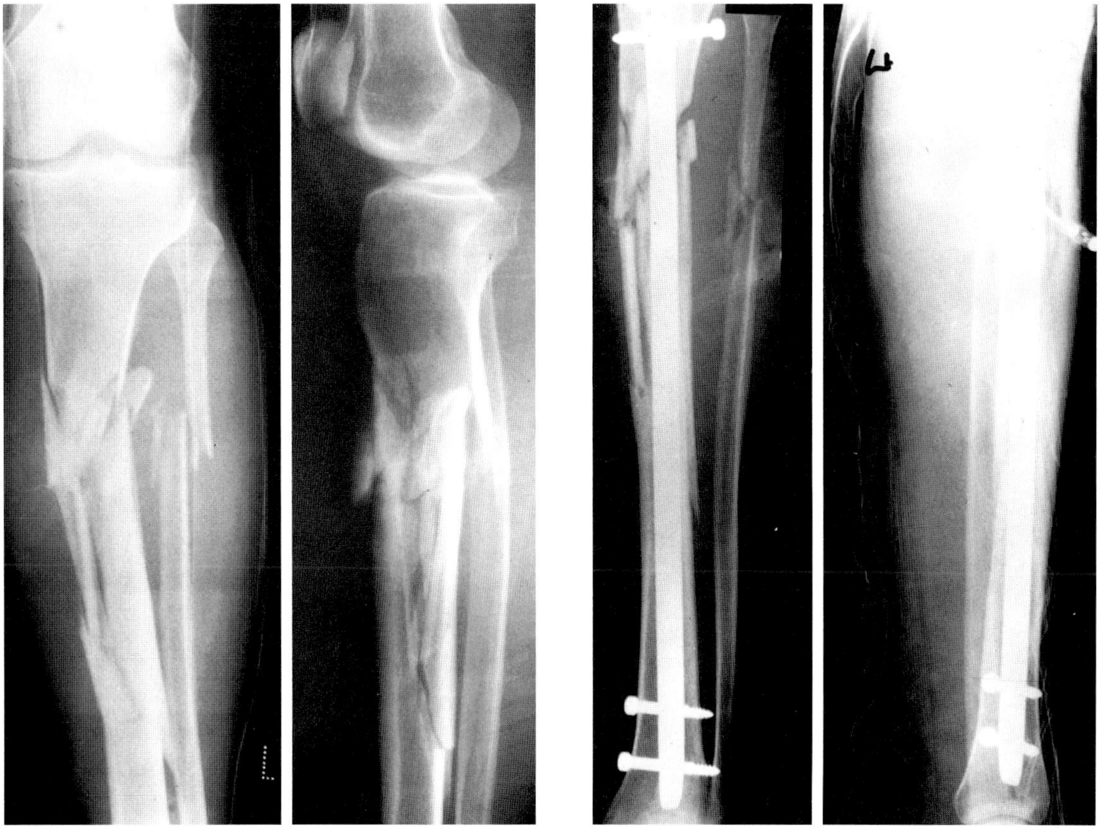

Figure 2.15

a A closed comminuted tibial fracture. A number of treatment methods could be used, but this type of fracture is most appropriately treated with a statically locked intramedullary nail.

b Nailing was undertaken on the day of admission and a good reduction was achieved.

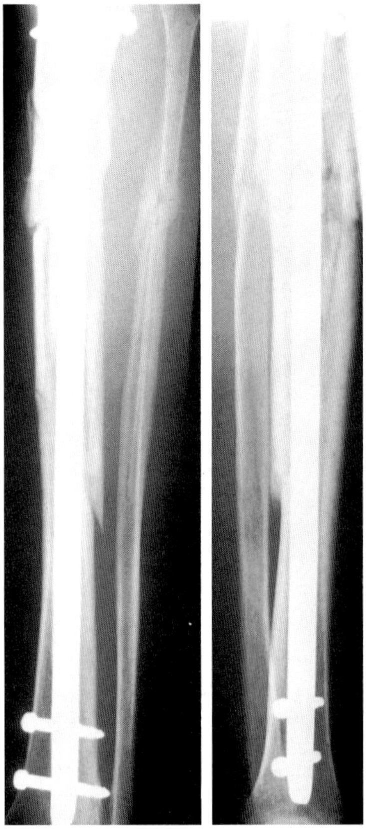

Figure 2.15 *continued*

c After 3 months the fracture is clearly uniting and the patient was bearing weight by this time. The fracture was clinically and radiologically united after 27 weeks.

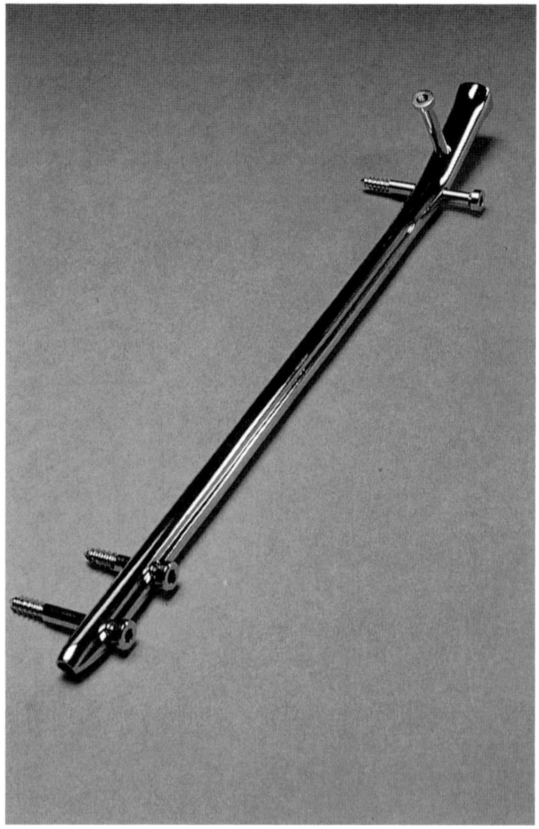

Figure 2.16

The Grosse-Kempf locking tibial nail. Two proximal and two distal cross-screws can be inserted. The nail is slotted throughout most of its length.

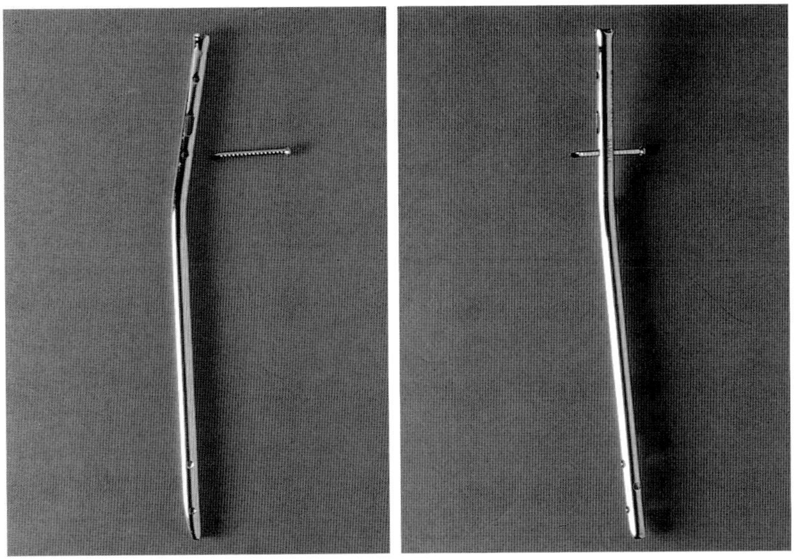

Figure 2.17

The AO locking tibial nail. This nail differs in design from the Grosse-Kempf nail in that the curve in the nail is more distal. There is no provision for an antero-posterior proximal cross-screw. There is a small proximal lip which has been placed in an effort to minimize the incidence of postoperative knee discomfort.

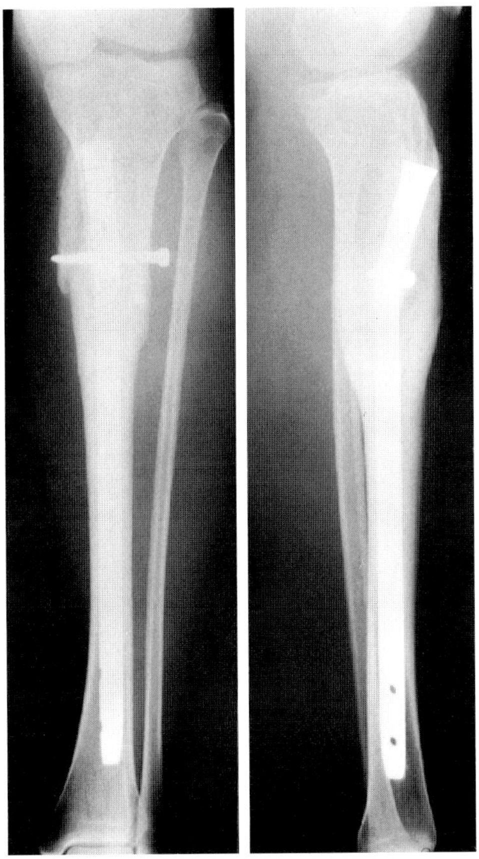

Figure 2.18

a A proximal dynamically locked nail. The use of this type of lock is more common in the femur than the tibia, as proximal tibial fractures that do not require a static lock are relatively uncommon. In this case, there has been some iatrogenic damage to the medial tibial cortex, but it was considered that a proximal lock would hold the fracture and this proved to be the case.

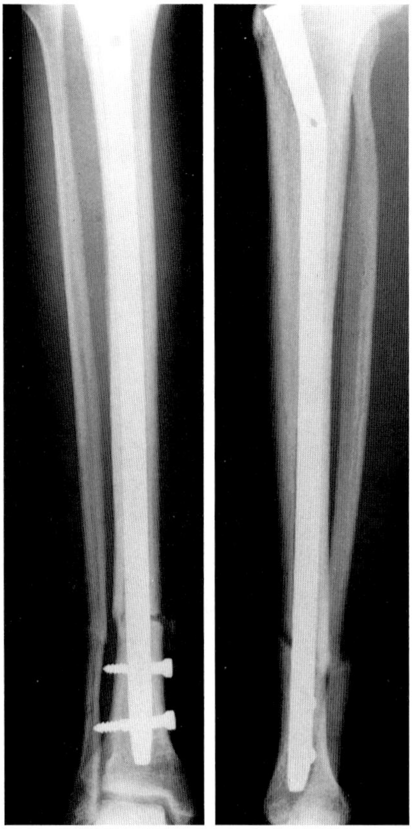

Figure 2.18 *continued*

b A distal dynamic lock. This is frequently used in the tibia where distal fractures are relatively common.

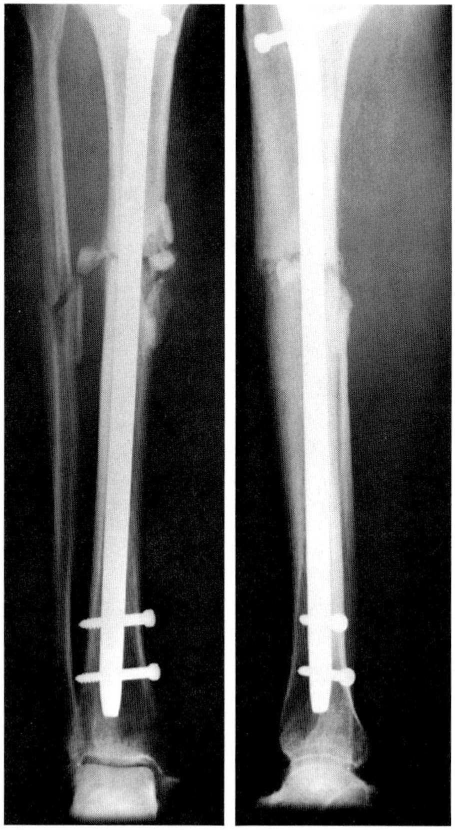

Figure 2.19

A static lock with locking screws placed proximally and distally should be used if there is any comminution or if the fracture is segmental. In this case, the comminution is relatively minor but the surgeon should resist the temptation to use a dynamically locked nail if there is any comminution. It is always safer to use a static lock if there is any doubt as to which mode to use.

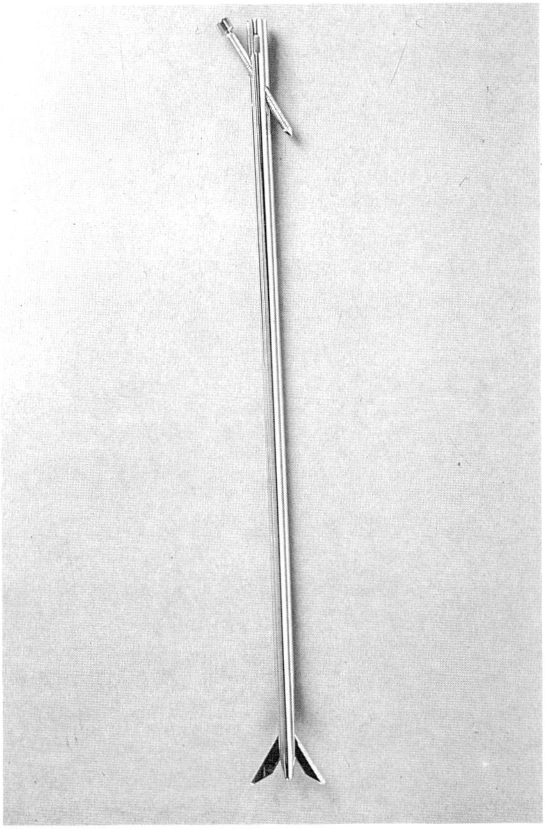

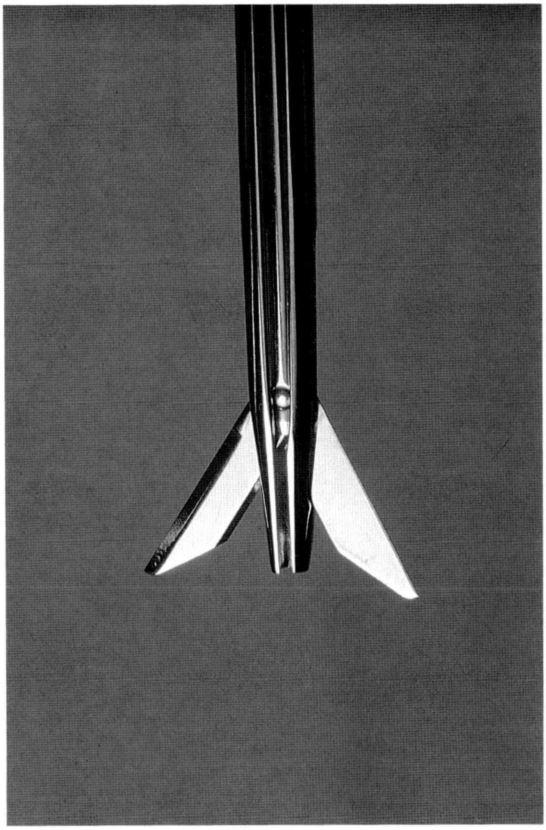

Figure 2.20

a A Brooker-Wills nail. A stainless-steel nail with an anterior bow and an anterior slot running the complete length of the nail. The design of the distal flanges means that it can only be used with a proximal dynamic lock or a static lock.

b Distal fixation is gained by the use of two flanges which are extruded from the nail by depression of a metal rod located within the nail. The flanges provide good distal stability but are occasionally difficult to retract during nail removal.

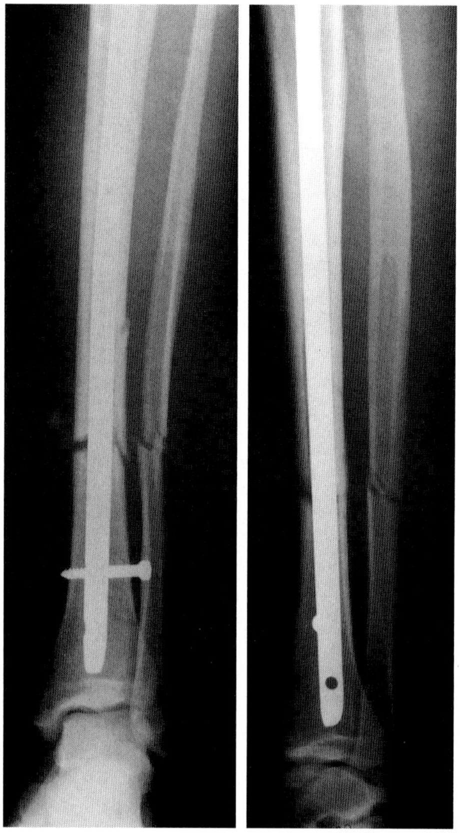

Figure 2.21

Reaming of the medullary canal produces a considerable quantity of bone which is extruded from the fracture site. It is likely that the osteogenic properties of this material enhance fracture union. Extruded bone can be seen medial to the fracture site.

CHAPTER 3 INDICATIONS FOR CLOSED NAILING

As with most other surgical techniques, there are no absolute indications for closed intramedullary nailing of the femur or tibia. All fractures can be handled by a variety of different methods and each surgeon must develop his or her own indications for the use of a particular technique. It is in fact important that orthopaedic trauma surgeons are conversant with all techniques of fracture fixation and are prepared to use whatever technique is indicated for a particular fracture. Once a surgical technique is selected, the surgeon must understand how to perform it correctly and be aware of the advantages and disadvantages associated with it. Closed intramedullary nailing, like other treatment methods, is associated with complications, but its advantages have encouraged many surgeons to adopt its use in the treatment of femoral and tibial fractures.

There are a number of situations where intramedullary nailing has been shown to be effective and is advocated by many surgeons. These are:

- Closed femoral diaphyseal fractures
- Aseptic non-unions of both femur and tibia
- Pathological fractures of both femur and tibia

Other possible indications for the use of closed nailing in the treatment of femoral and tibial fractures are more contentious, although the success of the locking intramedullary nail has meant that surgeons have expanded their indications to include:

- The treatment of closed displaced tibial fractures
- Tibial fractures associated with intact fibulae
- Open tibial and femoral fractures
- Subtrochanteric femoral fractures
- Infected non-unions
- Mal-unions

The use of intramedullary nailing in the management of open fractures is debated. Many surgeons will not accept internal fixation in the management of open fractures, particularly those affecting the tibia. However, others accept that intramedullary nailing can be used for Gustilo Type I and Type II fractures, although external fixation remains the treatment of choice amongst most surgeons for the Gustilo Type III fracture.

The treatment of open femoral and tibial fractures with an intramedullary nail is discussed in more detail in Chapter 11.

Pre-operative assessment

Certain femoral and tibial fractures are not suitable for intramedullary nailing and thus the pre-operative assessment should include a careful review of both the patient and the fracture to see if intramedullary nailing is the treatment of choice.

Position and type of fracture

Femoral intramedullary nailing is suitable for fractures below the lesser trochanter and above the level of insertion of the distal cross-screw. Figure 3.1a shows a Gustilo Type IIIb open proximal femoral fracture unsuitable for closed nailing with a conventional locking nail. This fracture was treated with interfragmentary bone screws and a plate (Figure 3.1b), although a reconstruction nail could have been used. The use of reconstruction nails is discussed in Chapter 20. As proximal fixation is mainly gained from insertion of the cross-screw into the lesser trochanter, careful inspection of the X-ray scans should be undertaken to see if trochanteric fixation is possible (Figure 3.2).

Distal femoral fractures can theoretically be stabilized if a distal cross-screw can be inserted. In reality, however, if the femoral fracture is very distal, it often communicates with the knee joint. Although intra-articular fractures can be fixed with a combination of an intramedullary nail and another treatment method (Figure 20.6), fractures such as the one illustrated in Figure 3.3 are better treated by alternative methods. The supracondylar femoral fracture should also be treated by other methods such as a blade plate.

The spectrum of tibial diaphyseal fractures is somewhat different to that of the femur. In the tibia, proximal diaphyseal fractures that do not involve the joint are relatively uncommon. This is probably fortunate as they are the most difficult tibial fractures to nail. Figure 3.4 illustrates an extra-articular tibial fracture that is difficult to treat with a locked intramedullary nail. In general, fractures within 8 cm of the tibial plateau are not suitable for nailing. Nailing of proximal fractures is discussed further in Chapter 7.

Distal tibial fractures that do not involve the ankle are much more common than the equivalent femoral fractures. In general, fractures that are within 5 cm of the ankle joint are not suitable for nailing. A low distal tibial fracture unsuitable for nailing is illustrated in Figure 3.5. Nailing of distal fractures is discussed further in Chapter 8.

In both bones, the surgeon must take great care to establish whether the fracture has an intra-articular extension (Figure 3.5) as these fractures are generally not suitable for closed nailing. The only other contraindications to nailing are the presence of an excessively narrow medullary canal or a fracture that is irreducible by closed means.

Soft tissues

The surgeon should always carefully examine any soft-tissue damage associated with a femoral or tibial fracture. Failure to do this may result in incorrect treatment and, in late osteomyelitis, non-union or soft-tissue damage. The use of intramedullary nailing in open fractures is discussed in Chapter 11 but some surgeons now accept that closed nailing provides a good treatment method for the stabilization of all grades of open femoral fractures. The alternative operative treatment that is currently recommended for the treatment of open tibial fractures is external skeletal fixation. Figure 3.6 shows the use of external skeletal fixation in the treatment of a Gustilo Type IIIb open tibial fracture. Currently this technique is more popular than intramedullary nailing in the treatment of severe open tibial fractures. Early results in Edinburgh, however, suggest that the use of intramedullary nailing for the treatment of such fractures may be associated with good results; but further research is required.

Even with closed fractures, the surgeon should examine the limb carefully for signs of degloving of the skin, as open treatment of a fracture under these circumstances may result in further skin damage or loss. The use of closed intramedullary nailing in the management of over two hundred closed tibial fractures was associated with full thickness skin loss in only one patient.

If there are signs of soft-tissue damage in the areas where surgical incisions will be placed during closed intramedullary nailing, the operation should be performed as soon as possible after admission so as to minimize the risk of bacterial contamination of the skin.

Other injuries

Multiply injured patients may often have their individual fractures treated differently than if those fractures had occurred in isolation. Closed intramedullary nailing is a very good technique for the treatment of isolated femoral or tibial fractures, but where a number of the major long bones in the lower limbs have been broken it may be a difficult and time-consuming technique to use. Under these circumstances, a surgeon may choose a different surgical technique such as external skeletal fixation, which is easier and quicker to apply. The surgeon may then elect to change to medullary nailing at a later date.

Bone shape

Infrequently, the surgeon may be faced with a femur or tibia which is unusually shaped. If this does occur it is usually secondary to a previous conservatively managed fracture, an example of which is shown in Figure 2.2. However, Figure 3.7 shows a proximal fracture in a pagetic femur in which there is a distal bow. Under these circumstances, a long intramedullary nail could not be inserted and a short Küntscher nail was used to stabilize the fracture which united without a problem. Alternatively an external fixation device can be used for such a fracture (Figure 3.8).

Bone quality

Intramedullary nailing is a suitable technique for bone of poor quality. Techniques such as plating and external skeleton fixation are less appropriate in elderly bone because of the problems of maintaining screw position. Moran et al (1990) particularly recommended femoral nailing for fractures in the elderly. In undeformed osteoporotic or osteomalacic bone, nailing is straightforward provided the correct surgical technique is followed. It is however wise to insert all possible cross-screws as there is an increased tendency for the cross-screws to back out of such bone.

Age and health of patient

As with other surgical procedures, age and health are usually not a bar to surgery. In fact, early surgery with the encouragement of postoperative mobilization as soon as possible is the optimal way to treat femoral and tibial fractures in the elderly patient. In this particular group, traction carries a high morbidity and is not only costly but very labour-intensive.

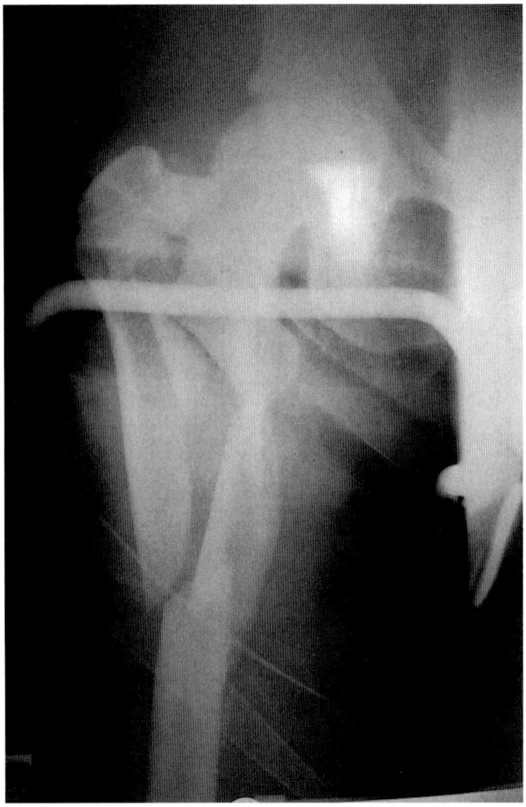

Figure 3.1

a Gustilo Type IIIb open proximal femoral fracture in a 22-year-old male following a road-traffic accident. The proximal location of the fracture above the lesser trochanter means that a conventional locking nail is inappropriate.

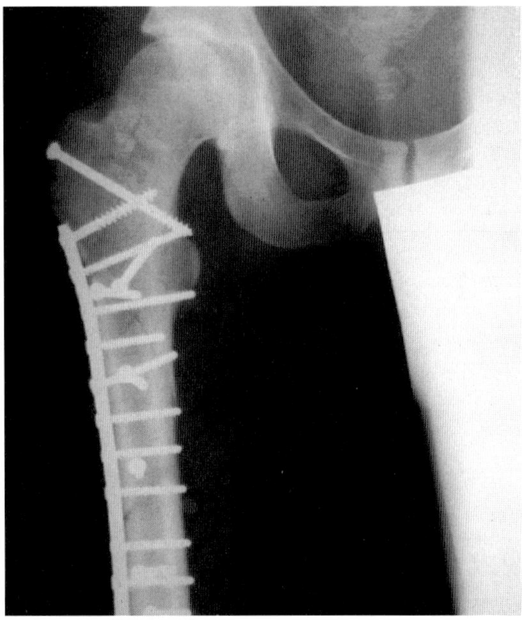

b The fracture was internally fixed with interfragmentary screws and a dynamic compression plate. The fracture united but Pseudomonas osteomyelitis developed.

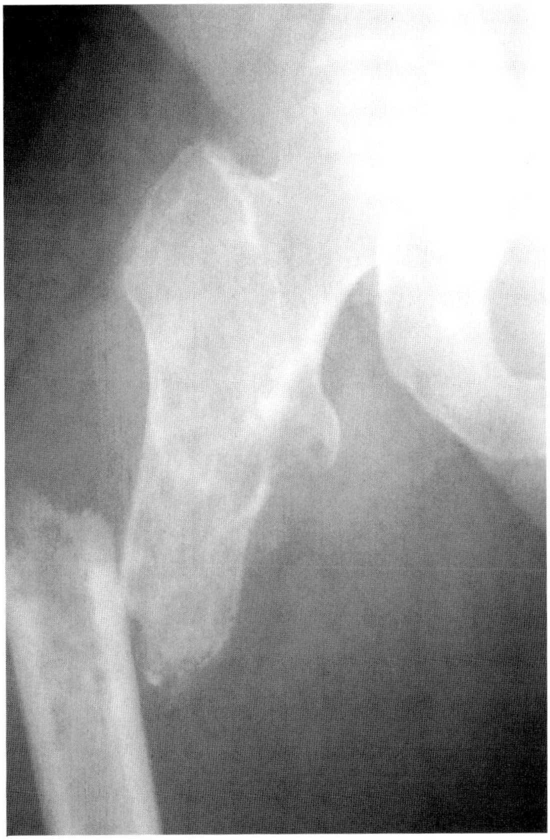

Figure 3.2

An intact lesser trochanter is essential for adequate fixation of the proximal cross-screw. This patient had metastatic bronchial carcinoma involving the lesser trochanter. Under these circumstances, a reconstruction nail or hip screw and side plate is preferable to a conventional locking femoral nail.

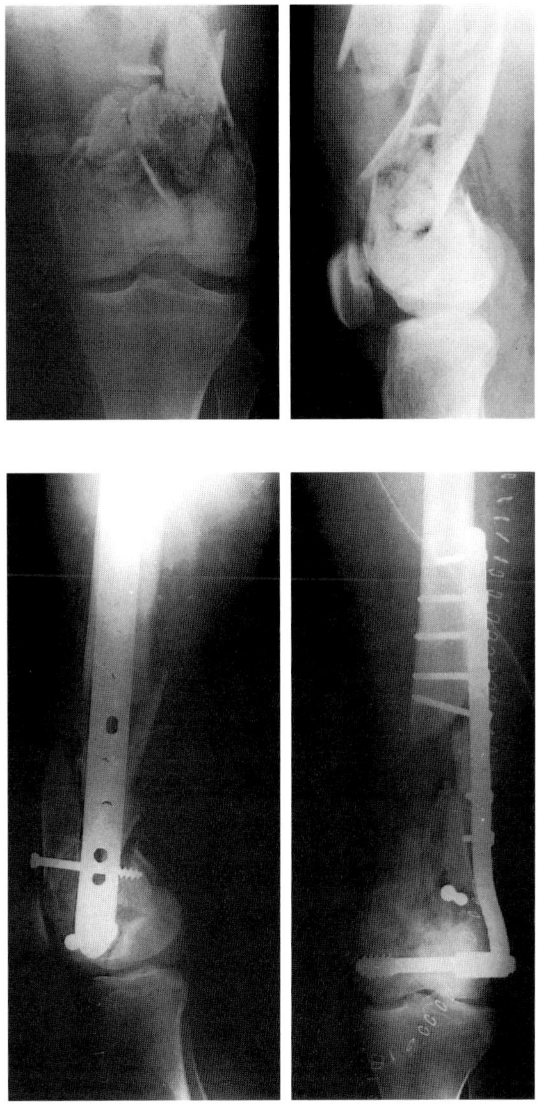

Figure 3.3

a Gustilo Type IIIb distal femoral fracture with an intercondylar extension. Christie et al (1988) illustrated a similar case where a statically locked intramedullary nail was used to stabilize such a fracture, but the technique is difficult.

b Most surgeons find that it is easier to use a femoral supracondylar fixation device for such a fracture. In this case, the fracture healed without subsequent bone grafting and good knee function was obtained.

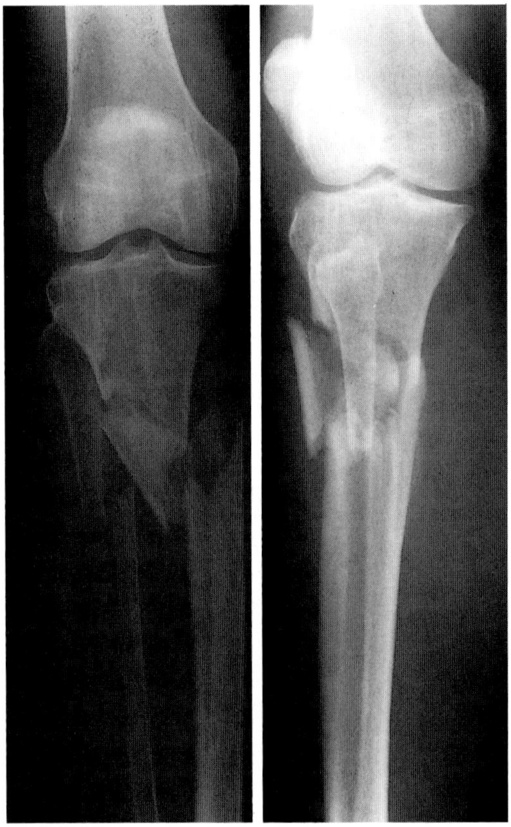

Figure 3.4

A closed proximal tibial fracture which is unsuitable for locked nailing. The lateral view in particular shows that the fracture is too proximal to allow for sufficient fracture stability to be gained.

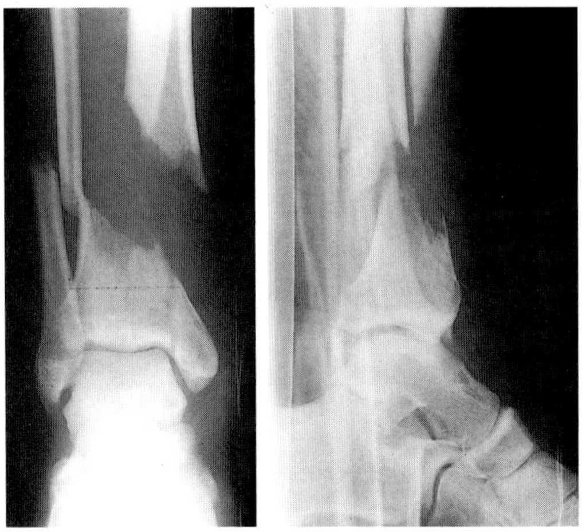

Figure 3.5

A distal tibial fracture that is unsuitable for nailing. Not only is the distal fragment too small to ensure adequate stabilization with a locking nail but there are multiple intra-articular fractures. This was a closed fracture with proximal migration of a 4 inch section of tibia which had been denuded of its blood supply. External skeletal fixation was used to treat this fracture.

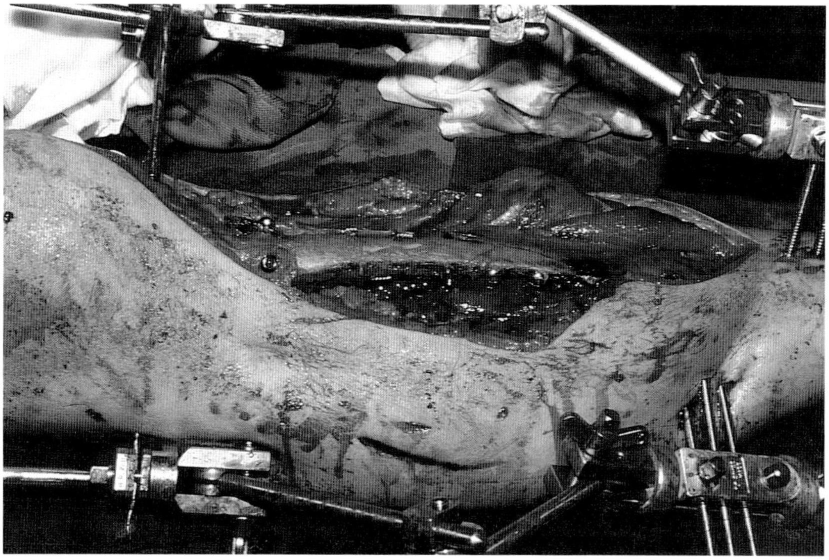

Figure 3.6

The use of a Hoffmann external fixation device to treat a Gustilo Type IIIb open tibial fracture.

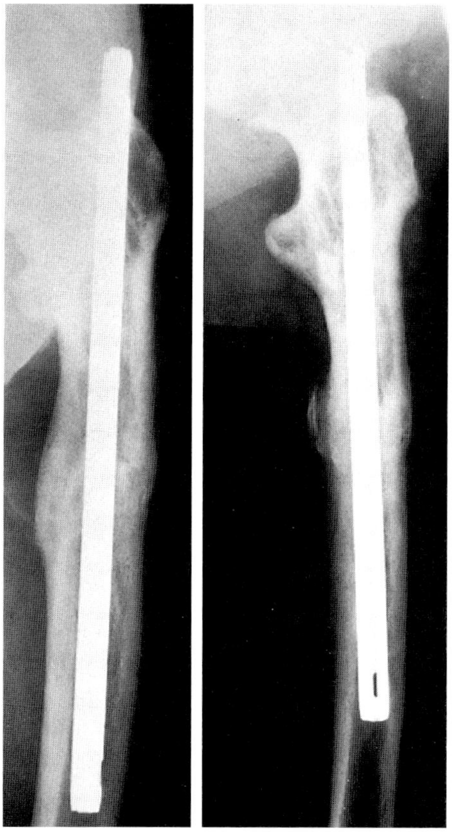

Figure 3.7

A proximal femoral fracture in a pagetic femur with a distal varus deformity. A Küntscher nail has been used to stabilize the fracture. Good contact between the nail and the endosteal surface of the cortex was obtained distal to the fracture.

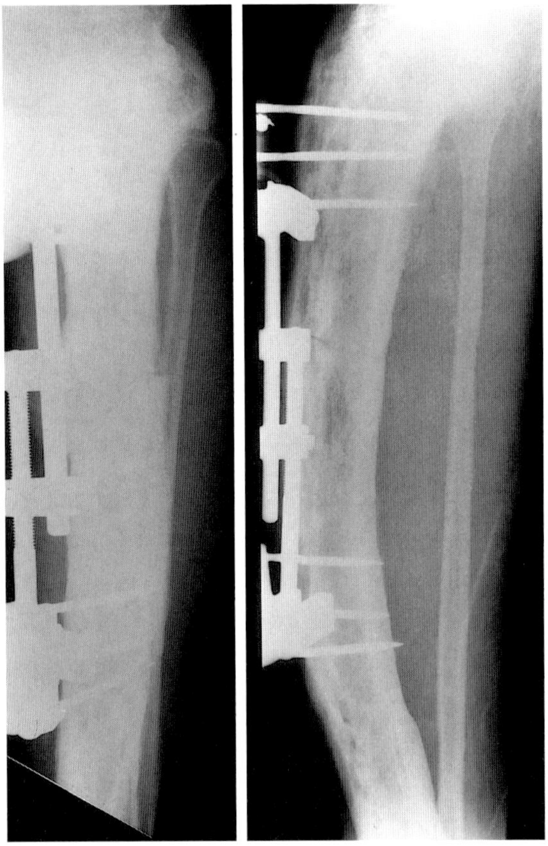

Figure 3.8

A fracture in a pagetic tibia of an 82-year-old lady. The use of an intramedullary nail would have meant multiple osteotomies in a somewhat frail patient. External skeletal fixation was used to treat this fracture which healed.

CHAPTER 4 CLOSED NAILING OF THE FEMUR

Preparation for surgery

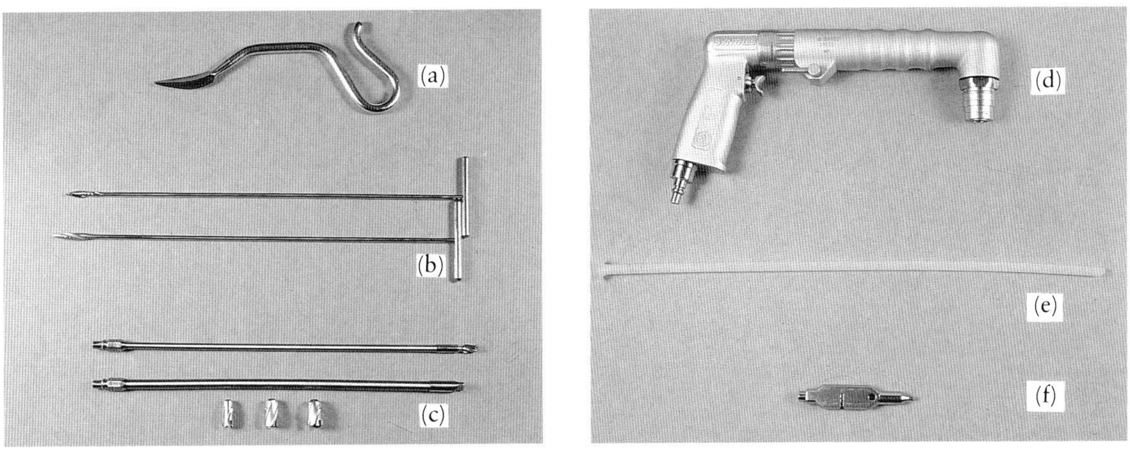

Figure 4.1

Prior to commencing closed intramedullary nailing of the femur it is important to have the correct equipment. Most nails require the use of power reamers such as those marketed by the AO group in addition to the specialized equipment appropriate for the nail. The essential ancillary instrumentation used to insert the Grosse-Kempf nail is illustrated:

(a) Bone awl to breech the femoral cortex
(b) Hand reamers
(c) Flexible intramedullary reamers and bits
(d) Power drill with reamer driving attachment
(e) Plastic tube to facilitate exchange of guide wires
(f) Guide wire holder

The use of many of these instruments will be detailed later.

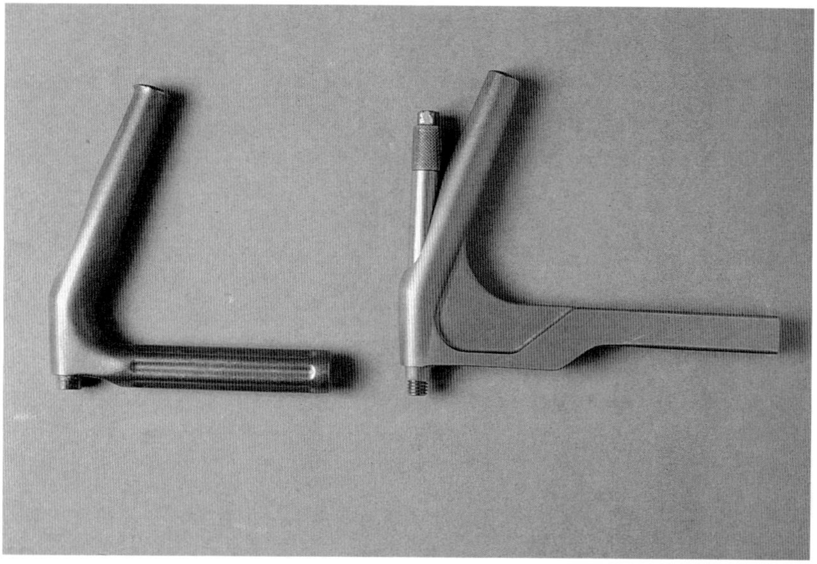

Figure 4.2

If a Grosse-Kempf femoral locking nail is to be used, particular equipment is required. The precise use of this instrumentation is detailed later, although much of it is obvious. As proximal and distal cross-screws may be used, drill bits of different diameters are required as well as a screwdriver and depth gauge. Figure 4.2 shows a Grosse-Kempf nail holder on the left and a proximal cross-screw targeting device on the right.

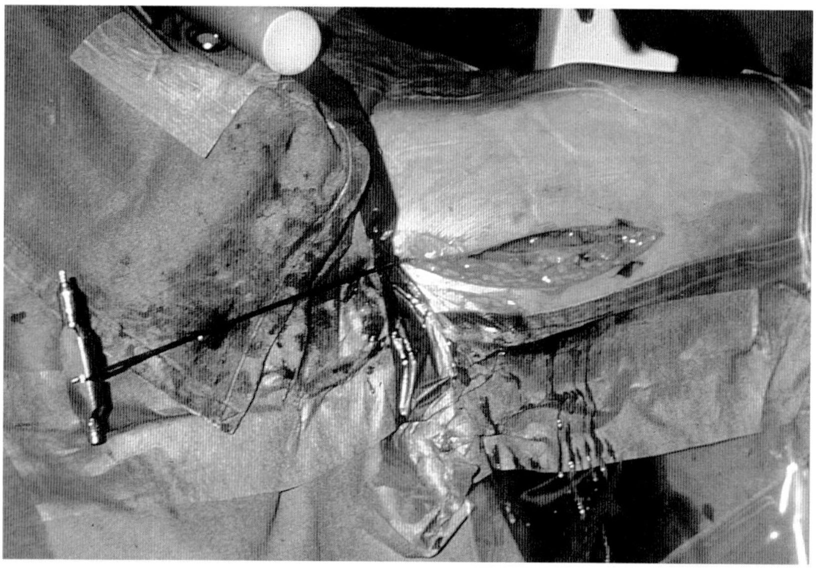

Figure 4.3

It is essential to have the correct guide wires before closed intramedullary nailing can be performed. The length of the guide wires must be such that they can be passed down the femoral medullary canal and still have sufficient exposed length to allow a femoral nail and introducer to be placed over them.

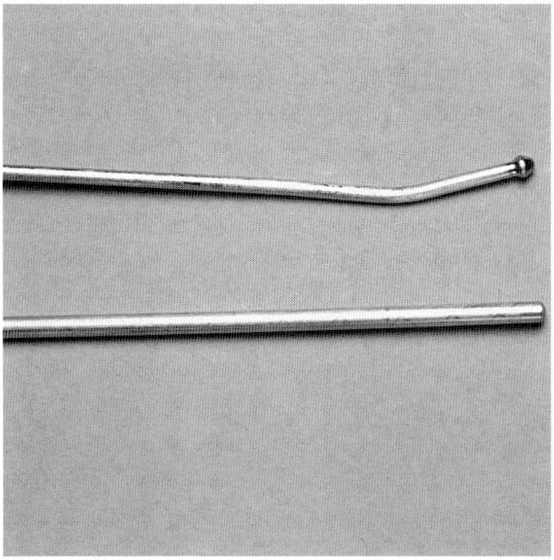

Figure 4.4

Two types of guide wire are necessary. Initial reduction and reaming is performed using an olive-tipped guide wire. This must be of sufficiently small diameter to allow the passage of flexible reamers over it. The olive tip aids removal should a reamer become stuck in the medullary canal. Fracture reduction is usually facilitated by bending the tip of the reamer by about 20 degrees approximately 2 cm from its tip. A straight olive-tipped guide wire is particularly useful in the reaming of very distal femoral or tibial fractures. The thicker straight guide wire is used to introduce the nail itself. It is graduated proximally to allow for accurate intra-operative calculation of the nail length.

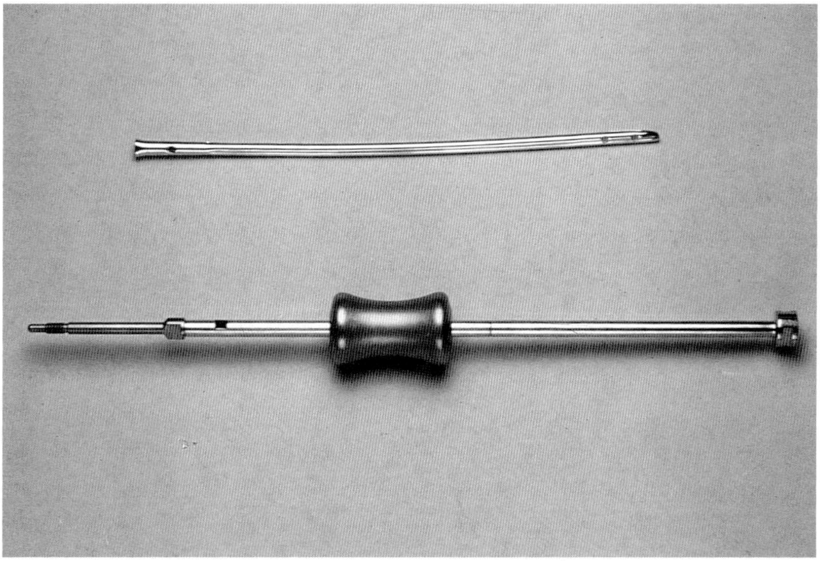

Figure 4.5

If an intramedullary nail becomes stuck in the femoral diaphysis, it can be very difficult to remove. Ideally the surgeon should avoid this complication by the use of correct surgical technique. However, it is important that a nail extractor be available at the time of surgery. The extractor for the Grosse-Kempf nail is shown here. Other extractors are similar, although they may use a hook to engage in a slot in the proximal nail instead of the screw-thread attachment shown here. Nail removal is discussed further in Chapter 19.

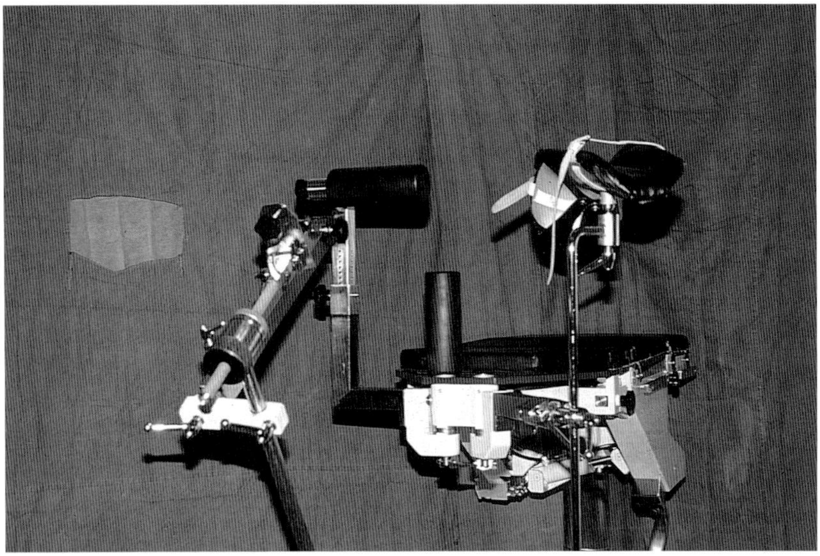

a

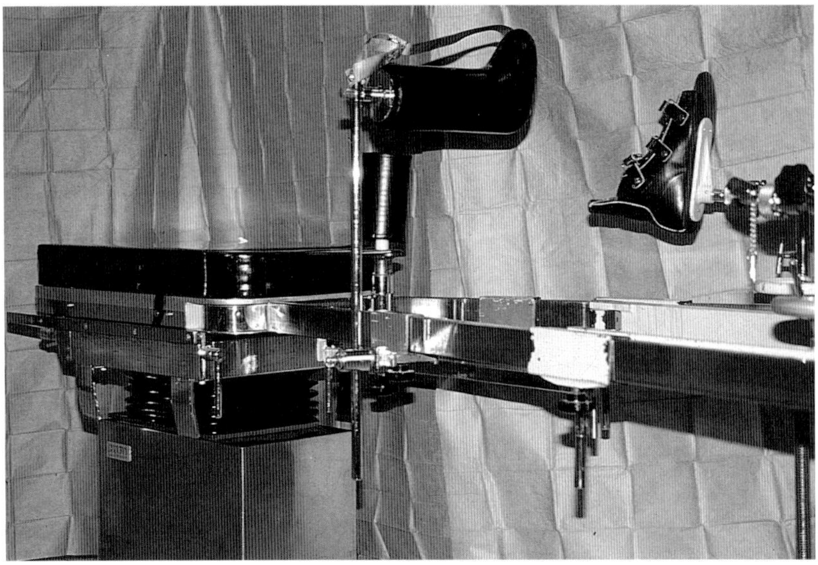

b

Figure 4.6

Before closed intramedullary nailing can be undertaken, it is essential to have an appropriate operating table. Many modern tables are suitable. Some are purpose-built for intramedullary nailing (Figure 4.6a) whereas others are regular operating tables that can be converted for nailing (Figure 4.6b). The particular attachments that are required depend on whether the lateral (Figure 4.8) or supine (Figure 4.9) position is preferred. Most tables are suitable for intramedullary nailing if minor alterations are made.

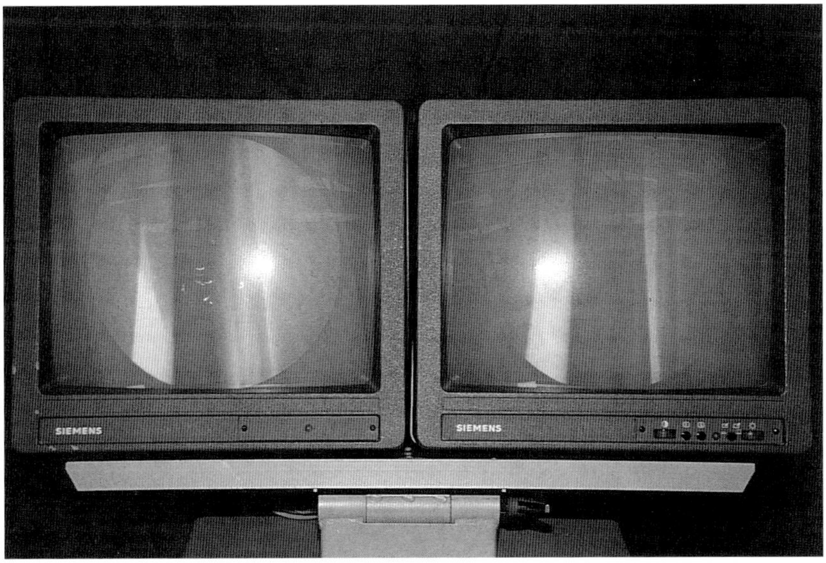

Figure 4.7

Most modern image intensifiers are adequate for closed nailing. It is preferable to have a second screen with a memory to allow simultaneous screening of both antero-posterior and lateral X-ray scans and to minimize radiation. It is essential to have a radiographer who is well trained in the use of the image intensifier.

Positioning of patient

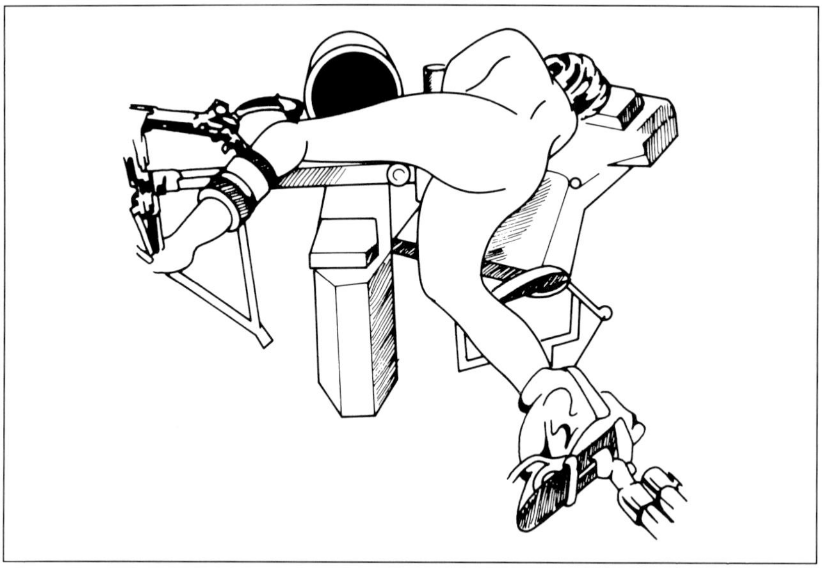

Figure 4.8

The lateral position provides easy access to the greater trochanter and, with the image intensifier placed in the position shown in Figure 4.8, good visualization of the femoral shaft can be obtained. Some surgeons prefer this position for nailing proximal femoral fractures, as the position of the femur compensates for the flexion of the proximal fragment. However, others find it more difficult to visualize the upper femur on the image intensifier in the lateral position. It may also be difficult to control the position of the distal fragment in distal femoral fractures with the patient in the lateral position. The fragment tends to drift into valgus. In addition, if distal cross-screws are required, the supine position provides for easier access.

However, each surgeon will develop his or her own technique and will usually adopt either the traditional lateral or supine positions.

One indication for the use of the lateral position is in patients with hip osteoarthritis. The flexion deformity associated with hip osteoarthritis makes the approach to the proximal femur difficult in the supine position. Surgeons that favour the supine position may have to approach the flexed hip from below in osteoarthritic patients (Moran et al, 1990). The lateral position permits hip flexion and therefore avoids this problem.

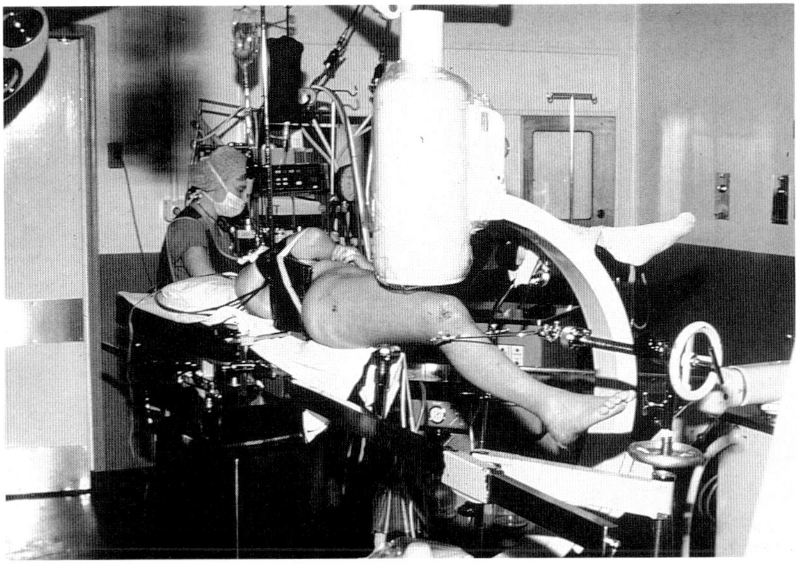

a

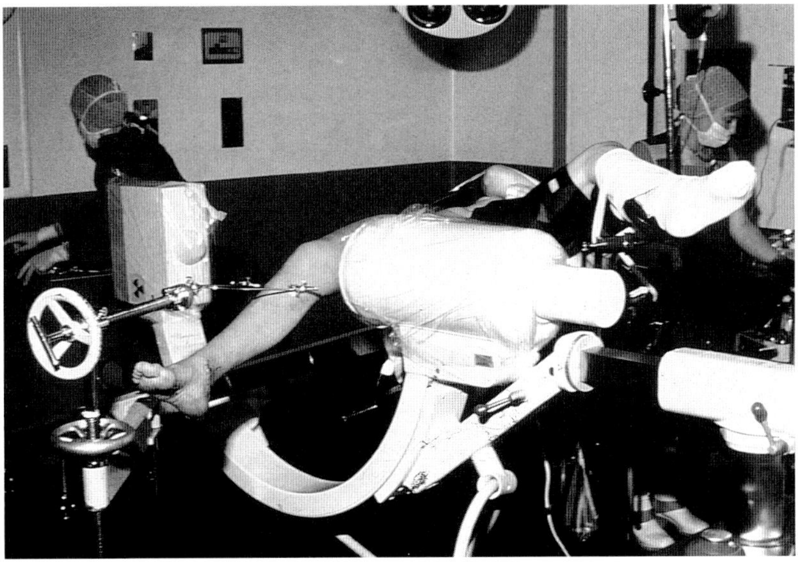

b

Figure 4.9

The supine position is preferred by many surgeons. The patient is placed supine on an orthopaedic table. Sufficient traction to reduce the fracture is applied to the leg, which is adducted to allow access to the greater tuberosity. This is important as, if the leg is not adducted, the difficulty in gaining access to the proximal femur may result in incorrect nail placement and considerable bony damage.

The other leg must not obstruct the image intensifier and is best positioned on a padded support with the hip flexed and abducted and the knee flexed. It should be well secured to prevent it falling off the support peroperatively. This is best demonstrated in Figure 4.9b. At all times the image intensifier must have good access in antero-posterior (Figure 4.9a) and the lateral planes (Figure 4.9b). It should be possible to visualize the complete femur without difficulty.

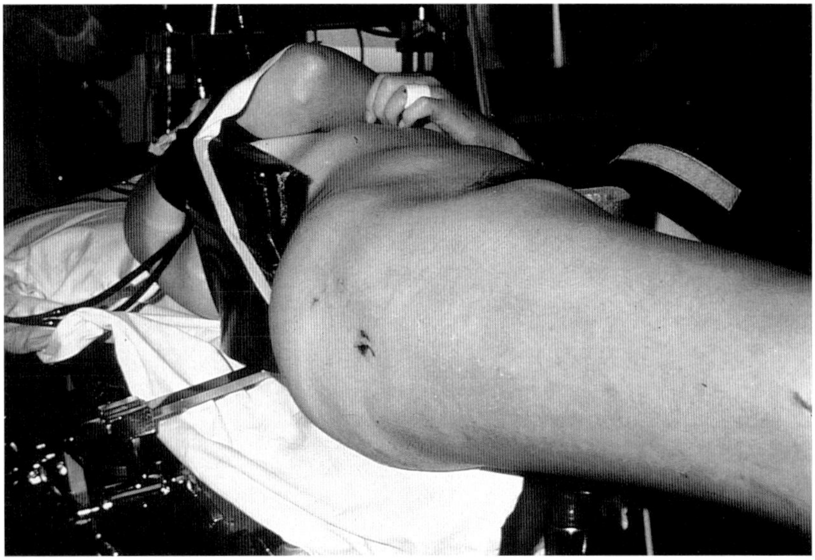

Figure 4.10

The importance of good access to the proximal femur cannot be overemphasized, particularly in fat or well-muscled patients. In addition to maximal adduction of the leg, it is useful to place a pad in the ipsilateral loin and thereby push the abdomen out of the way. This is usually adequate to provide good access, but occasionally it can be supplemented by placing a board under the thorax and abdomen and lying the patient away from the side of the fracture.

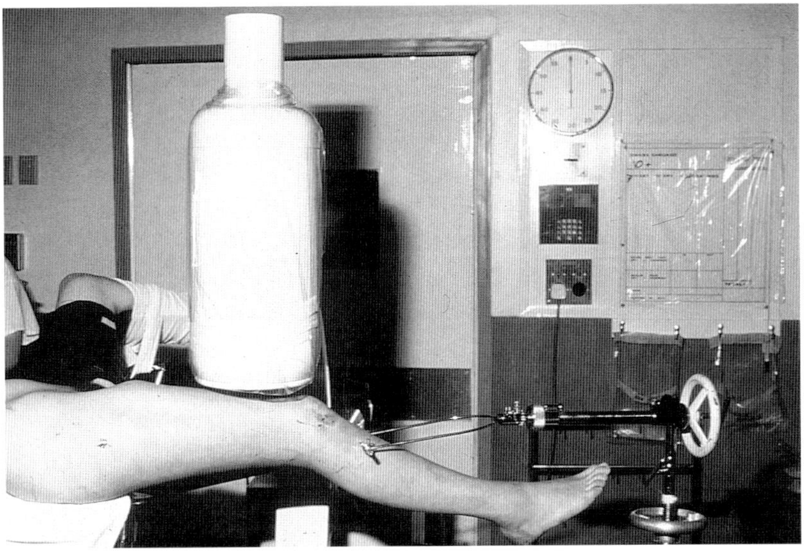

a

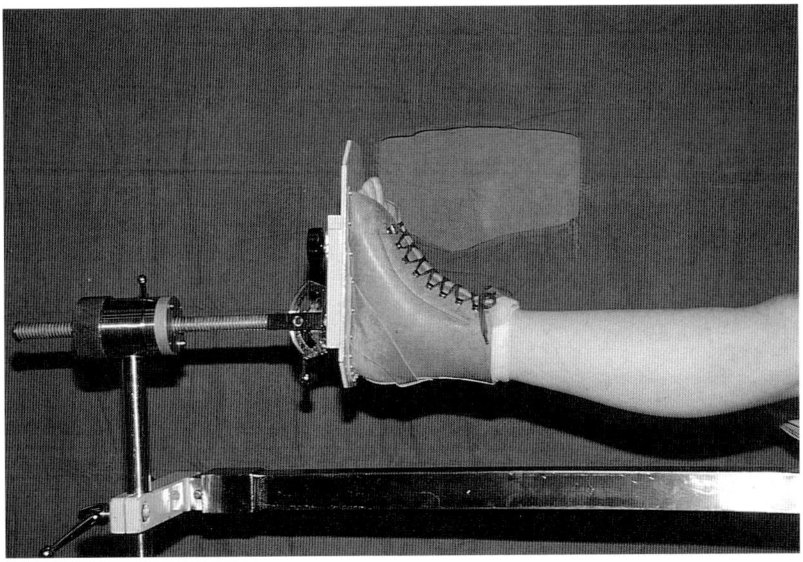

b

Figure 4.11

Traction can be applied through a skeletal pin (Figure 4.11a) or through an orthopaedic boot (Figure 4.11b). The choice between the two usually depends on the size of the patient and the time that has elapsed between the fracture and operation. If the patient is thin and is operated on soon after admission, then skeletal traction is not always required and the use of the orthopaedic boot may be satisfactory. However, should the patient be fat or well-muscled, or should there be a delay before surgery, then skeletal traction should be used in the ward and the pin retained at operation. If the fracture is more than 3 or 4 days old, or has shortened, then a skeletal pin is recommended as greater traction can be applied.

If a skeletal transfixion pin is used it can be placed in either the distal femur or the proximal tibia. A distal femoral pin provides for a more direct pull on the fracture, but in reality either position is usually satisfactory. If a femoral pin is used in a distal femoral fracture, care must be taken that the pin does not obstruct nail insertion.

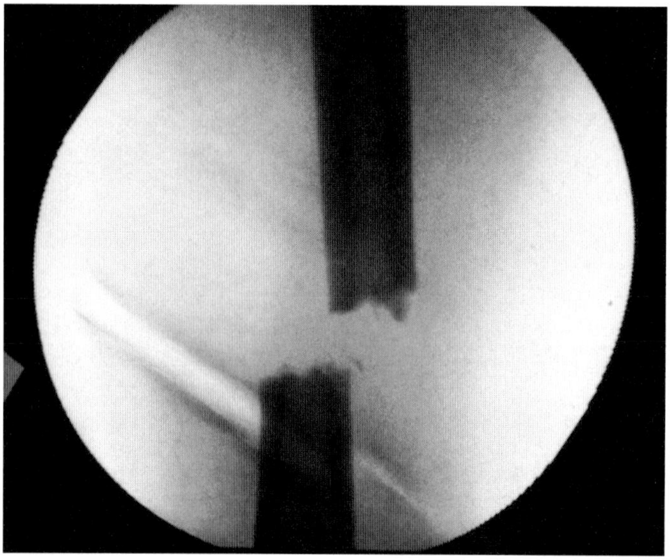

a

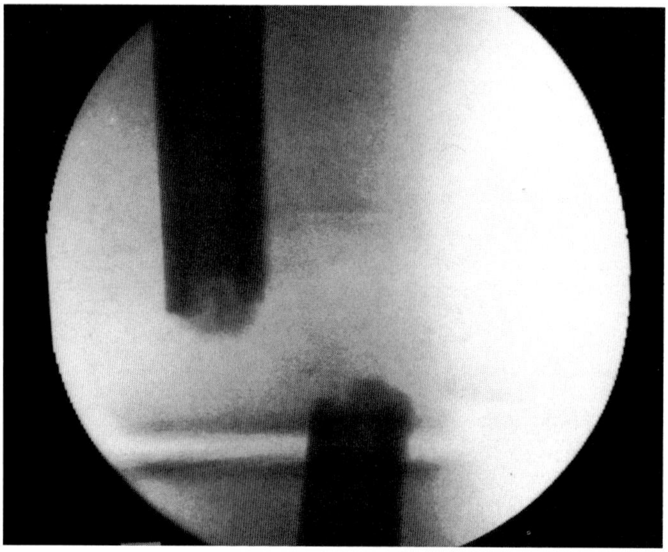

b

Figure 4.12

Once the patient is set up on the orthopaedic table, it is very important to check that the fracture can be reduced. Figure 4.12a and b show antero-posterior and lateral image intensifier views of a femoral diaphyseal fracture just below the isthmus. The patient is a 24-year-old woman with small muscles and relatively light traction though an orthopaedic boot has resulted in slight overdistraction of the fracture. Although some overdistraction is acceptable and may aid reduction, gross overdistraction should be avoided.

Despite the gap between the bone ends, reduction was achieved, although in this case it was obviously impossible to maintain the reduction until a guide wire was passed. If closed reduction cannot be obtained pre-operatively the operation should not proceed. Instead a different fixation method should be chosen. Usually an open nailing will be performed.

Pre-operative reduction of femoral fractures is usually straightforward but the maintenance of the reduced position peroperatively requires an experienced assistant. The assistant should be familiar with the technique that is required to reduce the fracture – the technique having been practised pre-operatively. Ideally the assistant should also be gowned and gloved to assist with fracture reduction.

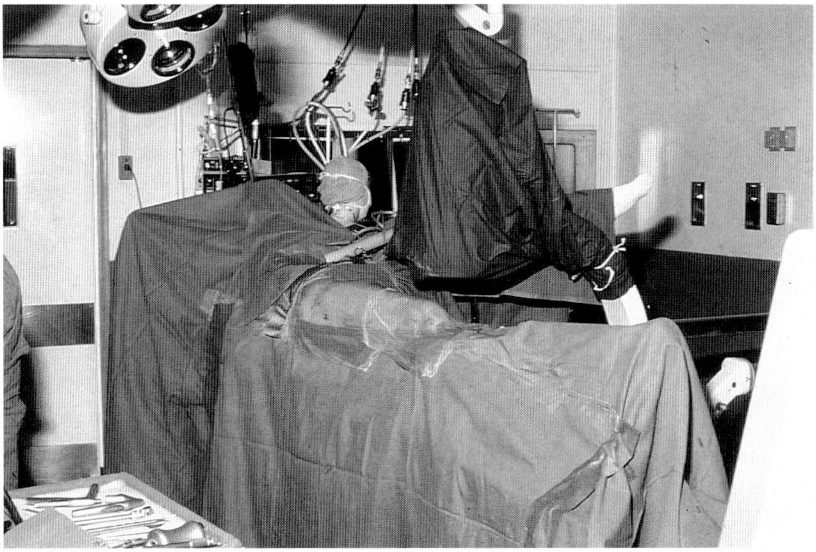

Figure 4.13

The patient should be draped to allow access to the whole femur in case distal cross-screws are required. As the lower end of the incision is level with the greater trochanter, the drapes should be placed to expose the skin between the iliac crest and the knee. Five extra large drapes are usually sufficient to cover the patient adequately. One extra large drape should be placed on the lateral side of the thigh between the thigh and the floor. This will ensure sterility when lateral views are taken with the image intensifier. The intensifier itself can be draped in the usual manner using a sterile bag which is tied tightly around the C-arm. Plastic adhesive squares are used to ensure that the drapes remain in position during the operation.

Alternatively a modified plastic hip drape can be used. This is suspended from a bar above the patient and dropped to the floor. The image intensifier is placed on the far side of the hip drape and does not need to be covered.

The surgeon stands at the greater trochanter and the image intensifier screen is conveniently placed at the foot of the table. The scrub nurse will usually stand beside the surgeon with the instruments located between the nurse and the intensifier screen.

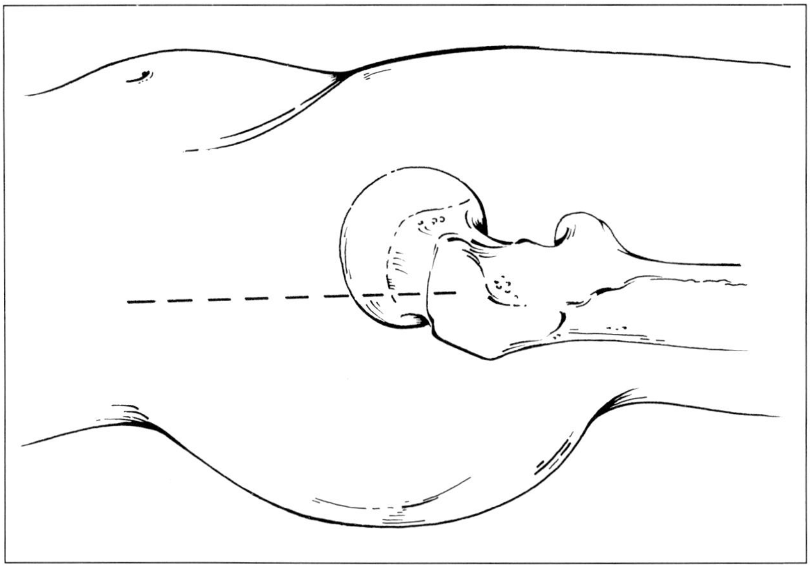

a

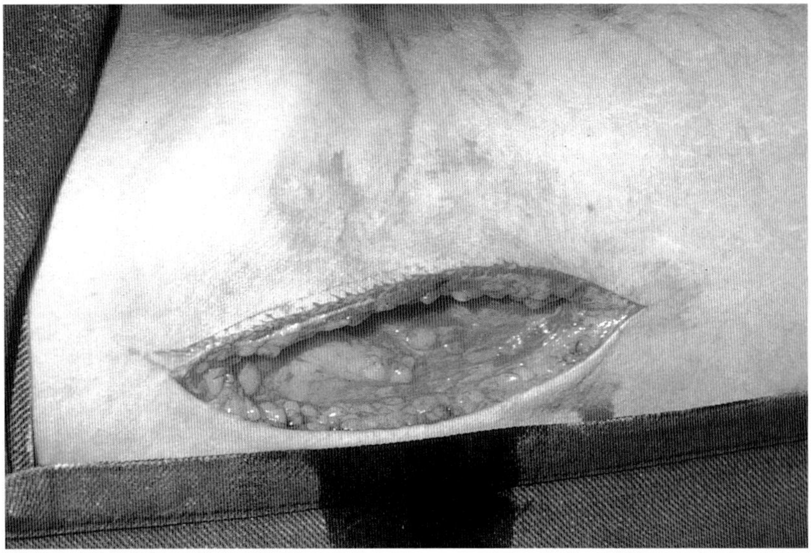

b

Figure 4.14

The incision for closed femoral nailing starts at the level of the greater trochanter and is carried proximally for approximately 10 cm (Figure 4.14a). The proximal location of the fracture is highlighted by the clinical photograph shown in Figure 4.14b, which illustrates the relative positions of the incision and the anterior iliac spine. The most common mistake regarding the incision is to centre it on the greater trochanter. This means that the incision will have to be extended proximally per-operatively to accommodate the instruments.

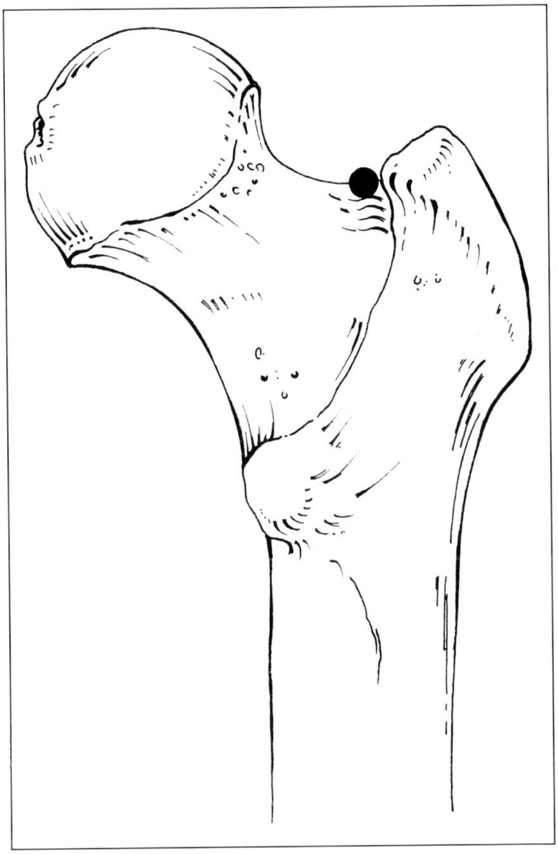

a

Figure 4.15

After the skin incision has been made, the subcutaneous fat and deep fascia are incised. Subsequent surgery is carried out by palpation rather than visualization of the relevant structures. There is debate about the optimal point of entry in the proximal femur. Some surgeons suggest that the tip of the greater trochanter is the correct location, whereas others feel that the more centrally located piriformis fossa provides more direct access to the femoral shaft. Figure 4.15a illustrates the location of the piriformis fossa which is palpated just medial to the greater trochanter. This location should be sought and a defect in the cortex made with the bone awl (Figure 4.15b).

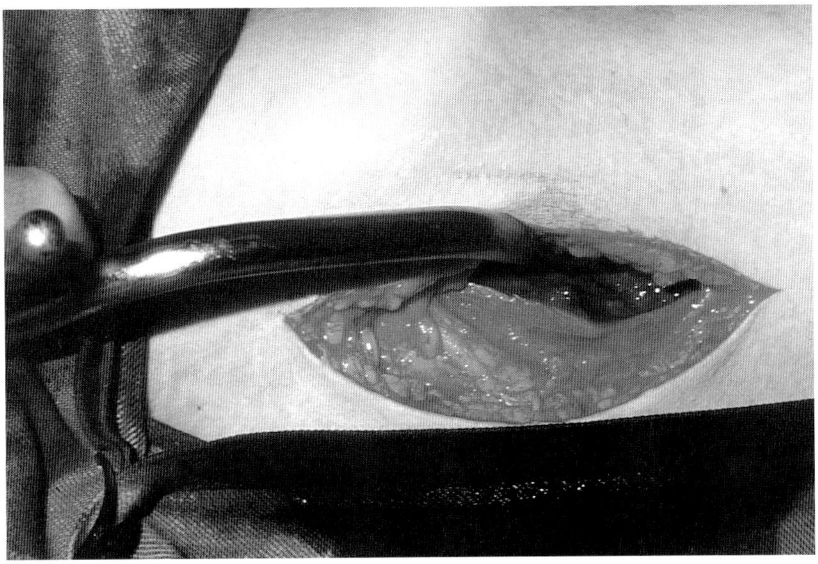

b

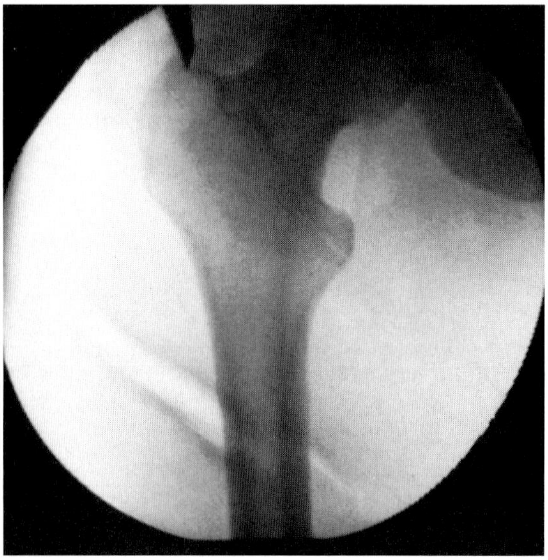

a

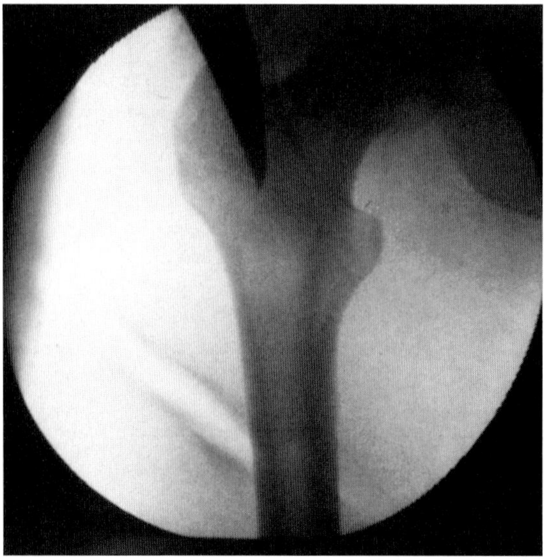

b

Figure 4.16

It is not always possible to place the tip of the bone awl exactly in the piriformis fossa, but usually a point between the fossa and the tip of the trochanter will be adequate. Figure 4.16a is a picture taken from the image intensifier which illustrates the use of a starting position just lateral to the fossa. If the starting position is too far lateral (lateral to the tip of the greater trochanter) then it will be difficult to pass a nail round the curve into the medulla and a proximal femoral fracture may ensue.

In addition, a lateral starting position often results in the nail twisting as it is passed down the femoral shaft. This may not matter if a straight Küntscher nail is used but, if the nail is contoured to match the bow of the femur, twisting the nail may result in bony damage. It will also ensure difficulty in placement of the distal cross-screws. If the starting position is too medial then not only is it difficult to pass the nail into the medullary canal but a femoral neck fracture may occur (Figure 23.15). The bone awl should be driven right through the cortex, as shown in Figure 4.16b.

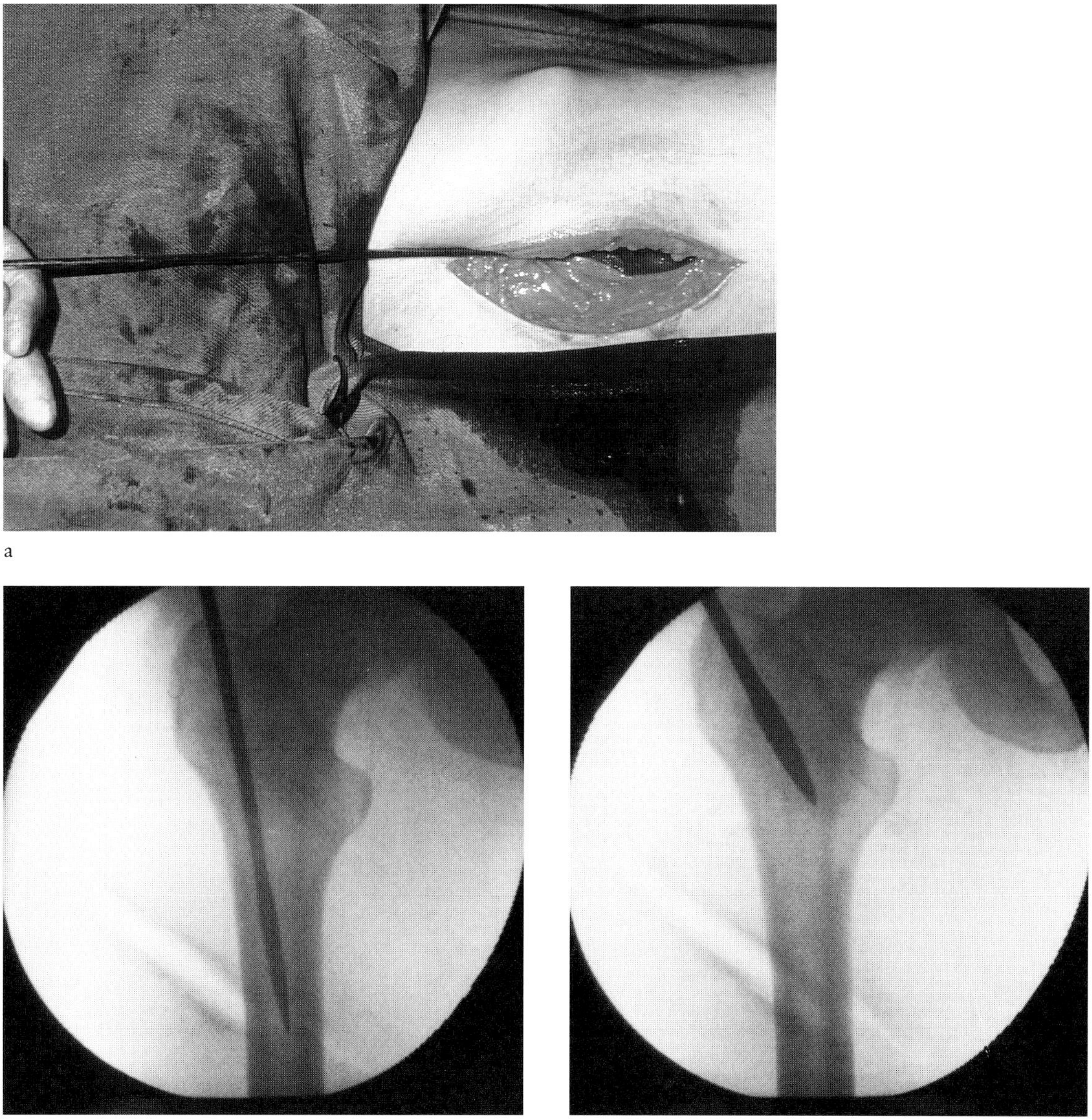

a b c

Figure 4.17

After removal of the bone awl, it is usually impossible to pass a guide wire down the medullary canal unless the metaphyseal bone is soft. In young bone, the metaphysis may be very hard and considerable effort is required to penetrate it. A small hand reamer is passed through the cortical defect into the medullary canal (Figures 4.17a and b). Care must be taken that the hand reamer is driven in the correct direction, as it is possible to perforate the medial cortex if the wrong direction is chosen (Figure 4.17c).

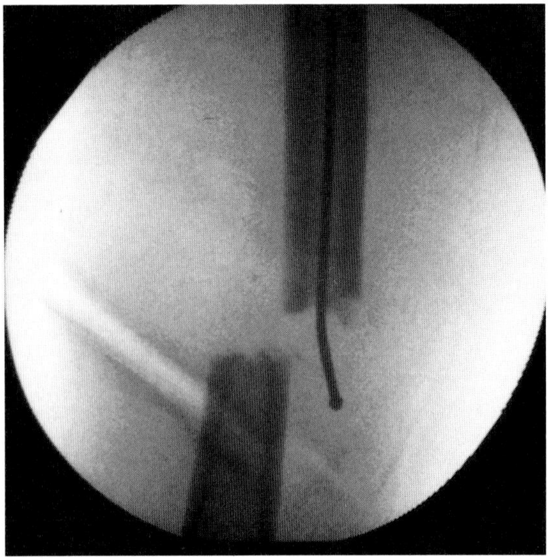

a

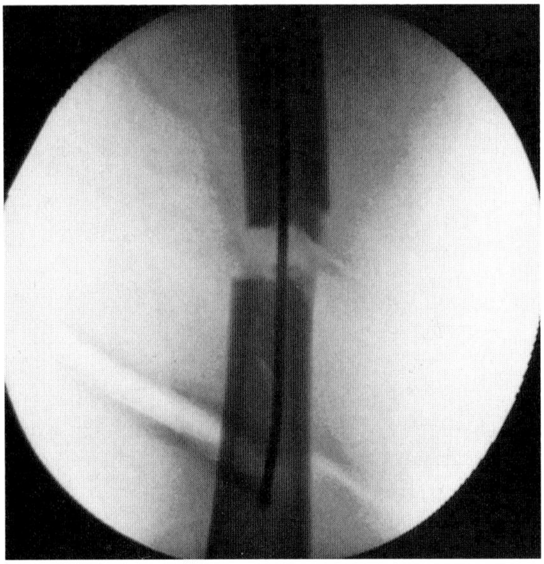

b

Figure 4.18

After removal of the hand reamer, an olive-tipped guide wire is passed down the medullary canal as far as the fracture site. If the fracture is undisplaced, a straight olive-tipped guide wire is used but if reduction is required, as shown in Figure 4.18a, the presence of the bend in the distal guide wire allows the surgeon to 'feel' for the distal fragment. By rotating the guide wire, it is usually possible to engage the distal fragment. An untipped guide wire should not be used at this stage as the olive tip permits removal of the reamers should they become stuck in the medullary canal. The fracture should be reduced by use of the same technique as practised pre-operatively and the guide wire passed into the distal fragment (Figure 4.18b). In cases where reduction is difficult, the screening mode on the image intensifier may be required. Screening time should be kept to a minimum to reduce radiation.

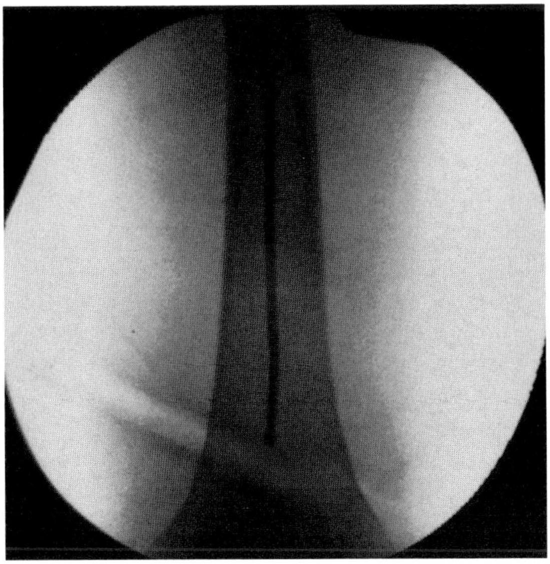

Figure 4.19

The olive-tipped guide wire should be passed into the centre of the distal fragment. The reamers and the nail will always follow the guide wire and therefore an eccentrically located guide wire will result in a mal-positioned nail (Figure 23.3). It is very important to be centrally located on the antero-posterior X-ray scan (Figure 4.19) as, if the guide wire is placed close to the medial or lateral cortices, a valgus or varus deformity will ensue. As there is a smaller distance between the anterior and posterior cortices than between the medial and lateral cortices any mal-position of the guide wire in the lateral X-ray scan is less critical. However, the surgeon should aim for a centrally located guide wire on both X-ray views.

The guide wire should be placed firmly into the metaphyseal bone of the distal femur to minimize the risk of it backing out later.

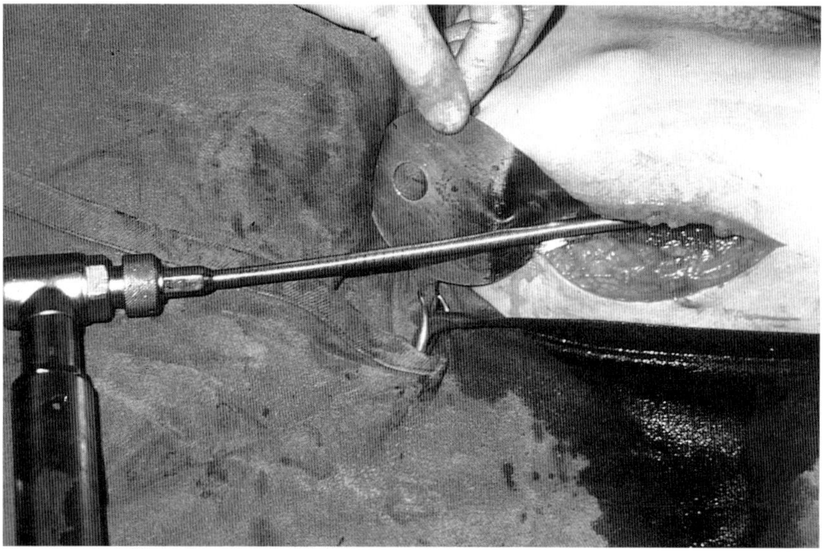

a

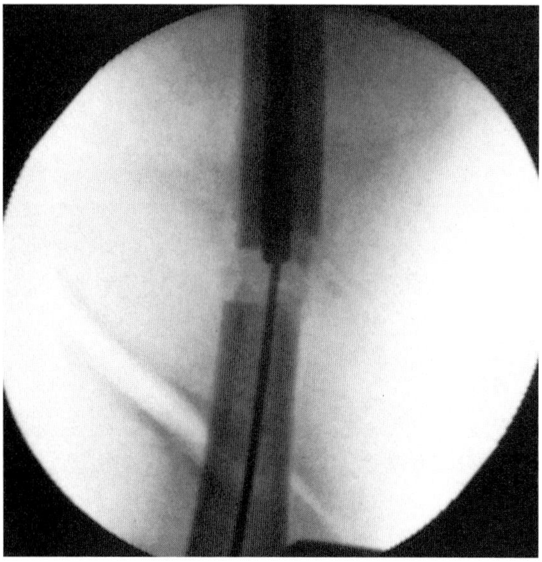

b

Figure 4.20

The reamers are introduced over the olive-tipped guide wire (Figure 4.20a). The initial reamer is end-cutting and enlarges the track to 9 mm. Subsequently side-cutting reamers are used to expand the track in 0.5 mm increments. The progress of the reamers can be checked on the image intensifier (Figure 4.20b). Care should be taken to ream the whole length of the femur. Failure to do this may result in distraction of the fracture or cortical damage as a nail is hammered into unreamed bone. Power reamers must be used. Hand reamers have no place in closed nailing of a fracture except initially to breach the proximal metaphysis.

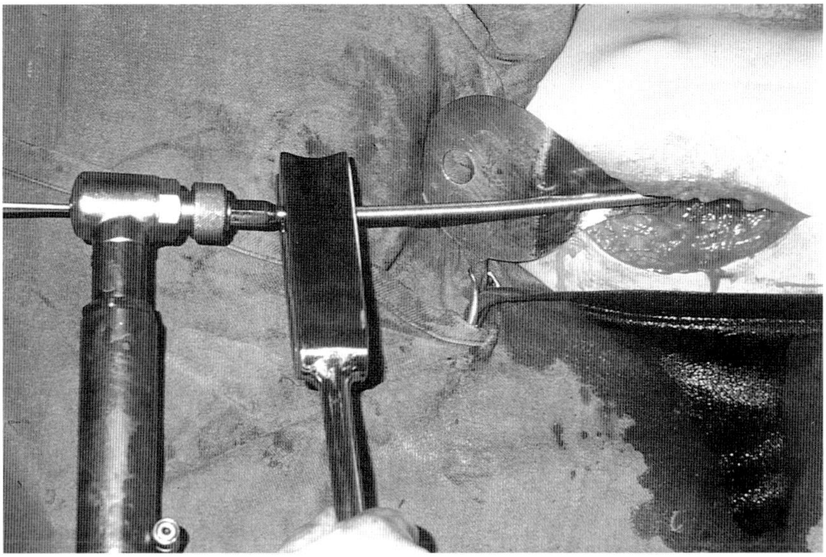

Figure 4.21

The internal diameter of patients' femoral medullary canals varies greatly but it is usually fairly easy to ream to about 12 mm. After this, care must be taken to prevent the reamer from sticking within the canal. Reamers should only be increased by 0.5 mm at a time and reaming should be undertaken slowly when the endosteal surface of the cortex is felt.

If the reamer does get stuck inside the medullary canal, a number of procedures can be undertaken to release it. Gentle use of the drill may free the reamer, although as the drill overheats it may lose power. A period of rest to allow the drill and the surgeon to cool may be necessary. The flexible drive of the reamer can be reversed by using either a drill or a spanner applied to the top of the reamer. However, some flexible reamers are made of coiled steel and reversal of direction may cause the reamer to uncoil.

A slot hammer can be positioned over the reamer against the drill attachments and the assembly tapped out. Care must be taken not to damage the drill. This method is illustrated in Figure 4.21. Alternatively the guide wire extractor can be placed on the guide wire and a slot hammer used. The olive tip on the guide wire engages in the reamer bit to facilitate removal.

If these manoeuvres are unsuccessful, open operative removal will be necessary. If the reamer is stuck at the fracture site, this may be relatively straightforward. However, if the reamer is stuck at a distance from the fracture then one fragment of the femur may have to be split to allow removal. This is rarely required however.

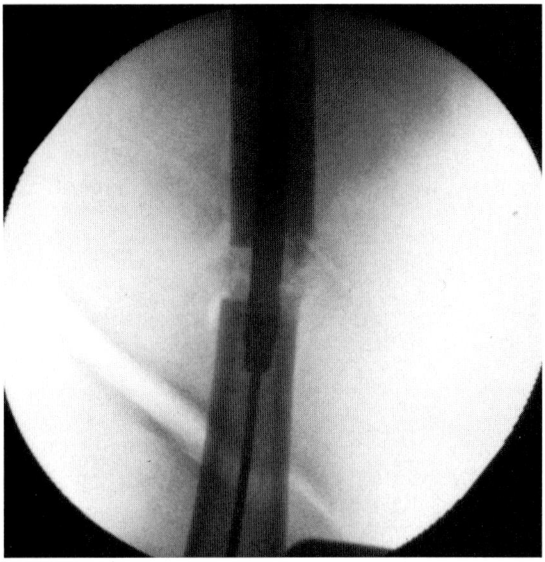

a

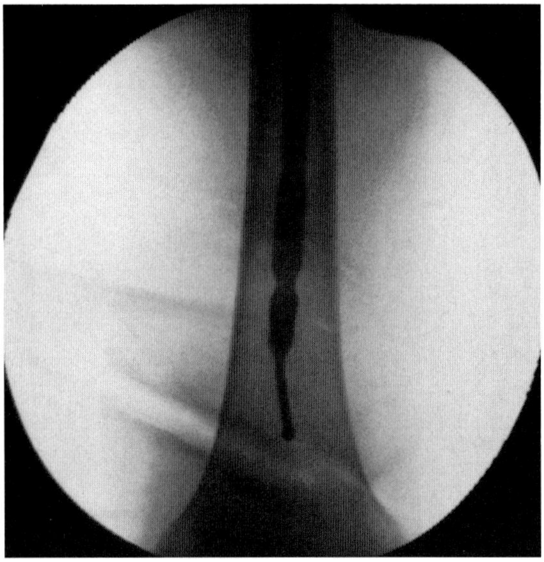

b

Figure 4.22

Reaming should always be carried out so that the resultant track in the medullary canal is 1 mm wider than the intramedullary nail that the surgeon proposes to use. If reaming is difficult, the surgeon may choose to ream only 0.5 mm more than the nail, but this is hazardous as the nail may stick and be impossible to remove. The surgeon should never merely ream to the same size as the nail. It is advisable to use at least a 12 or 13 mm nail in adult femora. If a smaller nail is used it may bend (see Figure 23.5) and be difficult to remove or replace. In older patients the medullary canal may be very wide and nails of 15 or 16 mm may be required. Care should be taken when reaming across the fracture site (Figure 4.22a) as there may be some cortical damage unless the fracture is properly reduced. The surgeon should always remember that the reamer can only be passed as far as the bend in the guide wire (Figure 4.22b). This does not matter in this particular fracture but in more distal fractures the surgeon might have to change to a straight olive-tipped guide wire to facilitate distal reaming.

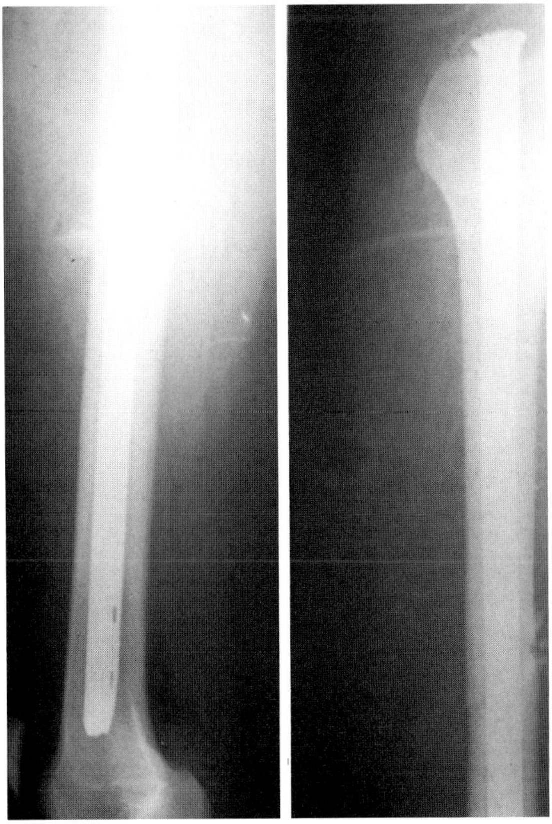

Figure 4.23

The decision as to the size of the nail depends mainly on the exact location of the fracture. In fractures located at or very close to the isthmus, as here, the surgeon will rely on contact between the endosteal surface of the cortex and the nail to achieve stability. He or she should, therefore, ream to a size that will ensure 2 cm of contact on each side of the fracture. If there is any doubt as to the stability of the fixation, cross-screws should be inserted.

If the fracture is proximal or distal to the isthmus it will be impossible to achieve stability merely by gaining good contact between the endosteal surface and the nail on both sides of the fracture. Therefore, the medullary canal should be reamed only until there is contact between nail and cortex in whichever fragment contains the isthmus. Obviously the surgeon should ream to allow at least a 12 mm nail to be inserted.

If there is comminution at the isthmus, there will be no contact between endosteum and nail. It is therefore sufficient to insert a nail of the appropriate size for the patient as proximal and distal screws will ensure stability.

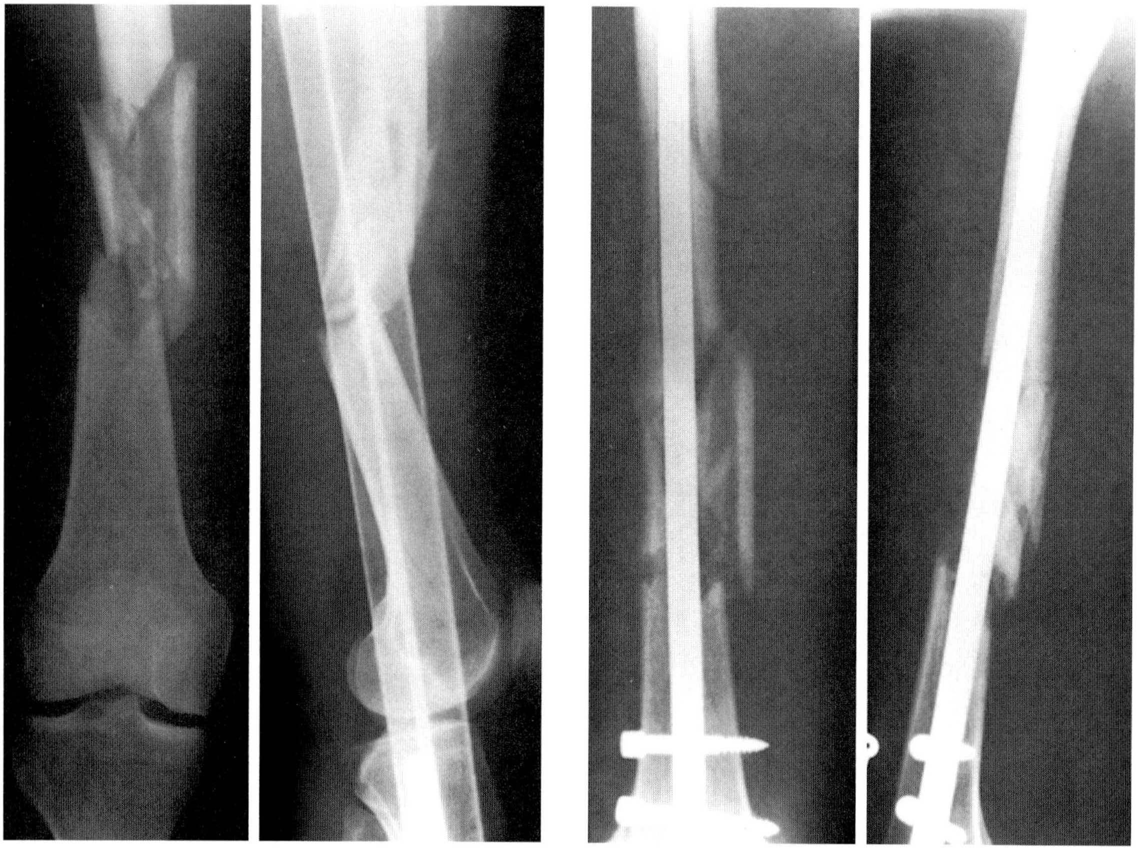

a b

Figure 4.24

When reaming a comminuted fracture, only the bone proximal and distal to the area of comminution need be reamed. Reaming of the comminuted area is unnecessary and potentially harmful to the muscle envelope around the femur. The reamer should be pushed through the comminuted area. Nailing of comminuted fractures is described further in Chapter 9.

Where there is a segmental fracture, the segment is frequently not intact (Figure 4.24a) and again it is usually sufficient to push the reamer through the damaged segment. After reaming, the nail is introduced in the standard manner (Figure 4.24b). However, where the central fracture segment is intact, reaming may cause the segment to spin and thus become devitalized. Under these circumstances, the segment may have to be held to prevent rotation. In the tibia this may be achieved by external pressure with the hand, but in the femur a skin incision should be made and a bone-holding forcep used. Nailing of segmental fractures is described in more detail in Chapter 10.

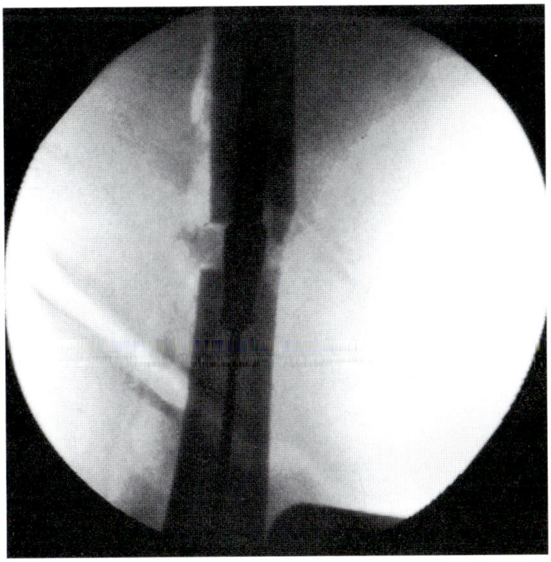

Figure 4.25

Reaming may be useful to aid fracture reduction. As progressively larger reamers are passed over the fracture site, gradual reduction will be achieved. However, it is important to reduce the fracture externally as the reamers pass across the fracture site. If this is not done, it is possible to ream the cortex eccentrically and therefore create cortical damage. This damage is often seen on the superior surface of the lower fragment as it sags downwards onto the guide wire under gravity. When this occurs, the lower fragment should be lifted by external pressure as the reamers are passed over the fracture site.

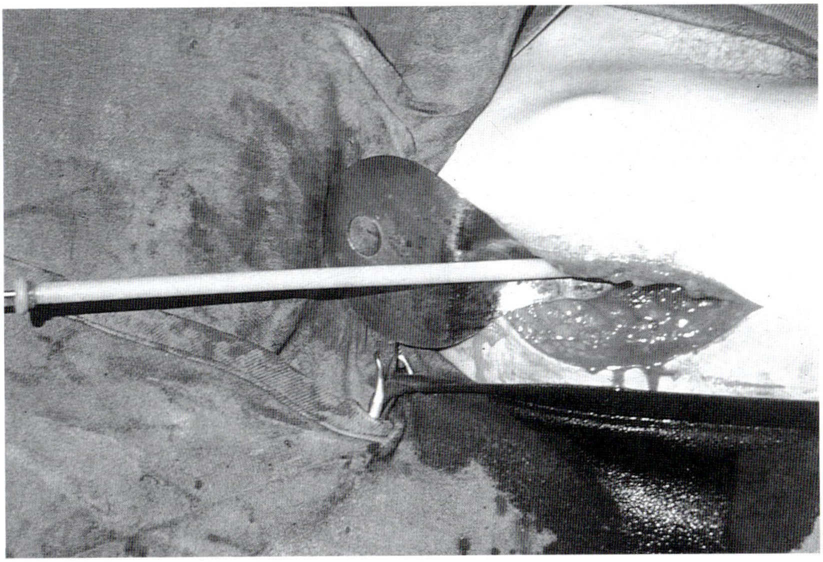

a

Figure 4.26

After the medullary canal has been reamed to the correct length and width, the reamers can be removed and the guide wire changed. To change guide wires without losing the reduction of the fracture, a flexible plastic sleeve should be used. The sleeve is passed down over the guide wire (Figure 4.26a) until it is across the fracture site. After positioning the sleeve, the olive-tipped guide wire is removed and the thicker, non-tipped guide wire passed down the femur (Figure 4.26b).

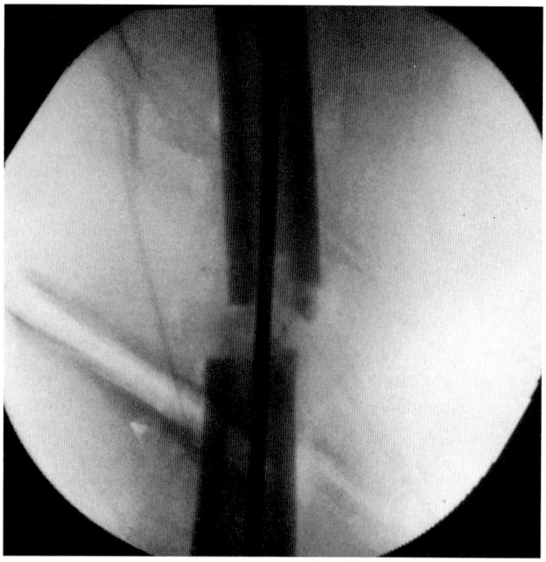

b

Figure 4.26 *continued*

Care must be taken in passing the plastic sleeve over the fracture site. Occasionally the sleeve will be obstructed at the fracture site and if the guide wire is removed at this time the fracture reduction will be lost. Most plastic sleeves have a small metal marker close to their tip to facilitate localization. The surgeon should check that the new guide wire is in the same position as the previous one.

A nail of the correct length should now be selected. Pre-operatively an approximate nail length can be calculated using an ossimeter or by measuring the contralateral femur if this is intact. This estimated length should be confirmed at the time of surgery.

If the guide wire is graduated, then assessment of nail length is straightforward. The guide wire is usually marked at 30 and 40 mm. A ruler is used to measure between these marks and the femur. Should the guide wire not be graduated, the length of the nail can be easily assessed by leaving the plastic sleeve within the femur and marking the point of entry of the wire into the sleeve. The length that the plastic sleeve protrudes from the femur can be measured and subtraction of this length and the length of the exposed guide wire from the total length of the guide wire will give the length of the nail.

Most modern intramedullary nails have a screw thread at the proximal end to facilitate removal. These nails can be placed into the femur so that the proximal end of the nail is flush with the femoral cortex. This minimizes the risk of late buttock discomfort. Other nails, such as the older Küntscher nail (Figure 1.1a) have a slot in the nail so that a hook may be used to remove it. Removal of these nails is facilitated by leaving the slot clear of the cortex. This must be considered when estimating nail length.

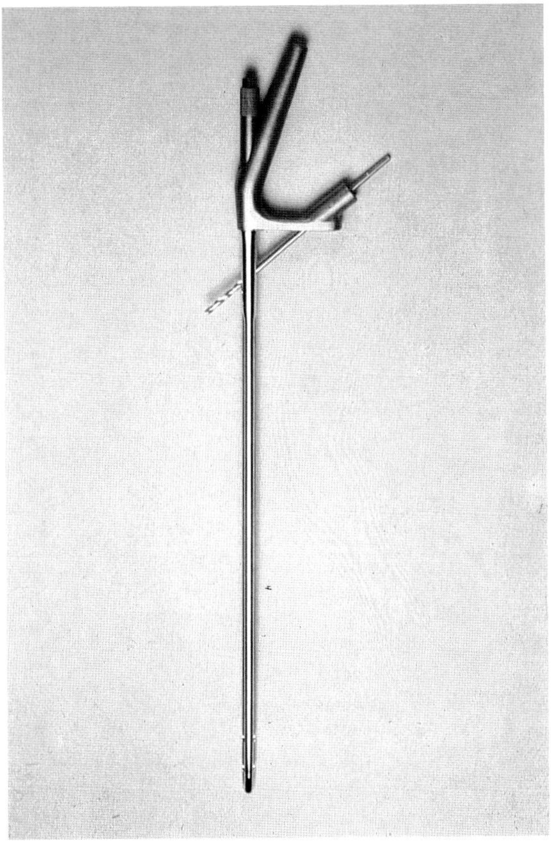

Figure 4.27

The nail can now be mounted on the appropriate introducer (Figure 4.2) and placed over the guide wire. If a locking nail with an oblique proximal screw is used, then care must be taken that the correct right- or left-sided nail is used. Non-locking nails, locking nails with a transverse proximal screw hole or locking nails predrilled with proximal holes in both directions are interchangeable between either femur. This figure shows a Grosse-Kempf femoral nail mounted on the proximal screw introducer. A drill bit illustrates the relationship between the introducer and the proximal screw hole.

The surgeon should assess whether a proximal cross-screw may be required. As the nail is passed into the femur, displacement may occur at previously undisplaced fracture lines. If this happens, proximal and/or distal cross-screws may be necessary. If the surgeon has not realized the potential need for proximal cross-screws the wrong introducer may have been used. As it is difficult to change the introducer after the nail has been hammered home, it is important to select the correct introducer initially.

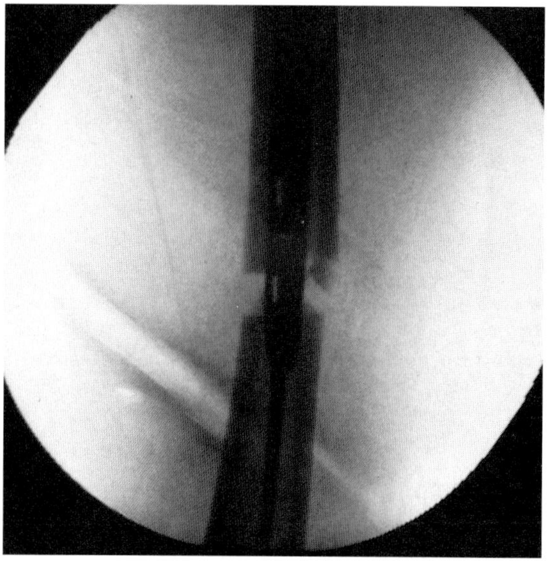

a

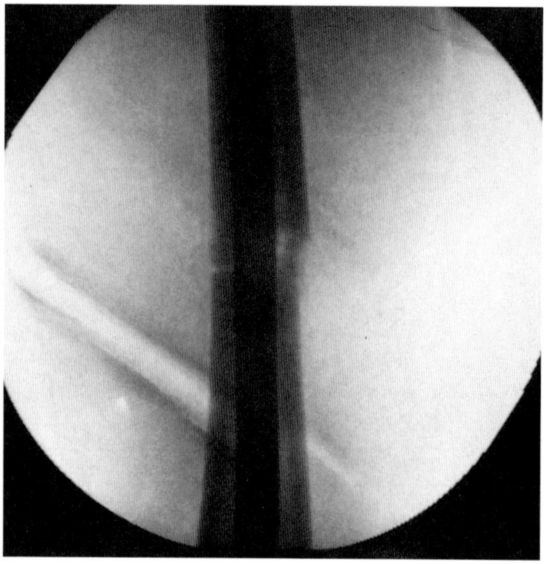

b

Figure 4.28

The nail can now be hammered into the femur. Initially it should be introduced so that the tip is just over the fracture site (Figure 4.28). The fracture should then be fully reduced and the nail hammered home. Excess traction should be slackened to facilitate reduction (Figure 4.28). The guide wire should be removed after the nail is across the fracture but before it is finally embedded in metaphyseal bone.

A problem that is frequently encountered is that the guide wire withdraws from the medullary canal as the nail is hammered home. Occasionally this can result in loss of fracture reduction before the nail is passed across the fracture. The surgeon should check that the guide wire is embedded in metaphyseal bone before the nail is inserted.

Care should be taken to avoid rotation of the nail during insertion. If the nail rotates significantly, the fracture site may displace and it will be difficult to place any distal cross-screws that are required. Sometimes, however, nail rotation is unavoidable, particularly if a lateral starting location is chosen.

Insertion of proximal cross-screws

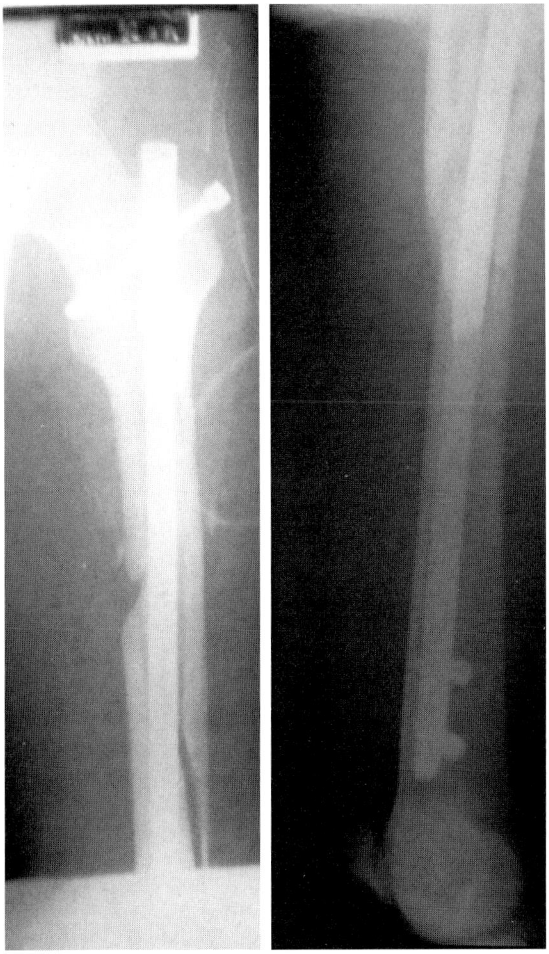

Figure 4.29

Proximal cross-screws are used when there is inadequate contact between the intramedullary nail and the endosteal surface of the cortex in the proximal fragment. This usually occurs when the fracture is above the femoral isthmus or when there is comminution or a segmental fracture. In the Grosse-Kempf system, the proximal cross-screw is obliquely placed between the greater and lesser trochanters, whereas in the AO nail the proximal cross-screw is transverse in orientation. The oblique cross-screw is preferred because of its greater adaptability in fracture fixation and because the more proximal entry hole creates less of a stress riser than the more distal entry point of the transverse proximal cross-screw.

With the Grosse-Kempf system the proximal cross-screw can be used to gain stability in a fracture in the subtrochanteric area, provided the lesser trochanter is intact. The nail in Figure 4.29 has not been hammered down sufficiently to allow the cross-screw to be placed in the centre of the lesser trochanter.

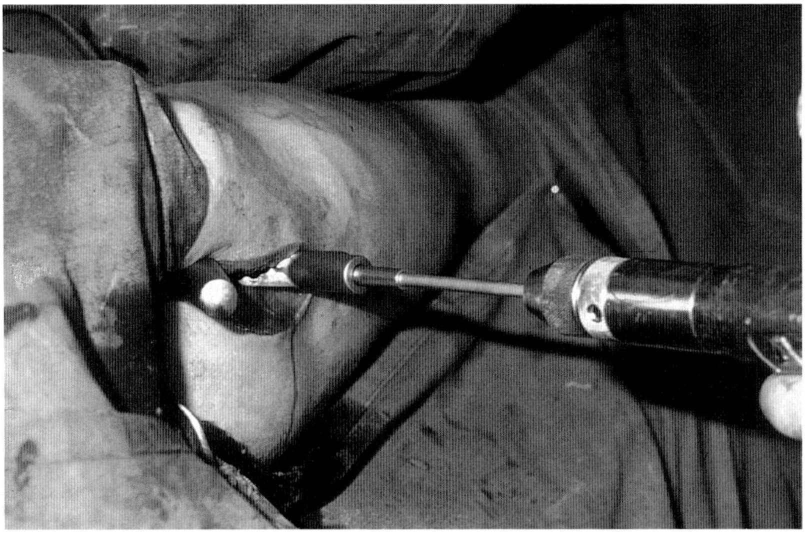

Figure 4.30

The proximal cross-screw is inserted in a standard manner. Initially a drill sleeve is inserted into the proximal screw jig and a 4.5 mm drill bit is passed down the drill sleeve. Both cortices of the femur are drilled and the bit is withdrawn. If the drill bit hits the metal nail, then a check should be made that the jig has not become loose on the nail. If this has occurred, the jig bolt should be tightened. If the proximal jig is loose, attempts to force the drill bit through the nail may result in breakage of the drill bit (Figure 23.13b).

A depth gauge is used to estimate the length of the proximal cross-screw. If necessary the position of the depth gauge can be checked with the image intensifier. A 6.0 mm drill bit is then used to overdrill the proximal cortex.

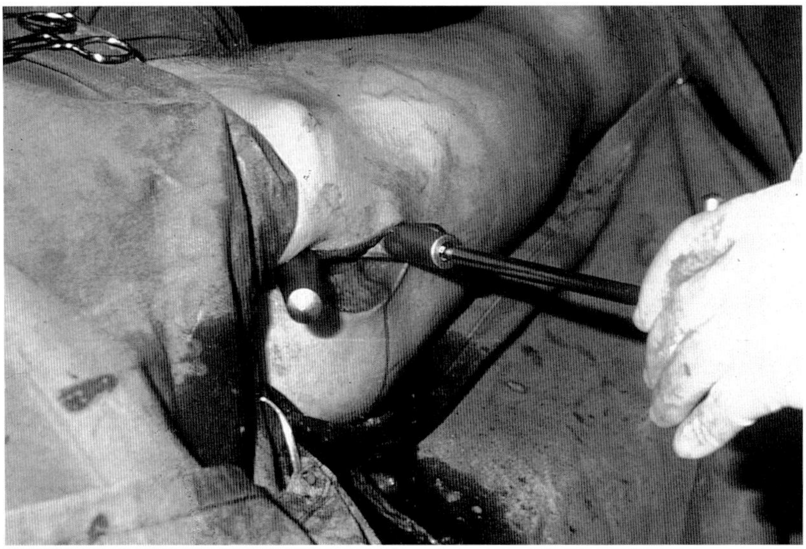

Figure 4.31

The correct length of screw is inserted. The screws are self-tapping and fully threaded.

CHAPTER 5 CLOSED NAILING OF THE TIBIA

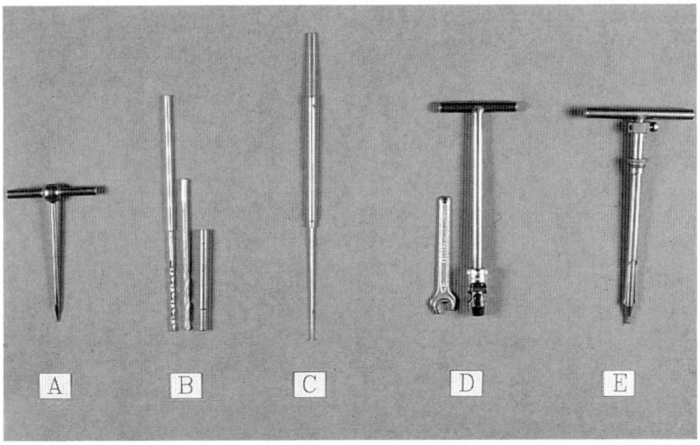

a

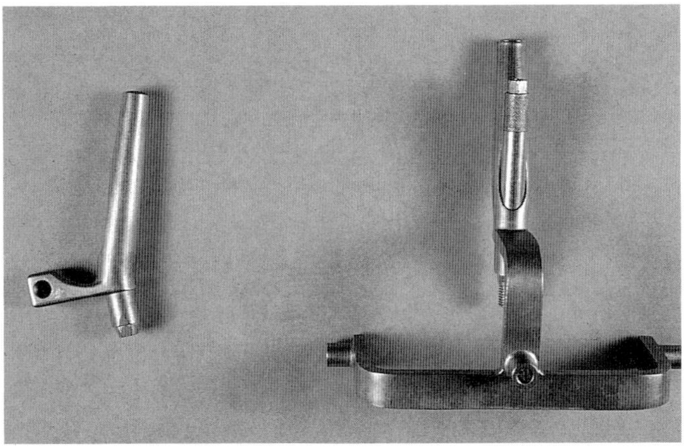

b

Figure 5.1

As with femoral nailing, a certain amount of equipment is required before intramedullary nailing of the tibia can be performed. In addition to the standard instrumentation required for femoral nailing illustrated in Figure 4.1, it is necessary to have specific equipment to permit the insertion of a tibial nail.

Figure 5.1a shows the equipment required to insert a Grosse-Kempf tibial nail:

(a) Bone awl
(b) Drill bits and drill sleeve
(c) Depth gauge
(d) Spanners
(e) Screwdriver

Figure 5.1b shows a tibial nail introducer and the proximal cross-screw insertion jig.

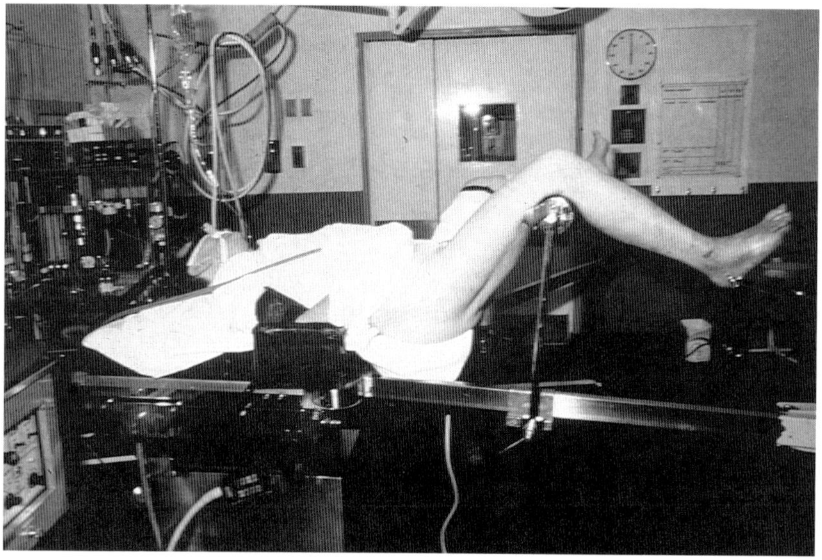

Figure 5.2

Despite the greater popularity of femoral nailing, closed nailing of the tibia is the easier procedure. As with femoral nailing, positioning of the patient is crucial. Unlike femoral nailing, however, only one position has gained popularity. As illustrated in Figure 5.2, the patient should lie on his or her back with the leg flexed over a padded circular support so that the angle of the knee is at least 90 degrees. The fracture can usually be reduced by application of traction to the foot through a calcaneal pin, inserted after the induction of anaesthesia. As with femoral nailing, traction can theoretically be applied through an orthopaedic boot, but a calcaneal pin is essential if there has been any delay prior to surgery or if distal cross-screws are required. If these are to be used, it is important to have access almost to the malleoli and an orthopaedic boot is contraindicated. Many tibial fractures are located below the isthmus and therefore a distal dynamic lock is frequently required.

Care should be taken in positioning the calcaneal pin as an incorrect position may lead to varus or valgus mal-alignment. It is important to place the transfixion pin at right angles to the calcaneus so that straight traction results in a direct pull on the fracture site. If the image intensifier shows a varus or valgus angulation secondary to the incorrect placement of the calcaneal pin, it should be replaced before the operation is started. The pin should be inserted under sterile conditions immediately pre-operatively. It can be removed postoperatively.

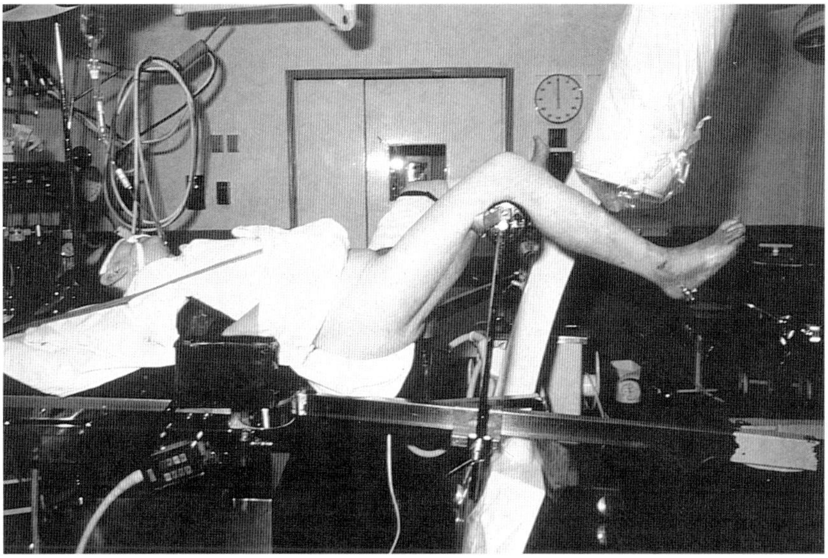

a

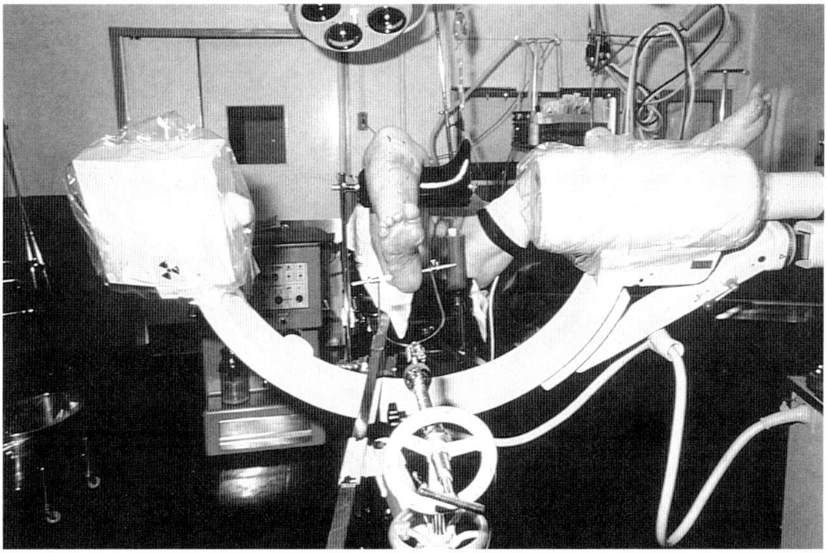

b

Figure 5.3

After positioning the patient correctly, the image intensifier should be used to visualize the fracture. As with the femur, it is important that the radiographer positions the intensifier so that, after draping, it can be moved easily between the antero-posterior and lateral positions. Figure 5.3a shows the position for an antero-posterior view of the fracture and the position for the lateral view is shown in Figure 5.3b. To obtain a good antero-posterior view it is important to angle the C-arm of the intensifier so that the beam is at right angles to the fracture. It is usually easy to get a good lateral view, but the radiographer should check pre-operatively that the beam can be set at right angles to the distal tibia as accurate orientation is necessary for the placement of the distal cross-screws.

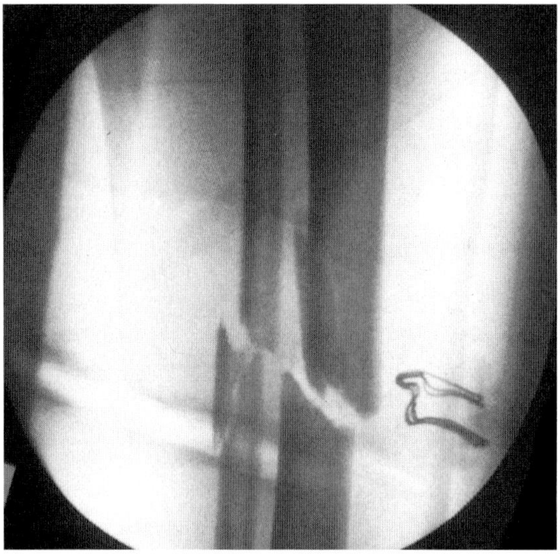

a

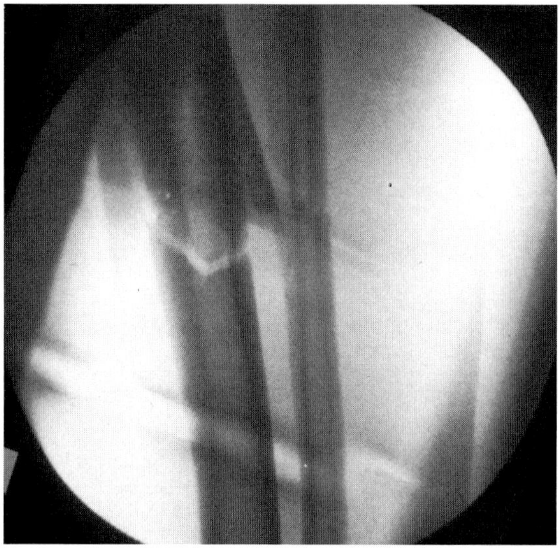

b

Figure 5.4

After the image intensifier has been set up and satisfactory views obtained the fracture should be reduced. This is usually easily achieved with straight traction but occasionally manipulation will be required. Sometimes the surgeon will be unable to reduce the fracture to a satisfactory position. Under these circumstances, closed tibial nailing should not be undertaken but some other method of fracture stabilization employed. As with closed femoral nailing, it is not important to maintain reduction prior to nailing but it is vital to obtain it and to be clear as to what manoeuvres are required to reduce the fracture during the operation. Figure 5.4 shows two views of a tibial fracture which has been reduced by straight traction.

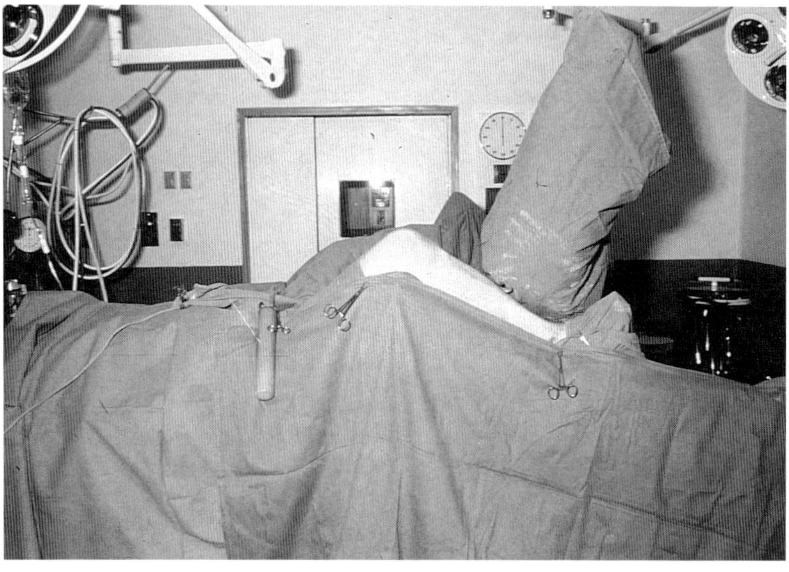

Figure 5.5

Draping of the leg should allow access to the whole tibia, particularly if the surgeon proposes to insert distal cross-screws. The upper drape can be wrapped around the lower femur to allow access to the knee and the lower drape wrapped around the calcaneal pin to allow access to the distal tibia. The image intensifier must be covered and it is useful to secure an extra large drape to the front of the table so that as the C-arm of the intensifier swings through into the lateral position it remains covered by sterile drapes.

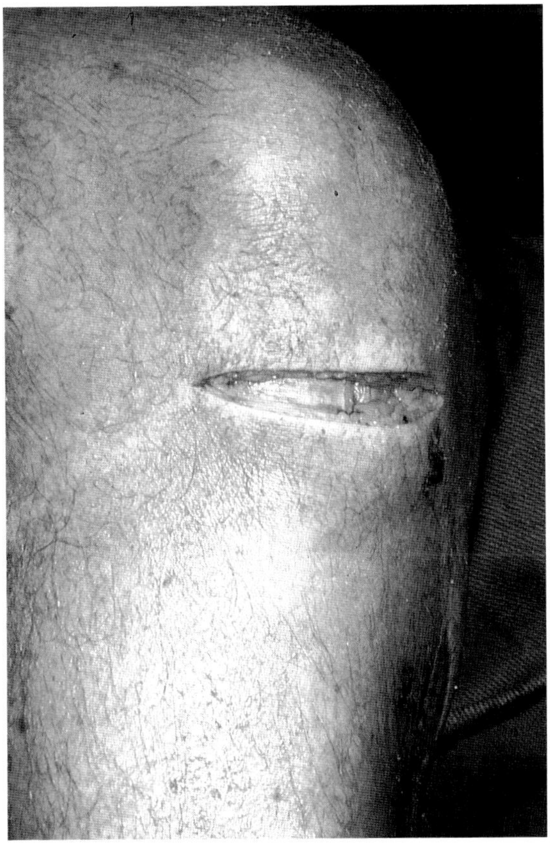

a

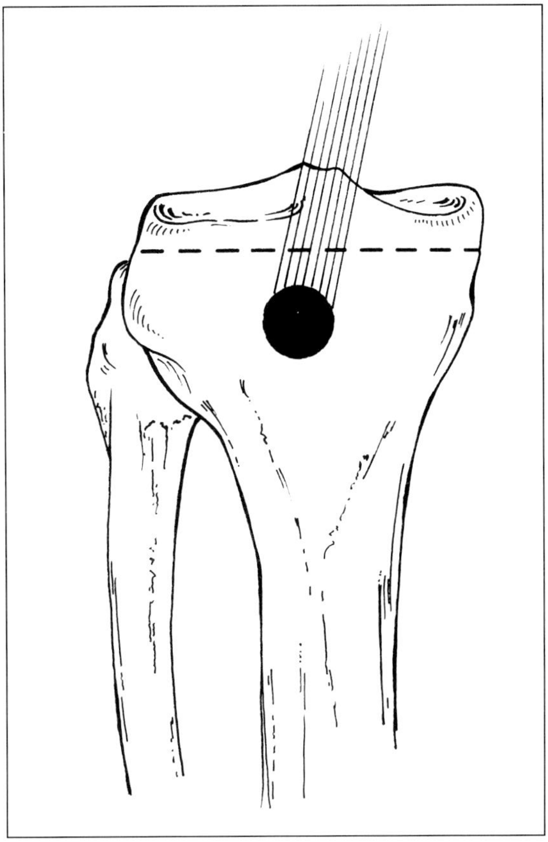

b

Figure 5.6

The incision should be transverse and lie approximately midway between the joint line of the knee and the tibial tuberosity (Figure 5.6a). A diagrammatic representation of the position of the incision is shown in Figure 5.6b. It is approximately 5 cm in length and, being parallel to Langer's lines, heals well. A vertical mid-line incision is recommended by some surgeons but this frequently causes cutaneous nerve damage, which results in hypoaesthesia on the lateral side of the leg. The vertical scar often heals with the formation of keloid and can be uncomfortable when knelt on.

After the skin incision has been made, access to the proximal tibia can be gained by either splitting the patella tendon or cutting down to bone just medial to the tendon. As the tibial tuberosity usually inserts lateral to the mid-line of the tibia, an incision made medial to the tendon is preferred since this allows access to the centre of the tibia without damaging the tendon.

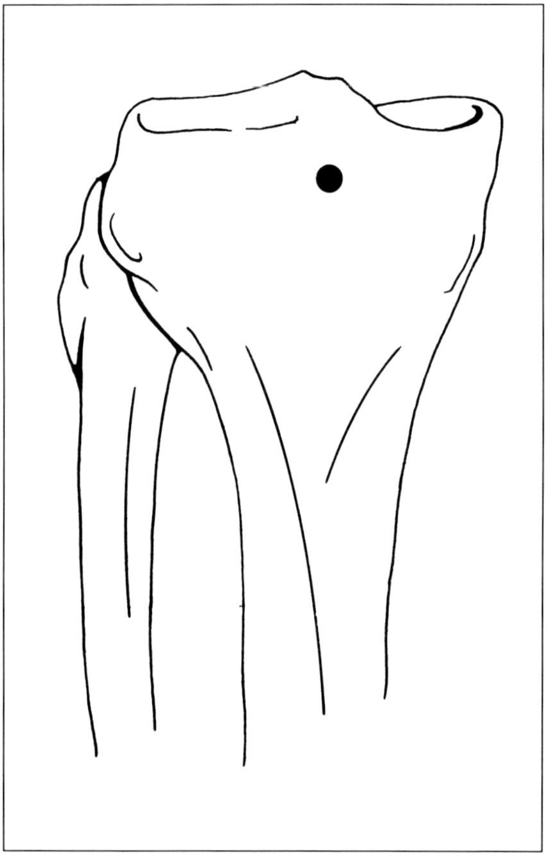

a

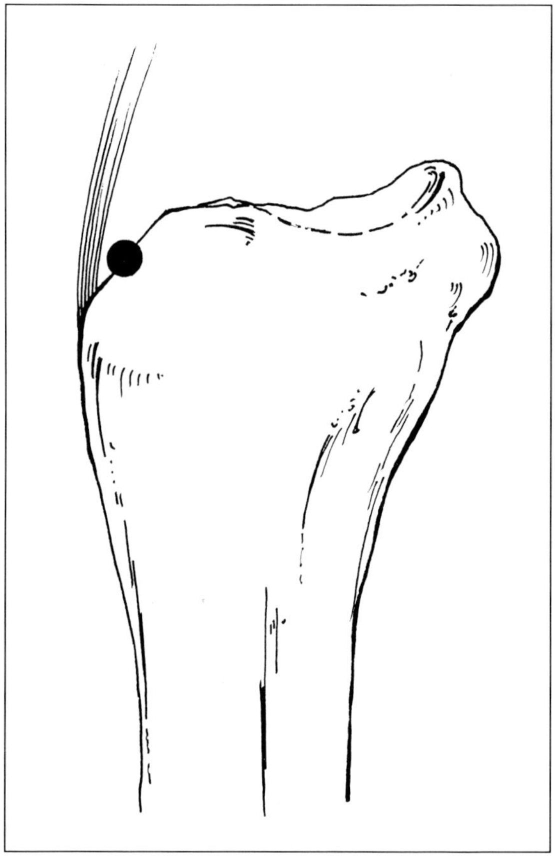

b

Figure 5.7

A large bone awl (Figure 4.1a) should be used to breach the proximal tibial cortex on the smooth cortical plane found between the joint and the insertion of the patella tendon. This is illustrated in two planes by the black dots shown in Figures 5.7a and b. The point of entry is not as crucial as that of the femur but it should be central in the tibia to permit easy access to the medullary canal. It is sited 1–1.5 cm below the joint line. If placed too high there is a risk of joint damage and if too low proximal comminution may occur.

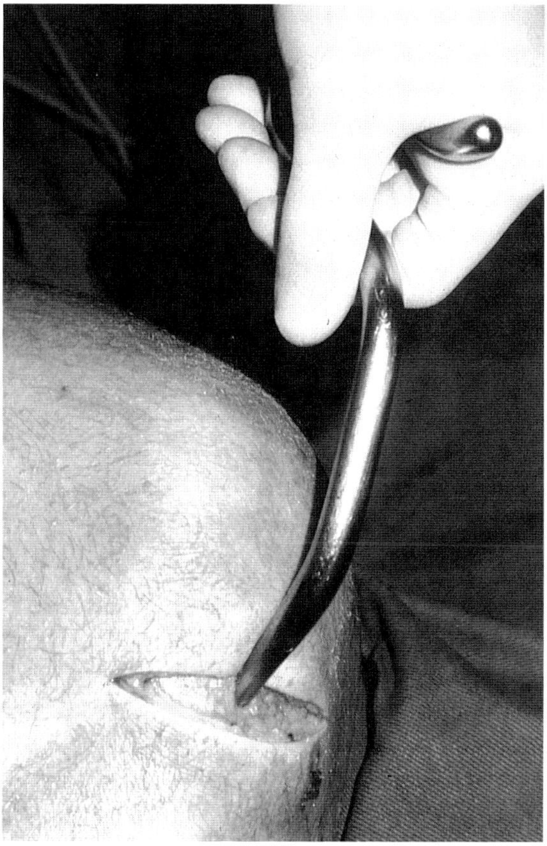

Figure 5.8

It is extremely important that the bone awl should be inserted in a curved manner so that its handle comes to be parallel to the tibial shaft. Failure to do this may result in penetration of the posterior cortex and possible arterial damage. This has been reported but it should never occur if the bone awl and subsequent hand reamers are used in the correct manner.

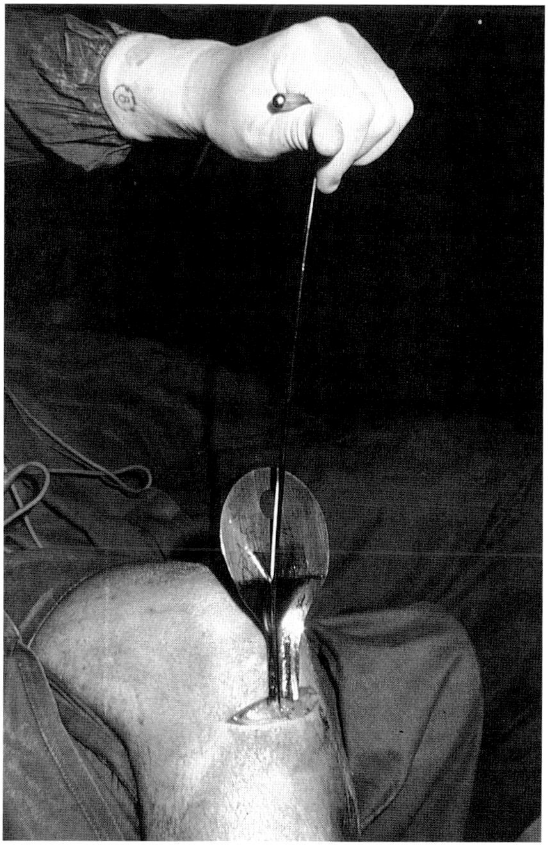

a

Figure 5.9

After the bone awl has been used to breach the tibial cortex, a hand reamer can be employed to penetrate the metaphyseal bone. Again, care must be used when passing this reamer into the tibia as it is relatively easy to pierce the posterior cortex if the wrong angle of entry is used. To facilitate the passage of the hand reamer into the medullary canal, it should be curved slightly (Figure 5.9a). This figure also illustrates the use of a tissue protector to prevent the reamer from coming into contact with the skin.

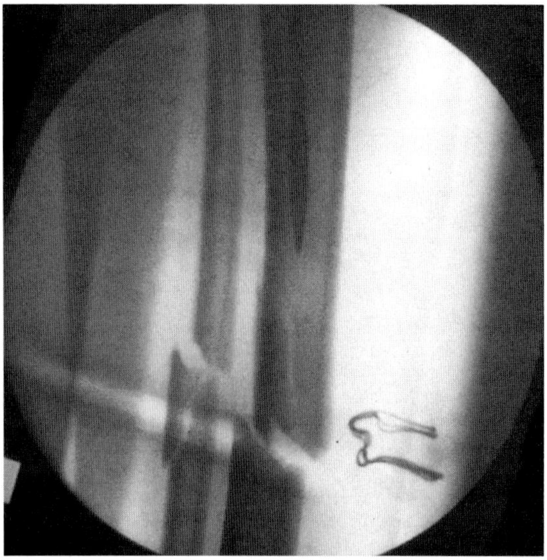

b

Figure 5.9 *continued*

The image intensifier can be used to visualize the reamer to check that it is correctly located (Figure 5.9b). Once the metaphysis has been penetrated there is no need to pass the hand reamer more distally.

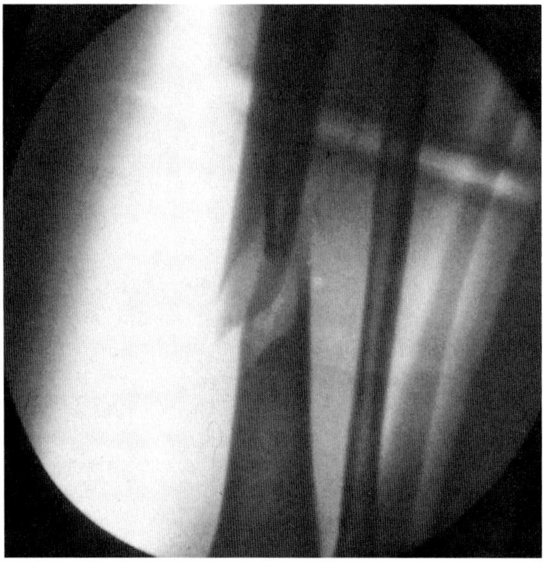

a

Figure 5.10

Following the removal of the hand reamer, an olive-tipped guide wire is passed into the medullary canal. As with the femur, the tip of the guide wire should be bent unless the fracture is well reduced. Figures 5.10a and b illustrate the use of a guide wire in a slightly displaced tibial fracture. Initially the guide wire is passed as far as the fracture site and the tip rotated to facilitate its passage over the fracture. Figure 5.10c shows the importance of rotating the tip of the guide wire in the correct direction. In this figure, it has been rotated so that it passes out of the tibia at the fracture site.

During the passage of the guide wire over the fracture, closed reduction must be carried out by the assistant. The intensifier should be used to pass the guide wire into centre of the distal fragment (Figure 5.10b) as passage down the medial or lateral cortex of the tibia will result in tibial mal-alignment.

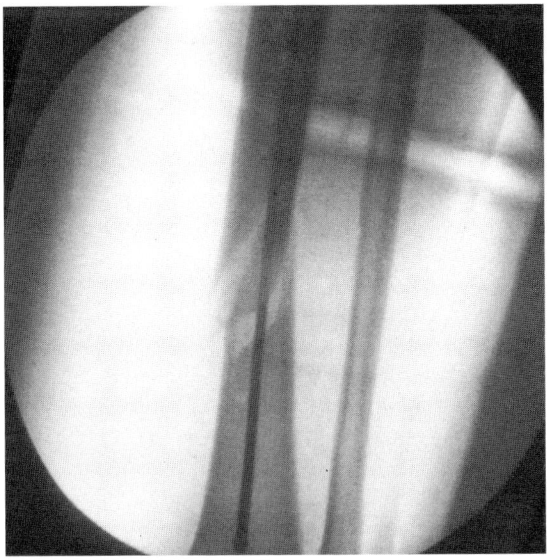

b

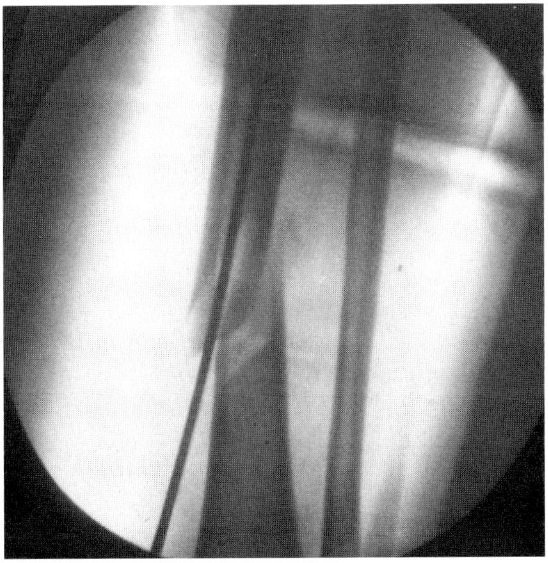

c

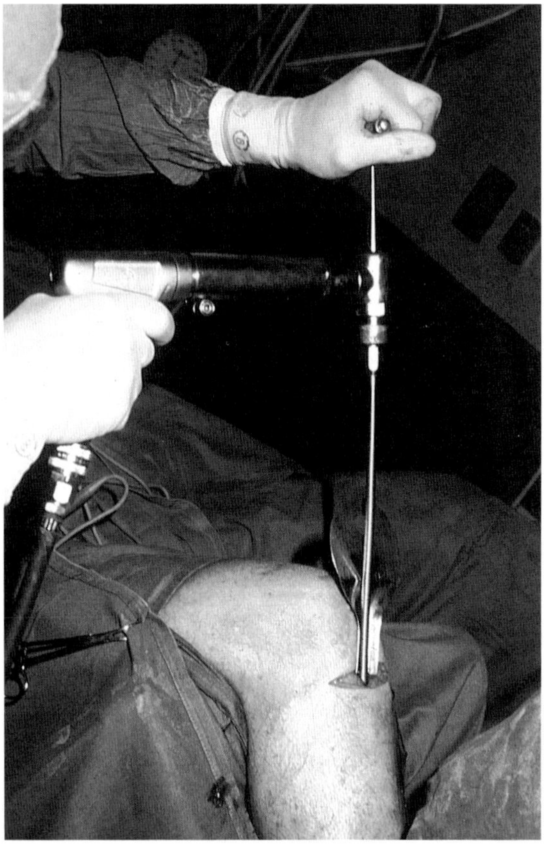

a

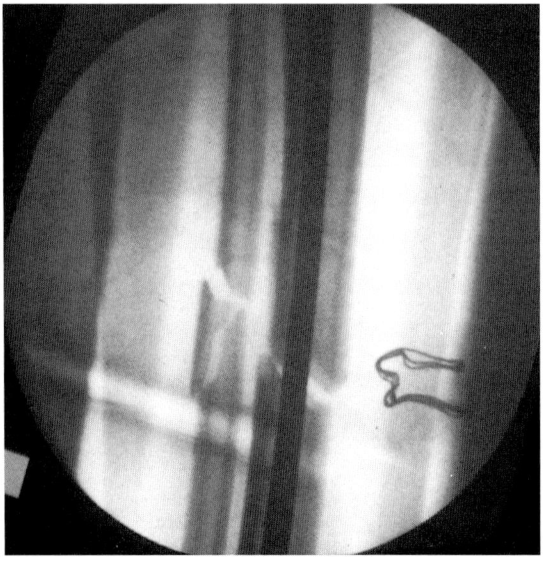

b

Figure 5.11

After the successful introduction of the guide wire, the tibia can be reamed (Figure 5.11a). As with the femur, the first reamer is an end-cutting reamer which should be passed into the medulla over the full length that the surgeon wishes to ream. It should always be remembered that the reamer can only be passed as far as the bend in the guide wire. Should the fracture be distal, then the bent guide wire should be removed and a straight olive-tipped guide wire passed into the canal. To facilitate this, a plastic sleeve should be used. Nailing of distal fractures is discussed further in Chapter 8.

If the fracture is displaced, it should be reduced by the assistant as each reamer is passed over the fracture site (Figure 5.11b). The criteria for reaming are the same as for the femur. If the fracture is at the level of the isthmus, approximately 1.5–2 cm on each side of the fracture should be reamed into a tube to take the nail. If the fracture is proximal or distal to the isthmus, the bone should be reamed until it will take an appropriately sized nail. In the tibia, a minimum diameter of 11 mm is recommended.

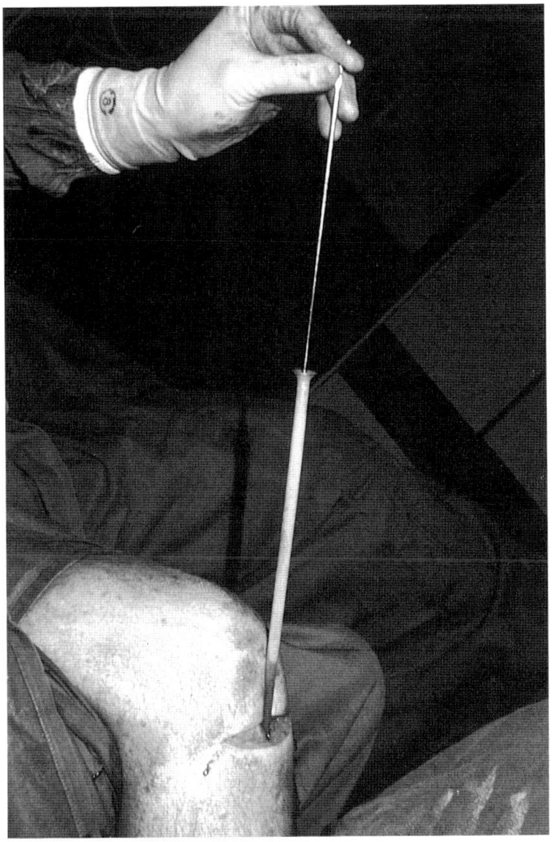

Figure 5.12

The tibia should be reamed to a size 1 mm greater than the diameter of the nail which is to be inserted. Failure to do this can result in damage to the tibia and in the nail becoming stuck in the area of the isthmus. After reaming, the olive-tipped guide wire should be changed to a thicker, graduated, straight guide wire. This is done in the same way as for the femur, using a plastic sleeve. The optimal length of the nail is best calculated peroperatively from the graduated markings on the second guide wire. Most tibiae will take nails 28–36 cm in length. The exact length can be calculated by measuring between the 30 or 40 cm marks on the wire and the nail insertion point in the tibia. When estimating the length of the nail it is important to ensure that the proximal end of the nail will be buried in the tibia to minimize the risk of postoperative discomfort. Alternative methods to assess nail length include the measurement of a second guide wire placed alongside the leg with both guide wires being visualized with the intensifier. In addition, pre-operative measurement of the normal tibia will help in the calculation of correct nail length.

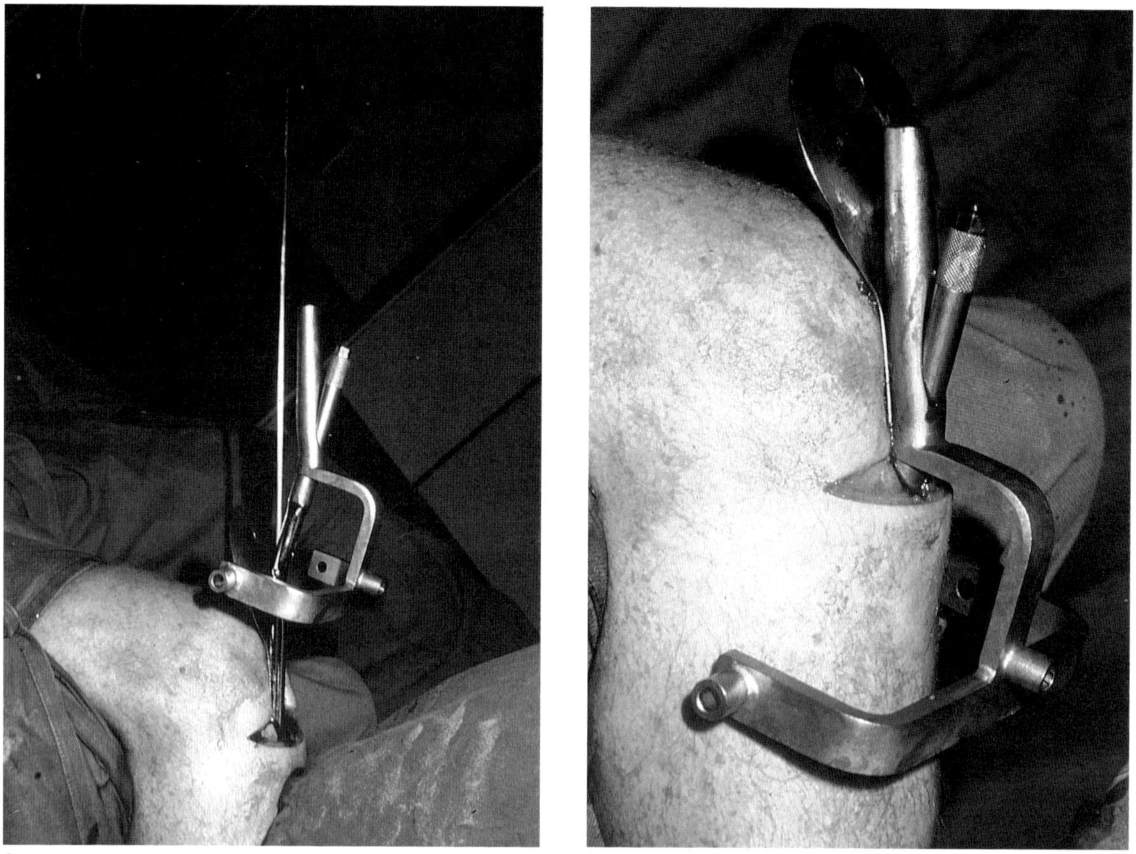

a b

Figure 5.13

The nail can be mounted on the ordinary insertion jig illustrated in Figure 5.1. However, if the surgeon feels that there is any likelihood of requiring proximal cross-screws the appropriate jig should be used. Figure 5.13a shows the insertion of a tibial nail using the proximal jig and Figure 5.13b shows the nail hammered into the tibia. The guide wire should be removed after the nail has been passed over the fracture. A tissue protector may be used to protect the skin during nail insertion. Figure 5.13b also illustrates the depth that the nail must be hammered into the tibia to bury its proximal end.

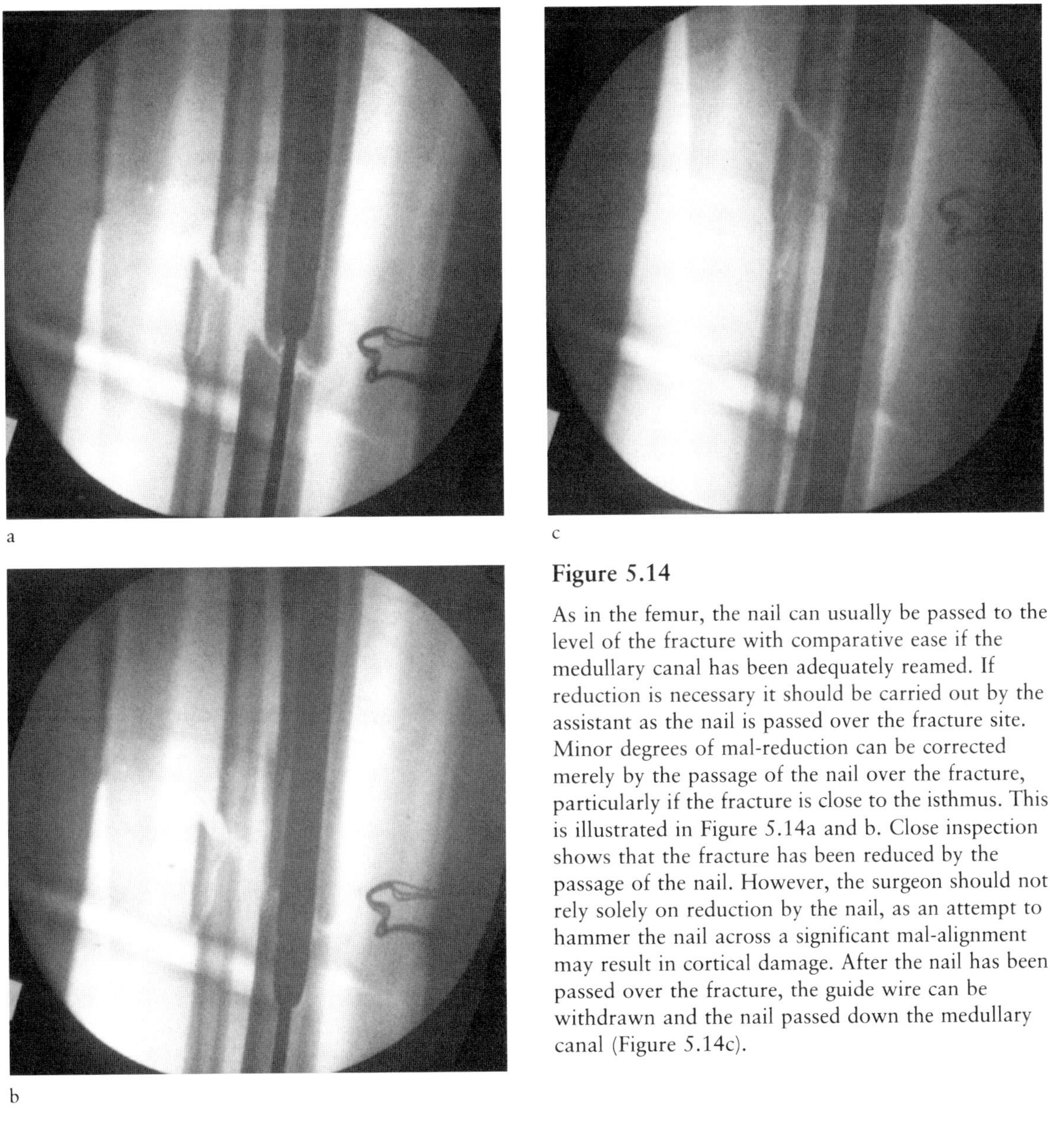

a

b

c

Figure 5.14

As in the femur, the nail can usually be passed to the level of the fracture with comparative ease if the medullary canal has been adequately reamed. If reduction is necessary it should be carried out by the assistant as the nail is passed over the fracture site. Minor degrees of mal-reduction can be corrected merely by the passage of the nail over the fracture, particularly if the fracture is close to the isthmus. This is illustrated in Figure 5.14a and b. Close inspection shows that the fracture has been reduced by the passage of the nail. However, the surgeon should not rely solely on reduction by the nail, as an attempt to hammer the nail across a significant mal-alignment may result in cortical damage. After the nail has been passed over the fracture, the guide wire can be withdrawn and the nail passed down the medullary canal (Figure 5.14c).

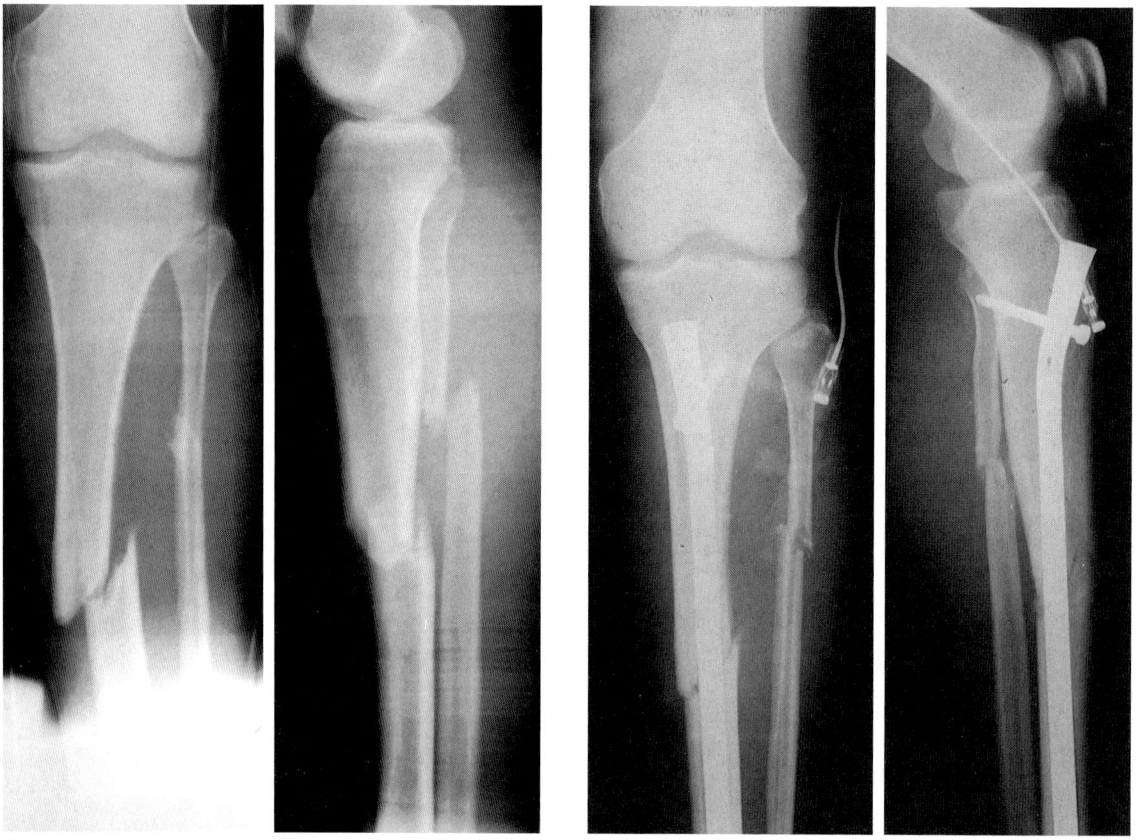

a b

Figure 5.15

Following insertion of the nail, the surgeon must decide if proximal cross-screws are necessary. The criteria for deciding this are the same as used for the femur. If the fracture is above the isthmus (Figure 5.15a), a proximal dynamic lock will be used (Figure 5.15b), but if there is comminution or the fracture is segmental, a static lock is indicated.

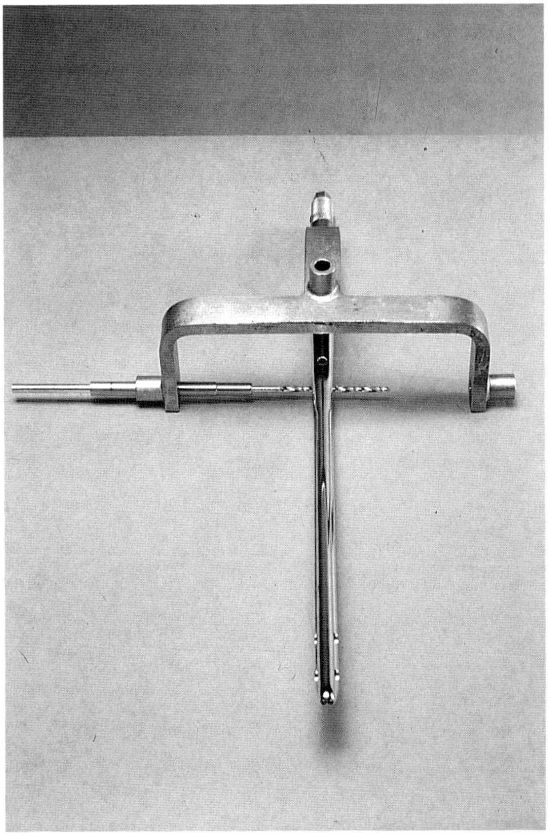

a

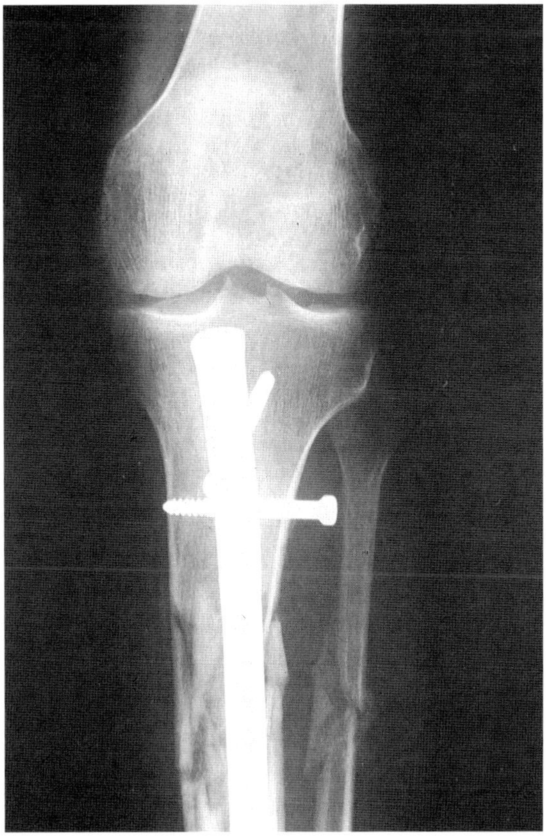

b

Figure 5.16

The jig for inserting proximal cross-screws is shown in Figure 5.13a and b. The jig will allow for the insertion of two proximal screws, one in the sagittal or antero-posterior plane with the other being inserted from either the medial or lateral side in the coronal plane. This is illustrated in Figure 5.16a, where the hole for the insertion of the antero-posterior screw is clearly seen and a drill bit marks the insertion point for the remaining screw. Both the proximal screws can be inserted (Figure 5.16b), but unless the proximal fragment is small, or the bone osteoporotic, sufficient stability will be gained from the insertion of only one of the screws. Usually it is easier for the surgeon to insert the antero-posterior screw, although occasionally the subcutaneous position of this screw gives rise to discomfort. Figure 5.16b shows that the laterally placed proximal cross-screw has not been fully inserted. Ideally this should be avoided, although screw loosening is very rare.

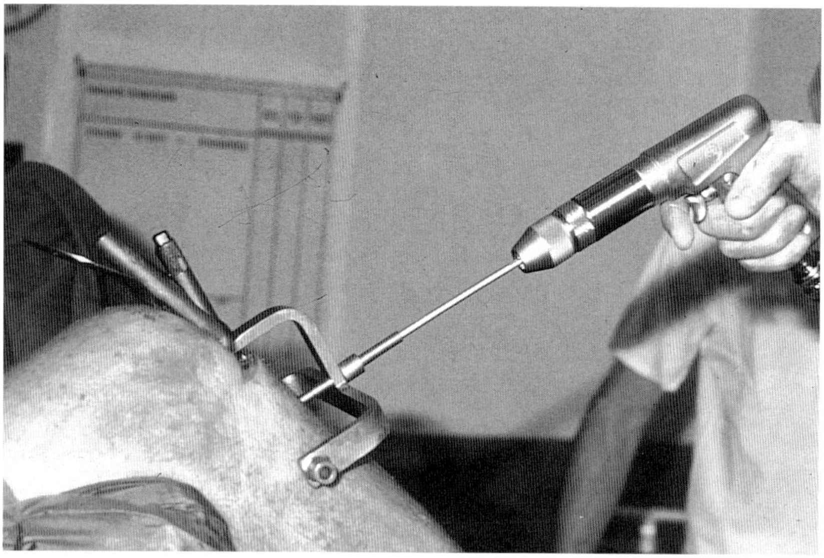

a

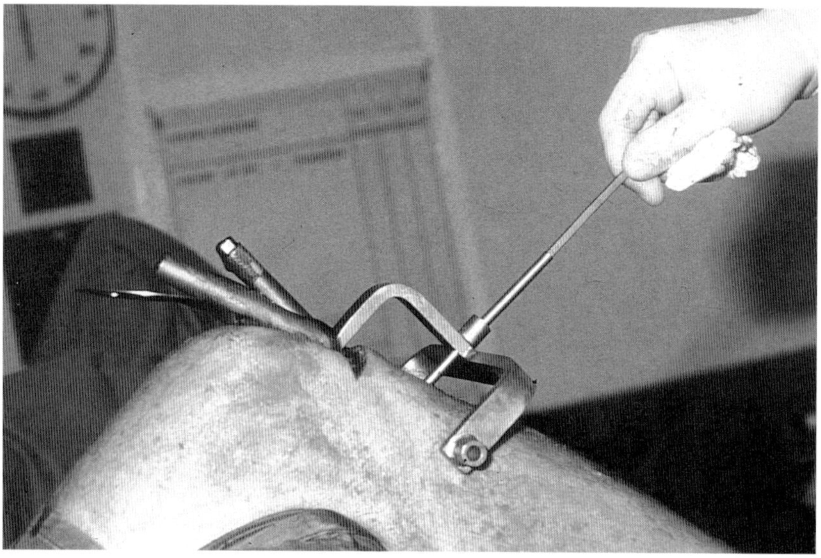

b

Figure 5.17

Insertion of the proximal screw is usually easily and quickly performed. After insertion of the nail, a drill sleeve is placed into one of the three channels on the jig (Figure 5.17a). Both tibial cortices are then drilled with a 3.5 mm drill bit, the bit passing through the nail. A depth gauge is then used to assess the exact length of the proximal screw (Figure 5.17b) and the 5.0 mm drill bit is used to overdrill the proximal tibial cortex.

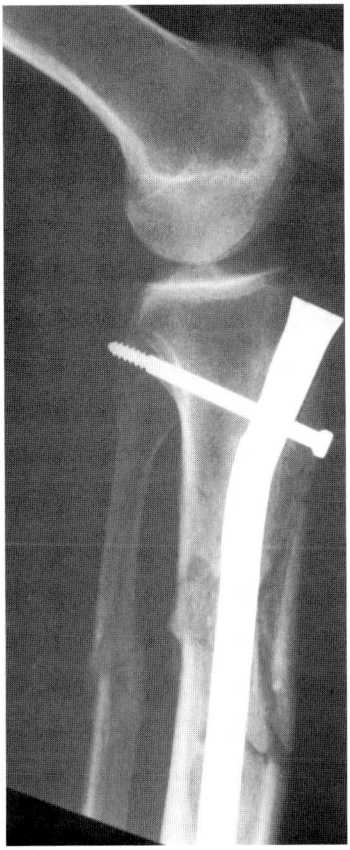

Figure 5.18

Care must be taken that proximal screws of the correct length are used. If too short a screw is used then complete stability will not be obtained. It is potentially dangerous to use too long a screw in the antero-posterior plane as it is theoretically possible to damage the vessels in the popliteal fossa, although this complication is rare. Thus care must be exercised in determination of the exact length of this screw. Ideally it should transfix both cortices with no significant protrusion into the soft tissues.

CHAPTER 6 DISTAL CROSS-SCREW INSERTION

The indications for the insertion of distal cross-screws are identical for the femur and tibia. They are required if the fracture is below the level of the isthmus such that inadequate contact is made between the nail and the endosteal surface of the cortex in the distal fragment. They are also required in all comminuted or segmental fractures. In the tibia in particular, many fractures are located below the isthmus and are associated with a rotational deforming force (Figure 6.1a). It is impossible to stabilize this type of fracture using an intramedullary nail unless distal cross-screws are employed. In such a case, one distal screw will provide good stability despite the relatively low position of the fracture (Figure 6.1b). The position of the fracture remained unchanged throughout the treatment and it was clinically united in 12 weeks (Figure 6.1c). Distal screws will be used in conjunction with proximal screws if the static locking mode is employed. This should always be used if there is any comminution or the fracture is segmental.

The insertion of the distal cross-screws is wrongly regarded by many surgeons as difficult and, because of this, many ingenious devices have been produced to assist the surgeon with distal cross-screw insertion. As the insertion of proximal cross-screws is relatively easy if the appropriate jig is used it would seem that the use of appropriately sized and shaped nail-mounted jigs could also aid distal cross-screw insertion. Such a jig designed for use with the Grosse-Kempf tibial nail is shown in Figure 6.2. As with the proximal jig, it is securely tightened on to the proximal end of the nail and the bar length is altered to bring an appropriately drilled distal block into alignment with the distal screw holes. The reason that this type of jig does not actually work is that the nails change shape on being passed down the medullary canal of either the tibia or the femur. Thus the distal screw holes do not end up correctly aligned with the siting block of the jig.

The concept of the nail-mounted jig remains popular however, and an attempt has been made to compensate for nail distortion in the design of the Russell-Taylor nail-mounted distal siting device (Figure 6.3). In this jig the distal siting block can be aligned in the image intensifier beam so as to line up the holes in the siting block with the distal nail holes. This and other similar devices can be used successfully but their design remains cumbersome and most experienced surgeons have discarded them.

An alternative to the nail-mounted jig is an image-intensifier-mounted system as shown in

Figure 6.4. The principle behind this type of device is also extremely simple. A metal gantry is attached to the image intensifier such that the intensifier beam passes through a siting hole of a size appropriate to receive a drill sleeve. The metal bar in which this hole is drilled is placed exactly at right angles to the intensifier beam. The position of the femur or tibia is adjusted so that the hole in the metal gantry is perfectly aligned with one of the distal screw holes. If this is done correctly, the surgeon will see a perfect circle where the beam passes through the siting hole and the superimposed distal screw hole. The drill sleeve is then secured in the siting hole and pressed up against the skin. An incision is made in the appropriate place through the skin and underlying tissues and the drill sleeve is advanced until it touches bone. The alignment of the gantry is then checked and, if satisfactory, the bone is drilled and the screw inserted. As with the more sophisticated nail-mounted jigs, these devices can be used although they are extremely cumbersome and time-consuming. Their use has been abandoned in favour of the free-hand technique by many experienced trauma surgeons.

Free-hand technique

The free-hand technique for insertion of distal cross-screws is identical for both the femur and the tibia. It is however somewhat easier in the tibia and it is with reference to the tibia that the technique will be described. The thickness of the soft-tissue mass around the femur makes the insertion of distal cross-screws more difficult. In the tibia distal cross-screws can be inserted from both medial and lateral sides, although the subcutaneous location of the anteromedial border of the tibia makes it easier to insert a distal screw hole from the medial side. However, either side can be used relatively easily and Figure 11.1 shows screws inserted from the medial side while Figure 6.1b shows a laterally inserted screw.

Unlike the tibia, the insertion of distal femoral cross-screws should only be undertaken from the lateral side. Not only does the equal bulk of the tissue found on medial and lateral sides of the femur make a medial approach unnecessary, but the medial location of the femoral vessels at the lower end of the femur makes a medial approach potentially hazardous. A lateral approach should be used in all cases.

The difficulty encountered in the insertion of distal cross-screws is in direct proportion to the thickness of the soft tissues overlying the bone. As it is important to be able to angle the initial probe that is used to mark the bone, so as to minimize the risk of radiation exposure to the surgeon, the size of the skin incision will vary with the location of the screw. Thus a lateral femoral cross-screw can be safely inserted through an incision of between 1 and 2 cm, while the medial tibial cross-screw needs only a stab incision.

To prepare for distal cross-screw insertion using a free-hand technique, the C-arm of the intensifier is placed in the lateral position with the beam exactly at right angles to the bone. The position is shown in Figure 5.3b. The C-arm and the position of the leg should be adjusted until one screw hole appears as a perfect circle. Frequently the nail rotates slightly during insertion and it helps greatly to have an operating table which has a compensatory tilting mechanism to allow the patient to be rotated to regain alignment of the nail within the intensifier beam. The screw insertion should not be started until one of the distal screw holes appears as a perfect circle.

The holes in the distal part of the nail appear elliptical if they are incorrectly lined up in the intensifier beam. If the nail is correctly rotated and the intensifier beam is not at right angles to the nail, the holes will appear elliptical in the transverse plane. This is shown in the upper hole in Figure 6.5 and in both holes in Figure 6.6. Should the rotation of the nail be incorrect but the image intensifier be correctly placed, the ellipse appears in the longitudinal plane. This is illustrated in Figure 6.7 where the tibia has been purposely rotated to an excessive degree following the insertion of the first screw. Incorrect rotation is verified by the relative positions of the tibia and fibula. Once one of the holes appears as a circle on the intensifier screen, the distal screw can be inserted.

A sharp-pointed object is placed on the skin so that it lies in the centre of the circle on the intensifier screen (Figure 6.8a and b). The pointer used should be long enough to allow the surgeon's hands to be kept out of the intensifier beam. A sharp Steinmann pin mounted on a T-handle is a satisfactory instrument. The bone awls that are supplied with the intramedullary nailing instruments are usually somewhat short and the surgeon risks hand irradiation. Once the pointer has been lined up in the centre of the circle, a skin incision of appropriate length can be made with the centre of the skin incision being the mark made on the skin by the pointer.

Exactly the same procedure is now undertaken with regard to the bone. The metal pointer is placed on the bone so that the tip is in the centre of the circle seen on the intensifier screen (Figure 6.9a and b). Once this is done, the surgeon makes a small depression on the surface of the bone with the pointer. To facilitate this and subsequent drilling, the C-arm of the intensifier should be lowered, but under no circumstances should the radiographer be allowed to adjust the position of the C-arm in any other way as once the position of the image is lost it is difficult to regain. If the C-arm is dropped, the image can be regained by merely raising the C-arm at any time during the procedure.

If the nail has rotated during insertion, it may be necessary to make a depression on the posteromedial or posterolateral angles of the tibia. This can be very difficult as the pointer and the drill bit may slide on the bone. If possible, the surgeon should try to prevent rotation of the nail during insertion.

The surgeon then inserts the 3.5 mm drill bit (4.5 mm in the femur) into the cortical depression (Figure 6.10) and drills through both cortices and the intervening hole in the nail. This is not difficult if the initial starting point has been correctly situated. The surgeon's choice of the correct angle through the tibia may be facilitated by following the orientation of the C-arm of the image intensifier.

It is usually apparent if the drill bit has passed through the nail as the screw hole is partially filled when seen on the intensifier screen. It is worthwhile removing the drill bit from the drill when the surgeon feels that the bit has passed into the nail hole (Figure 6.11a). If the intensifier image shows that the drill bit has passed through the nail hole, the drill can be reattached and the bit passed through the distal cortex. If there is doubt about the position of the drill bit, the leg can be rotated. If the drill bit is seen to lie within the screw hole on both internal rotation (Figure 6.11b) and external rotation (Figure 6.11c), then it is correctly located and the surgeon can proceed.

The length of the cross-screw is determined in the standard manner using a depth gauge and the proximal cortex is overdrilled with the larger drill bit (5 mm in the tibia and 6 mm in the femur). The screw of the correct length is then inserted using the screwdriver (Figure 6.12). It is important that the screw be inserted so that the head is against the proximal cortex or there may be tissue irritation from the head of the screw.

Once the cross-screw has been inserted it is useful to check that it is correctly located. This is easily done by repeating the lateral view on the image intensifier. The screw is correctly placed if the hole in the nail is filled (Figure 6.13). An antero-posterior view can be useful in determining whether the screws are of the correct length. However, care should be taken in interpreting the position of the screws from an antero-posterior X-ray scan as, if the screw is located just behind the hole, it may appear to be correctly located on the scan. Such a situation is shown in Figure 6.14.

If both distal screws are to be inserted then the process should be repeated after the image intensifier is realigned opposite the second hole.

After both screws have been inserted, the image intensifier will show both holes in the nail to be filled (Figure 6.15).

A number of devices have been invented to assist the surgeon in free-hand placement of distal screws; one of these is shown in Figure 6.16. This is a plastic siting device of sufficient length to keep the surgeon's hand out of the X-ray beam. Within the distal part of the device is a circular hole which is aligned between the X-ray beam and one of the distal screw holes. Once the siting device has been correctly aligned, a Kirschner wire or small drill bit can be passed through the siting device to penetrate the proximal cortex of the femur just opposite the distal screw hole. This type of device is of limited use as it prevents the surgeon from using both hands for the insertion of the Kirschner wire or drill bit. If the assistant uses the siting device, then the surgeon has to rely on the assistant to hold the device in the correct position.

Another possible modification is the use of cannulated screws which can be placed over a pre-inserted guide wire. It is obvious that the guide wire must be placed centrally in the distal nail hole or the screw will not pass easily through the nail.

Many trauma surgeons have abandoned all the various types of distal targeting or siting devices and use a variant of the free-hand method described above, taking particular care to keep their hands out of the X-ray beam.

Requirements for distal cross-screws

It is often assumed that two distal cross-screws should be used. The rationale for this is that the use of two screws will prevent rotation of the distal bone fragment in the sagittal plane. This however does not occur and in over 500 femoral and tibial nailings in Edinburgh carried out over the last five years there has been only one case where there has been displacement of the distal fragment because only one distal cross-screw was inserted; this is shown in Figure 23.9. One distal cross-screw provides adequate stability for the distal fragment unless the bone is of very poor quality. The management of distal diaphyseal fractures is discussed in Chapter 8.

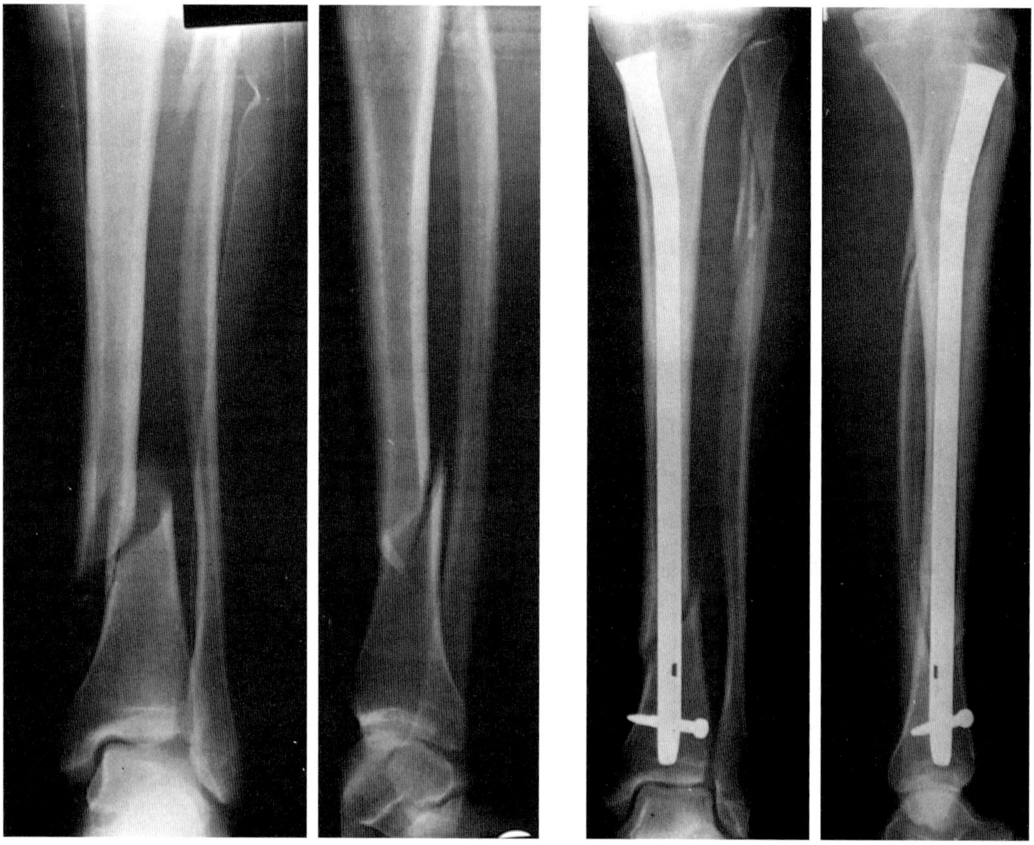

Figure 6.1

a A spiral fracture of the distal third of the tibia. This fracture is seen commonly following football injuries and is well treated by a distally locked intramedullary nail.

b A good reduction has been obtained and one distal cross-screw has been inserted.

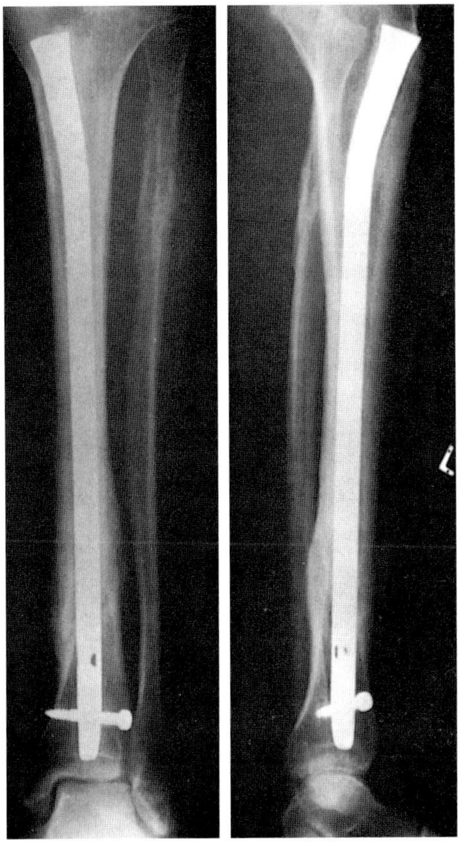

c After 12 weeks, the fracture was clinically united. There was no loss of fracture position and one distal screw was adequate to hold the fracture.

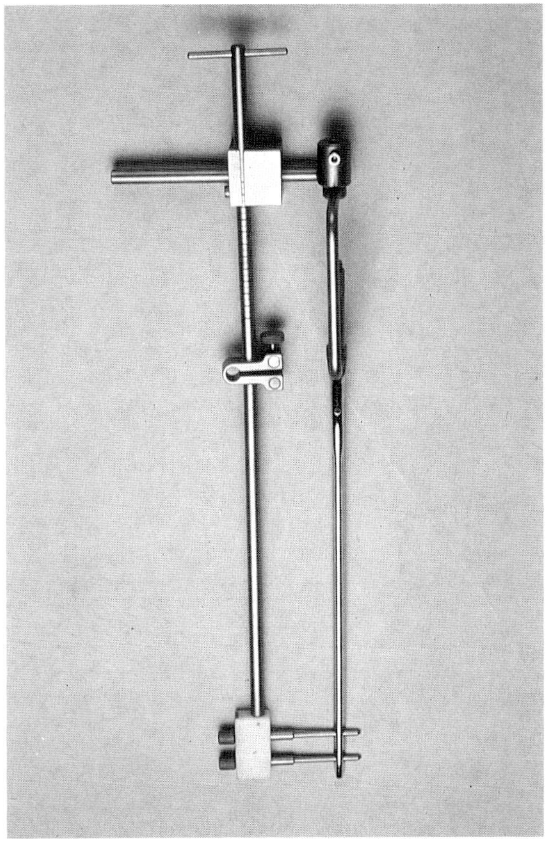

Figure 6.2

A nail-mounted distal cross-screw insertion jig suitable for the Grosse-Kempf nail. The jig allows for alteration of nail lengths. Nail deformation during insertion negates the usefulness of this device.

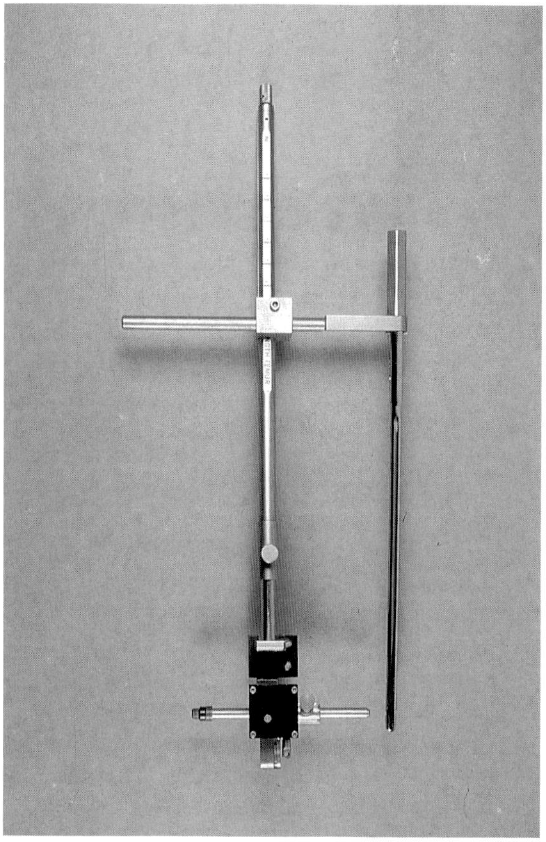

Figure 6.3

The Russell Taylor nail-mounted jig carries a multi-adjustable siting device which allows the surgeon to line up the distal screws after the nail has been inserted. However, devices such as this are a little awkward to use.

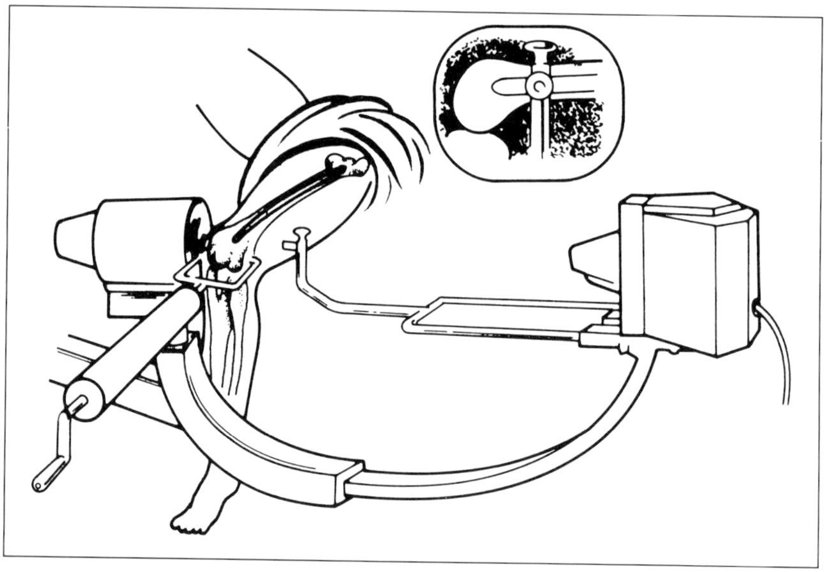

Figure 6.4

A diagrammatic representation of an image-intensifier-mounted jig. Such devices are useful but are frequently time-consuming to use.

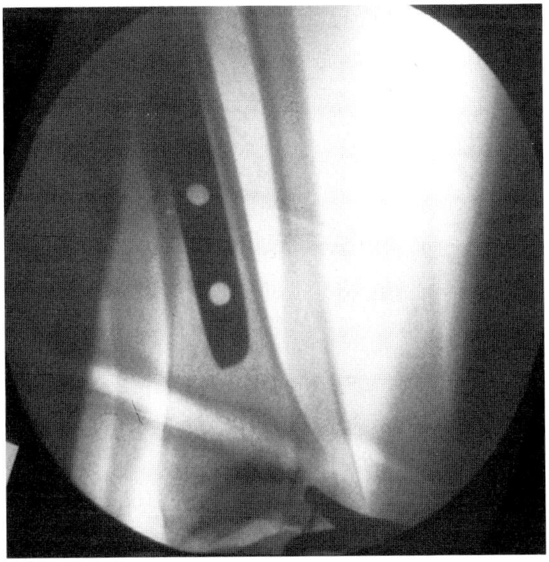

Figure 6.5

The free-hand insertion of the distal screws is only possible if the distal nail holes are correctly lined up in the intensifier beam. In this image-intensifier view, the lower screw hole appears as a perfect circle. The upper screw hole appears as an ellipse as it is not correctly lined up in the intensifier beam.

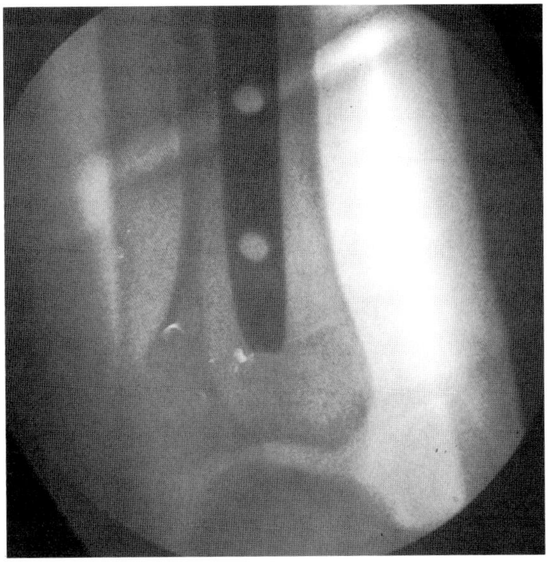

Figure 6.6

Both distal screw holes appear as ellipses as neither screw hole is lined up in the beam correctly.

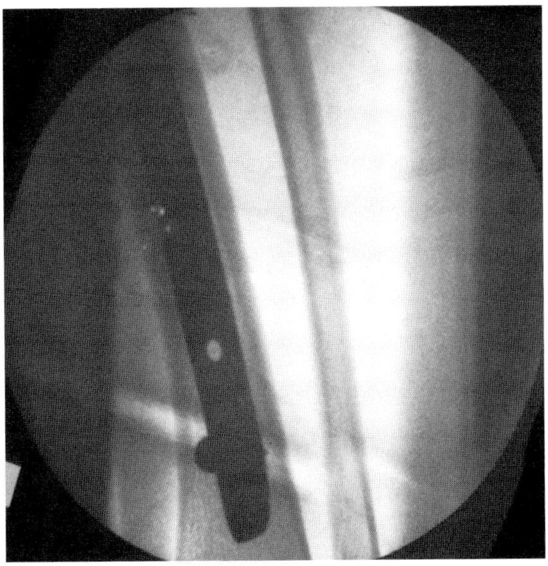

Figure 6.7

Here the screw hole is lined up at 90 degrees to the intensifier beam but the leg has been rotated to illustrate the elliptical appearance of the distal screw hole associated with such a rotation. If the nail has rotated significantly during insertion, it may be necessary to rotate the operating table in the opposite direction to permit distal cross-screw insertion.

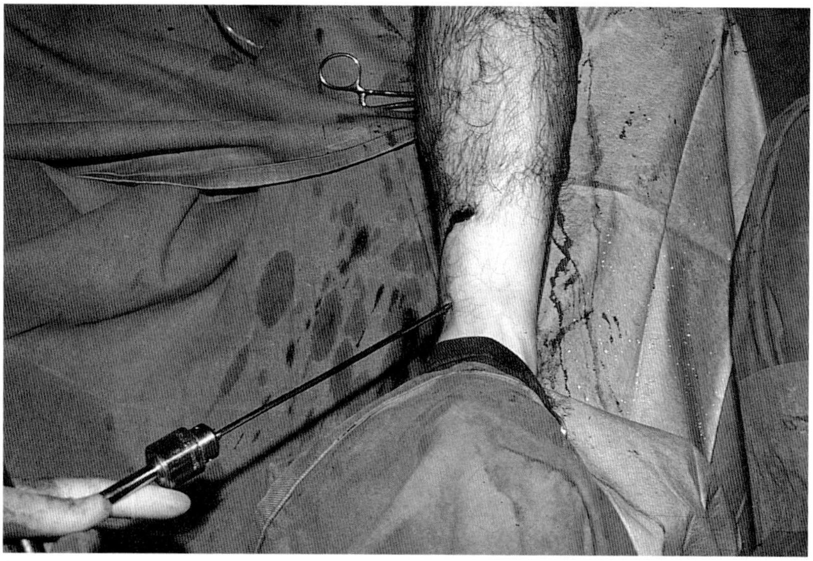

a

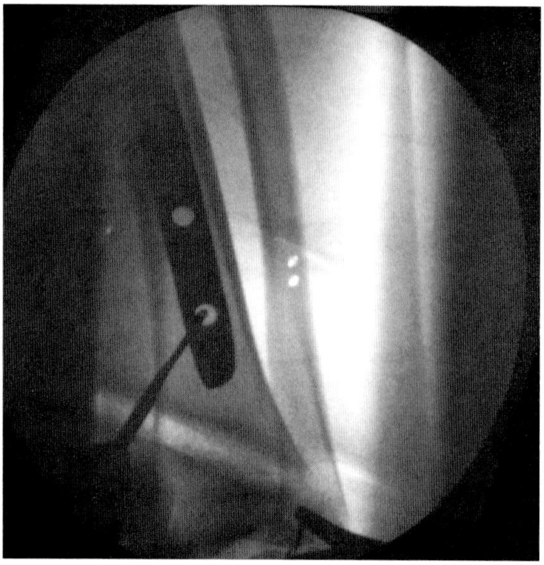

b

Figure 6.8

a Surgeons should be careful not to irradiate their hands during distal cross-screw insertion. The easiest way to avoid radiation is to use a long, sharp-pointed pin to indicate where the skin incision should be placed.

b The sharp-pointed pin or awl is lined up so that its point is central in one of the distal nail holes. A skin incision is made at the tip of the pointer.

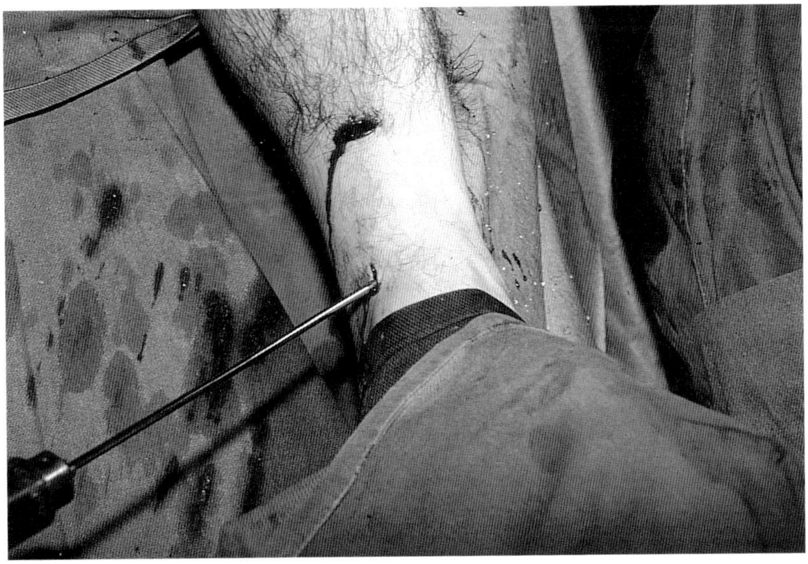

a

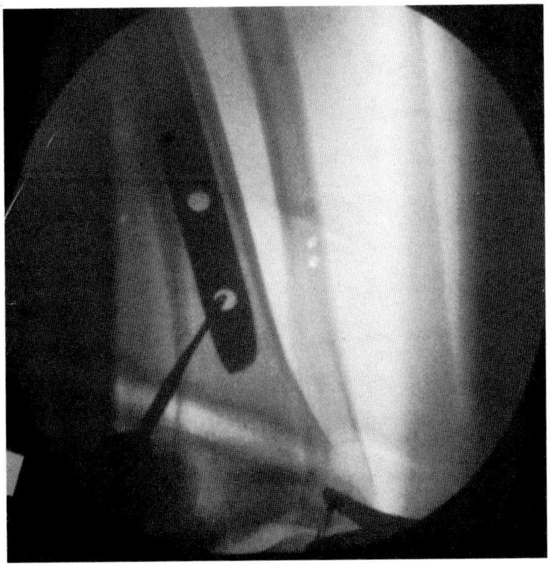

b

Figure 6.9

a The same process is repeated with the pointer placed on bone.

b Again the pointer is located centrally within the distal nail hole image and the bone is marked so that the surgeon can find the position again.

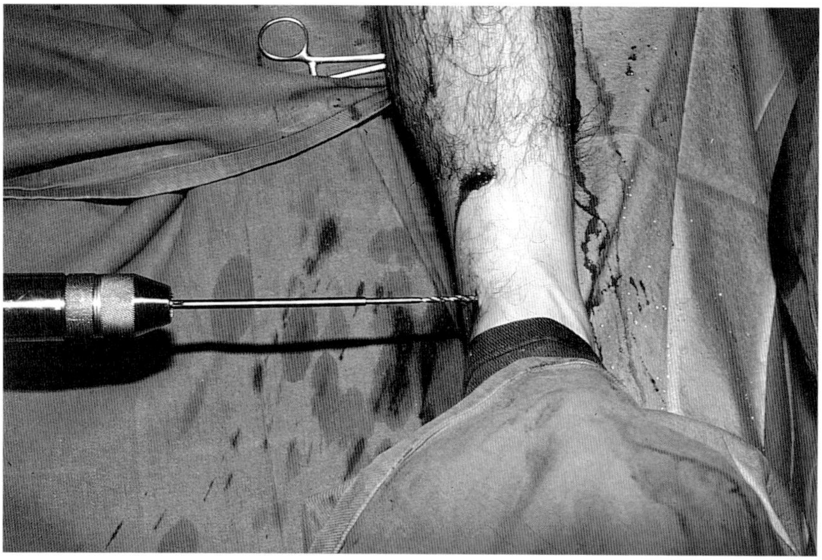

Figure 6.10

The drill bit is placed in the small cortical depression made by the pointer. The angle of the C-arm of the image intensifier can be used to assess the correct angle for distal cross-screw insertion.

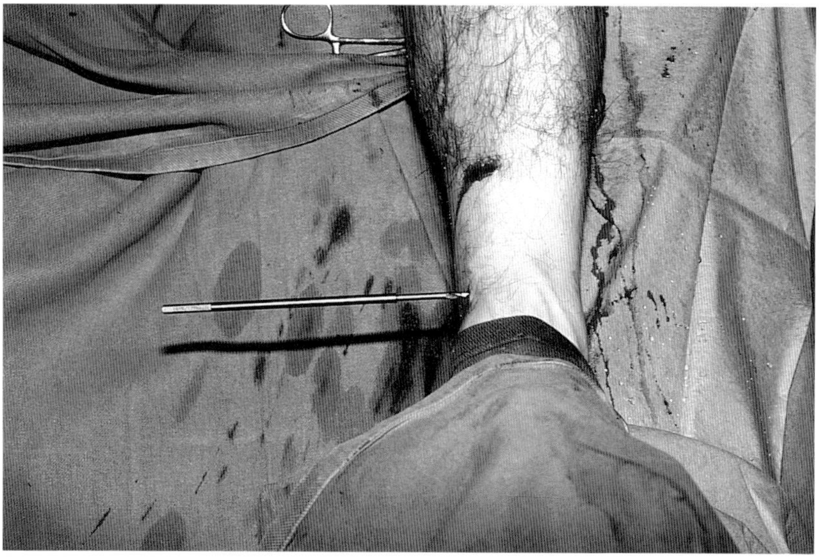

Figure 6.11

a Once the surgeon thinks that the drill bit has passed through the proximal cortex and the nail the drill can be removed. The image intensifier will show whether the drill bit is within the nail.

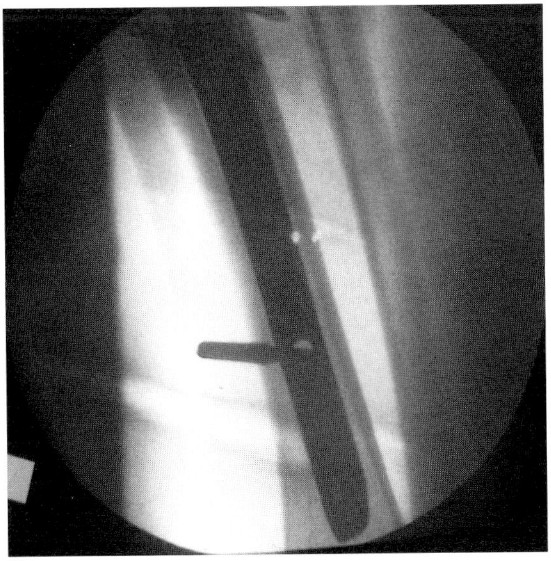

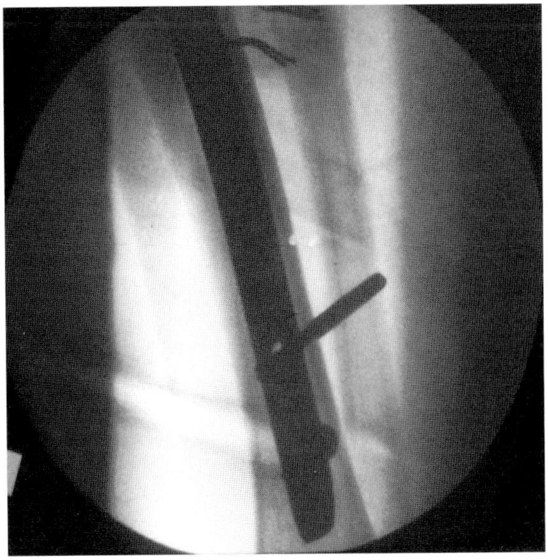

Figure 6.11 *continued*

b If there is doubt as to whether the drill bit is within the nail hole, the leg can be rotated.

c Internal and external rotation will show that the drill bit lies within the nail hole. If it does not, the drill bit must be removed and the process repeated.

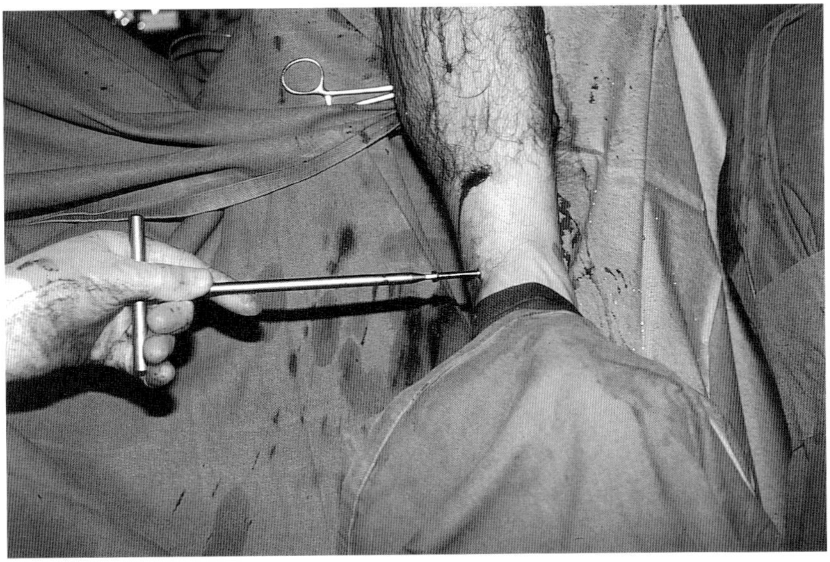

Figure 6.12

Distal cross-screws, like proximal screws, are self-tapping and are usually easily inserted. Care must be taken to ensure that the screw follows the drill hole, particularly in osteoporotic bone.

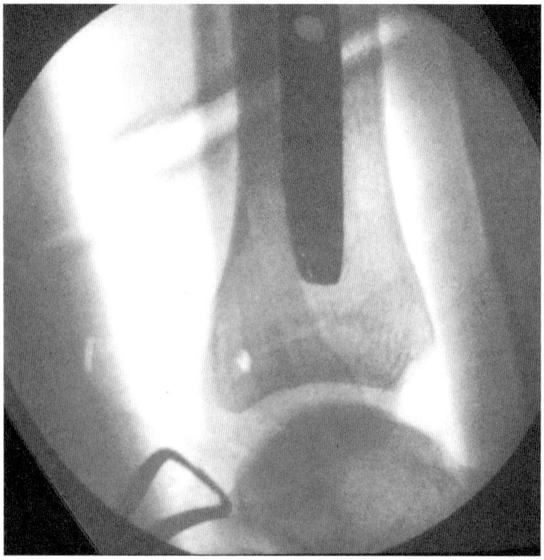

Figure 6.13

Once the screw is inserted properly, a lateral image-intensifier view will show obliteration of the screw hole in the nail.

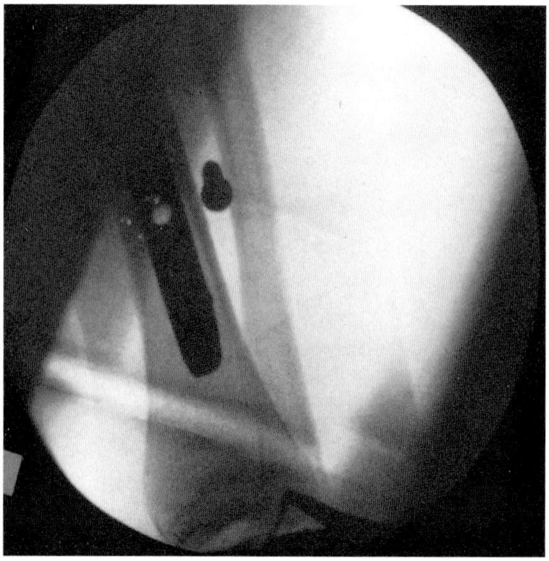

Figure 6.14

Care must be taken to ensure that the distal cross-screws are within the bone and nail, particularly if only one distal cross-screw is used. This is best seen on the lateral view.

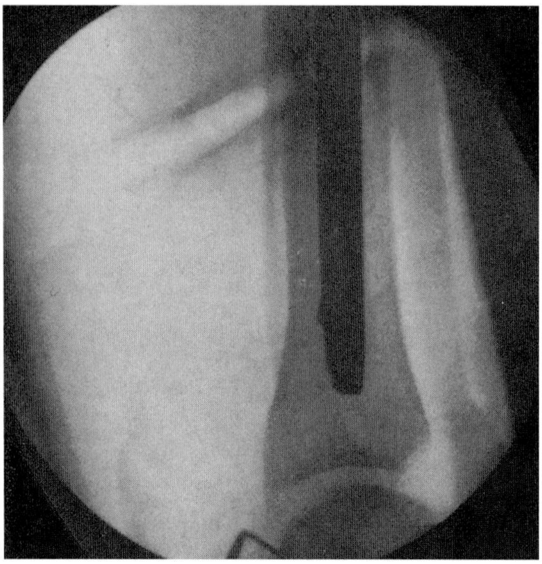

Figure 6.15

Once all distal cross-screws have been inserted, the lateral view can be used to check whether they have been correctly inserted and the antero-posterior view can be used to check the length of the screws. Any screw that is too long or too short should be replaced with one of the correct length.

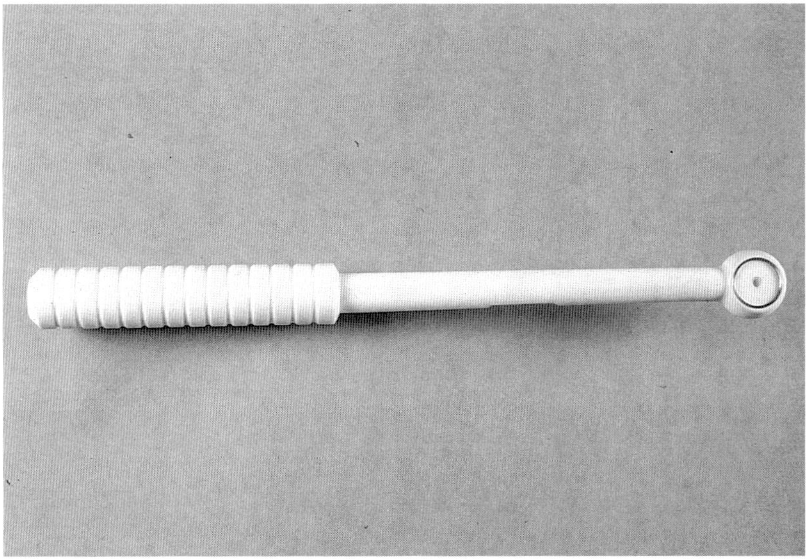

Figure 6.16

A plastic distal siting device, invented by Dr Dietmar Pennig (Münster, Germany). This is designed to facilitate the insertion of distal cross-screws using a free-hand technique.

CHAPTER 7 NAILING OF PROXIMAL FRACTURES

Femur

Locking femoral nails can be used to stabilize any proximal femoral diaphyseal fracture that leaves the lesser trochanter intact. The ideal position for the proximal cross-screw is shown in Figure 7.1. If the cross-screw is placed above the lesser trochanter, a stress riser may be created in the femoral neck and a femoral neck fracture may ensue (see Figure 23.15). Proximal femoral fractures that are either above the lesser trochanter or result in detachment of the lesser trochanter are not suitable for treatment with a conventional locking femoral nail. Such fractures may be treated with a reconstruction nail where the proximal screws are passed upwards and medially into the femoral neck and head (see Figure 20.2). The use of reconstruction nails is discussed in Chapter 20. A number of hip screw and side plate systems also exist for the treatment of such fractures.

Proximal femoral diaphyseal fractures are nailed according to the method detailed in Chapter 4 and are usually easily treated with a proximal dynamically locked nail or statically locked nail depending on the degree of comminution. However, because of the unapposed action of the hip flexors, the proximal femoral fragment may be pulled into flexion (Figure 7.2a and b). Unfortunately straight traction will not reduce such a proximal fragment and it can be very difficult to bring down the proximal fragment without actually opening the fracture. Some surgeons prefer the patient to be in the lateral position (see Figure 4.8) for proximal fractures but, if the supine position is adopted, the easiest method of reducing the proximal fragment is to insert a short Küntscher nail into the proximal femur and use the nail as a lever. The starting position for the bone awl is found in the usual manner and the awl is inserted (Figure 7.3). A hand reamer is passed down through the metaphysis to allow for the subsequent passage of a guide wire (Figure 7.4). A short Küntscher nail is then inserted into the entry point which can be reamed up to the correct size if necessary (Figure 7.5). Pressure on the nail reduces the fracture (Figure 7.6) and allows the passage of a guide wire down the shaft of the Küntscher nail (Figure 7.7) and across the fracture site (Figure 7.8). The guide wire is then passed down the femur and nailing can be undertaken in the standard manner. Obviously the flexible guide wire will not maintain reduction of a proximal fracture but appropriate pressure on the locking nail as it is inserted will facilitate the reduction of the proximal fragment prior to the nail being hammered across the fracture site.

Tibia

Proximal tibial diaphyseal fractures are fortunately relatively uncommon. Analysis of 250 tibial diaphyseal fractures treated by intramedullary nailing in Edinburgh has shown that only 5 per cent of such fractures occurred in the proximal third of the bone. Figure 3.4 illustrates a proximal tibial extra-articular fracture which would be virtually impossible to nail. It is unusual to see a more proximal fracture than the one illustrated in Figure 3.4 without there being articular involvement.

Nailing of proximal tibial fractures can be extremely difficult for a number of reasons. The proximity of the fracture line to the point of entry of the nail means that the short length of bone between the fracture and the nail entry point is subject to considerable stresses during nailing. This commonly results in some anterior comminution of the proximal fragments. The most common position for iatrogenic fracture of the proximal fragment is in the mid-line anteriorly. This fracture is inconveniently located just above the antero-posterior screw hole, thus rendering the antero-posterior cross-screw useless. A medial or lateral cross-screw must be used to gain proximal stability.

Proximal tibial comminution may be more extensive than just an anterior fracture as is shown in Figure 7.9, where an anteromedial section of the tibia has been raised following insertion of the nail. Fortunately the lateral cross-screw has gripped both the lateral and medial cortices to give some stability but an antero-posterior cross-screw could not be used. The fracture healed well and the patient subsequently regained full knee movement (Figure 7.9b).

The second problem associated with the nailing of proximal fractures is that the stability gained by the proximal screws may be poor. As with distal cross-screws, only one proximal screw is required under normal circumstances to stabilize the proximal fragment but, when proximal fractures are treated, the use of two proximal screws is mandatory. Despite this it may be difficult to control the fracture. Figure 7.10a shows a segmental tibial fracture with an undisplaced proximal fracture. Following nailing the proximal fracture has opened medially and the fracture is in slight valgus (Figure 7.10b). It might well have been preferable to use closed external fixation to hold this fracture. Surgeons inexperienced with locking nails should be careful with high proximal third tibial diaphyseal fractures and they may be wise to choose another treatment method.

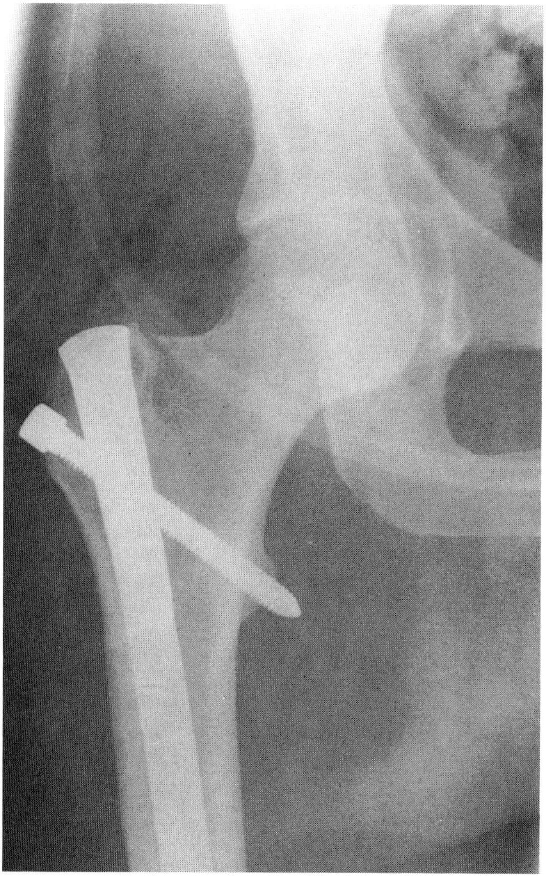

Figure 7.1

The proximal cross-screw of a locking femoral nail. This has been correctly inserted and is of the correct length. A proximal screw in the Grosse-Kempf system is fully threaded and must be screwed through the proximal hole in the nail.

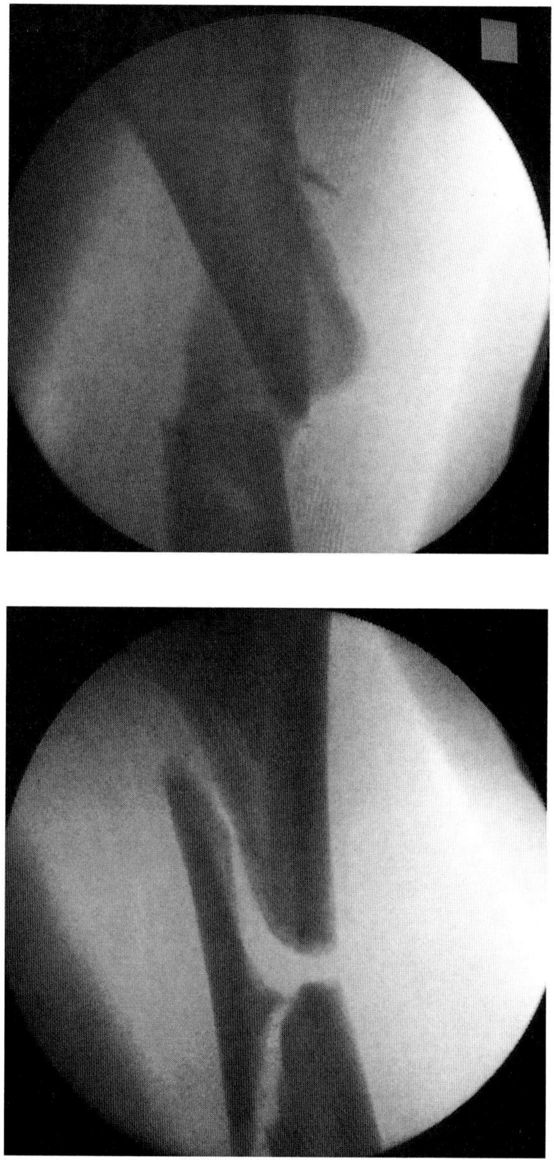

Figure 7.2

a The unopposed action of ilio-psoas often causes irreducible flexion of the proximal femoral fragment.

b The antero-posterior view shows that the butterfly fragment is below the level of the lesser trochanter and therefore a locking femoral nail can be used to stabilize this fracture, if the fracture can be reduced.

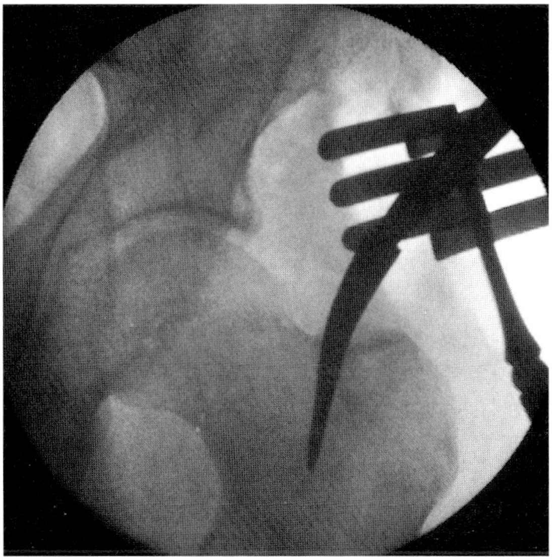

Figure 7.3

A bone awl is inserted into the piriformis fossa.

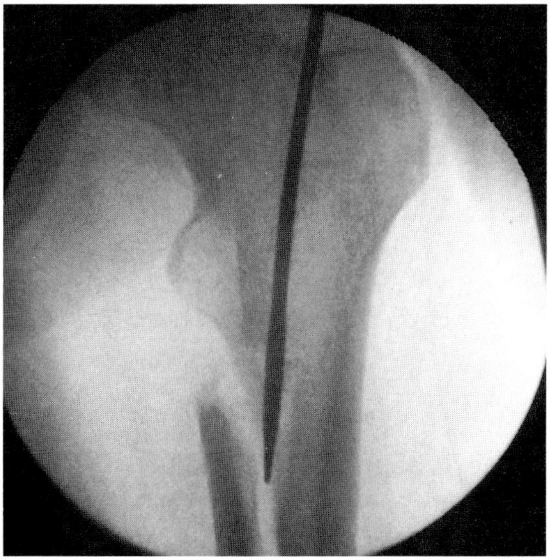

Figure 7.4

A hand reamer is used to breach the proximal metaphysis. The reamer should be bent so that it creates a proximal track aligned with the medullary canal of the femur.

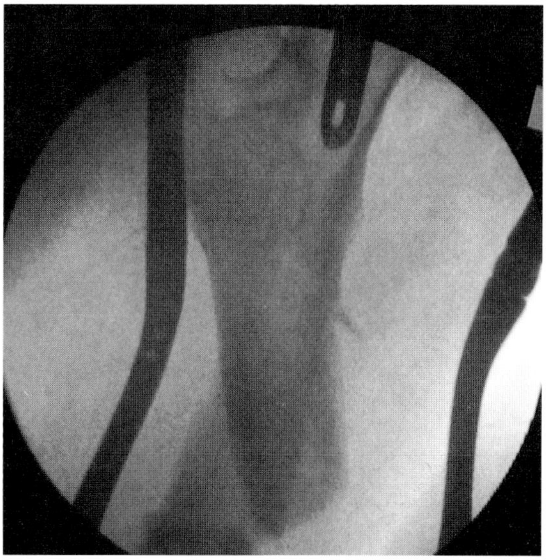

Figure 7.5

A small diameter Küntscher nail can be placed into the proximal cortical defect and hammered in for 1–2 cm to ensure stability.

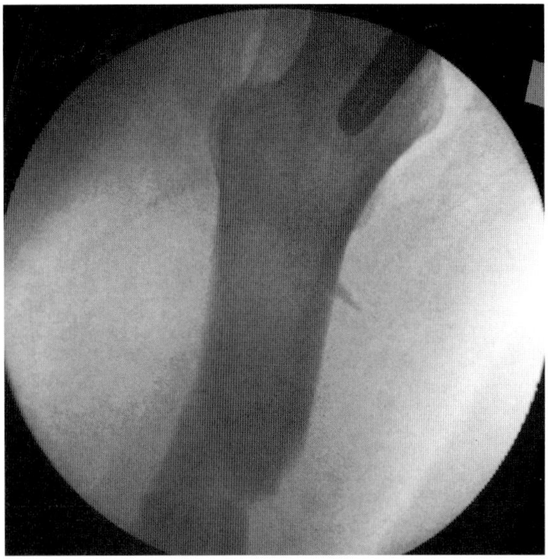

Figure 7.6

The Küntscher nail can then be used as a lever to reduce the fracture.

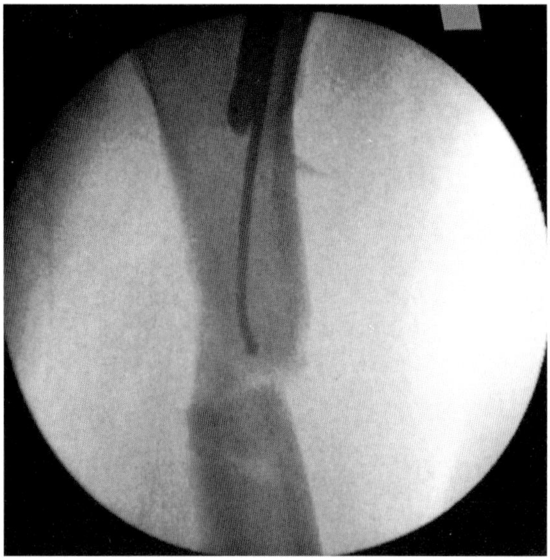

Figure 7.7

A curved olive-tipped guide wire can then be passed down through the Küntscher nail into the proximal fragment.

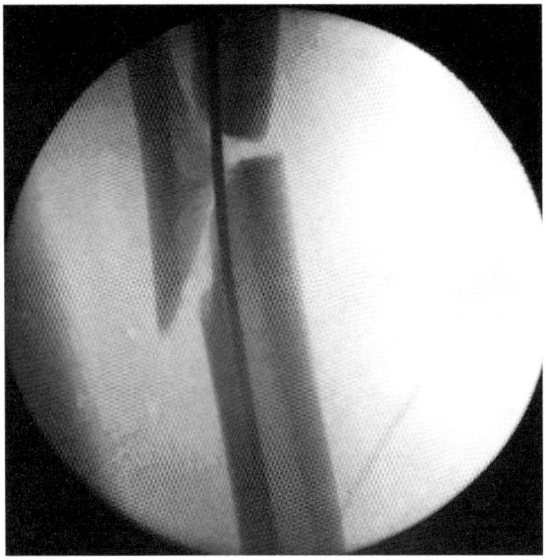

Figure 7.8

It is important to elevate the Küntscher nail to facilitate the passage of the guide wire across the fracture site. The Küntscher nail can then be extracted and the femur reamed. When the locking nail is inserted into the femur, it can be used to lever the proximal fragment into a reduced position before it is hammered over the fracture site.

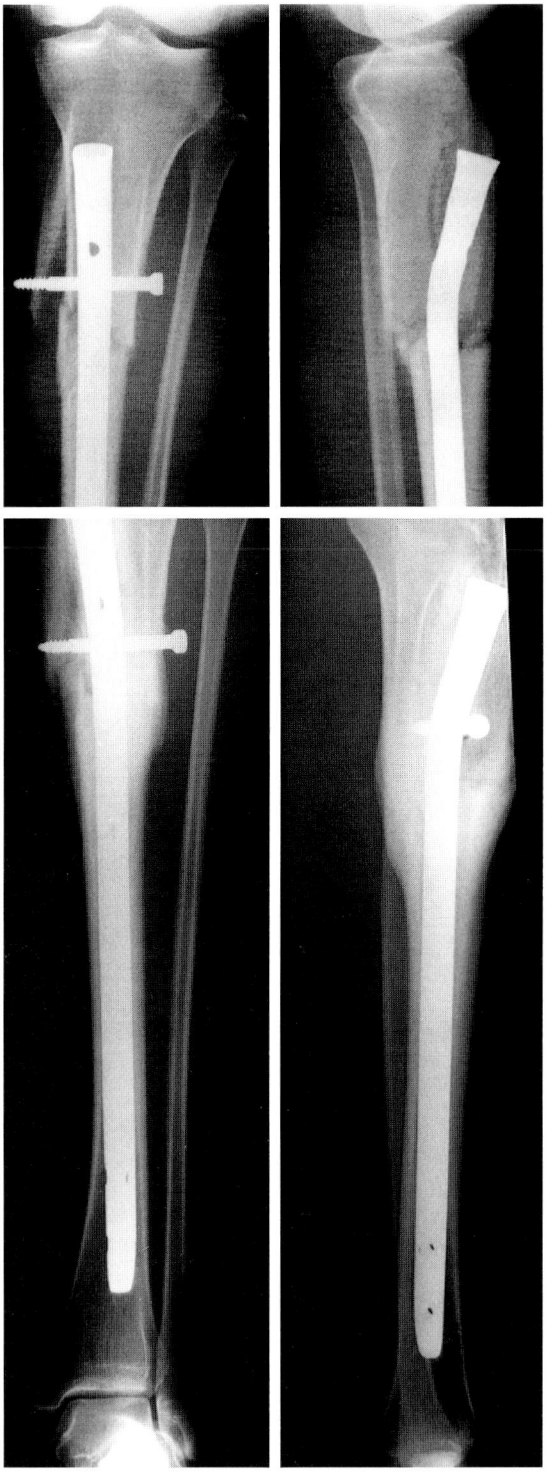

Figure 7.9

a Proximal comminution after the insertion of a nail into a proximal tibial fracture. Proximal comminution can be difficult to treat. In this case sufficient stability was obtained, but if there is extensive comminution even the use of both proximal screws will not ensure proximal stability.

b This fracture healed without the use of a plaster cast or other treatment method, but if there is significant proximal comminution another treatment such as closed external fixation should be used.

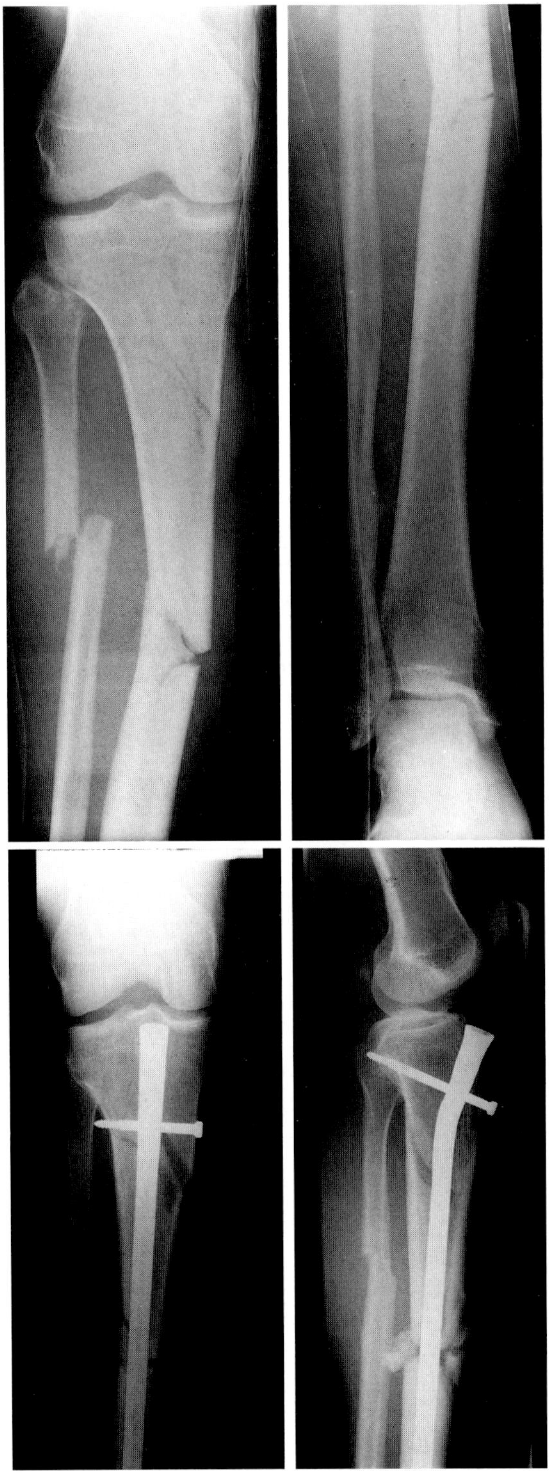

Figure 7.10

a A proximal tibial segmental fracture. The proximal fracture is undisplaced prior to intramedullary nailing.

b During nailing, the proximal fracture displaced slightly, resulting in slight valgus angulation. Despite the use of two cross-screws there was inadequate stability to control the fracture and still permit knee flexion. This patient was placed in a long leg cylinder for 6 weeks before knee mobilization could be commenced.

CHAPTER 8 NAILING OF DISTAL FRACTURES

Femur

Unlike the tibia there are few distal femoral fractures where there is doubt as to the role of closed nailing. Intramedullary nailing is not in general indicated for supracondylar fractures (Figure 8.1), distal femoral epiphyseal fractures or intercondylar fractures (Figure 8.2). A combination of techniques including intramedullary nailing can be used to treat intercondylar or condylar fractures (Christie et al, 1988), but many surgeons would probably use a supracondylar fixation device. Most other distal fractures can be nailed if a surgeon has experience. There are no particular technical problems in nailing distal femoral fractures, although the nail should, of course, be placed as far distally as possible remembering the presence of the femoral intercondylar notch. To facilitate distal nail placement, any distal femoral traction pin should be placed anteriorly to allow the nail to pass posterior to it. Figure 8.3 shows a distal femoral fracture which represents the limit of conventional closed nailing.

Tibia

Distal tibial fractures are much more common than distal femoral fractures. Fractures of the distal third of the tibia form approximately 51 per cent of all closed and Gustilo Type I tibial fractures seen in the Edinburgh Orthopaedic Trauma Unit (Court-Brown, Christie, McQueen, 1990). Any distal tibial fracture that is extra-articular can be treated by a locking nail if it is possible to insert one distal cross-screw with good contact between the screw in both bone cortices. In practice, this means that all fractures proximal to 5 cm of the ankle joint can be nailed. Most fractures that are within 5 cm of the ankle joint are intra-articular and should be treated by other methods. An example of a distal tibial fracture that would not be appropriately treated with a locking nail is shown in Figure 3.5.

Distal tibial fractures can be nailed relatively easily if the basic guidelines outlined in Chapter 5 are followed. There are, however, a number of technical points that the surgeon should be aware of.

Guide wire placement

It is important to place the guide wire in the middle of the distal fragment as seen on the antero-posterior view of the image intensifier. With middle third diaphyseal fractures the longer distal fragment tends to encourage the nail to take up in a central location distally. In distal third diaphyseal fractures, however, if the guide wire is placed down the medial or lateral aspects of the distal fragment, the fragment will tend to be displaced into varus or valgus as the nail is inserted. The guide wire must also be placed into the subchondral bone just proximal to the articular surface if adequate stability is to be achieved. The surgeon should always remember that if a curved guide wire is used to facilitate initial fracture reduction, the reamer can only be passed as far as the curve in the guide wire. If the surgeon wishes to ream into subchondral bone he or she must change from a curved guide wire to a straight olive-tipped one. The alternative is to ream the subchondral bone inadequately and to attempt to hammer the nail through this bone. This may well cause local damage and result in fracture site distraction.

As a curved guide wire will be used initially the surgeon will have to change from the curved to the straight guide wire. A 9 mm end-cutting reamer is passed down the medullary canal after insertion of the curved guide wire. The plastic tube is then inserted, as shown in Chapter 4, and the guide wires exchanged. Once the straight olive-tipped guide wire has been passed down into the correct position in the subchondral bone the 9 mm reamer is then used once again to ream through the subchondral bone as far as the olive. Conventional further reaming is employed and the nail is hammered down into the subchondral bone.

Numbers of cross-screws

Surgeons frequently insert two distal cross-screws in the belief that this will stop rotation in the sagittal plane. It is usually unnecessary to use two cross-screws as displacement of the distal fragment after insertion of only one distal screw is extremely rare, having only occurred in Edinburgh in one patient with particularly soft bone (Figure 23.9). It should be understood that distal fragment stability does not solely depend on the cross-screw, the main function of which is to preserve bone length and prevent axial rotation and angulation. There are strong ligamentous and capsular attachments around the ankle joint and these, combined with the penetration of the nail securely into the subchondral bone along with any contact between the proximal and distal fracture fragments, will help to stabilize the distal fragment (Figure 8.4).

Modification of nail length

If two cross-screws are to be placed into a small distal fragment or if a particularly small distal fragment is to be stabilized with one cross-screw the surgeon may wish to cut off the tip of the nail so that it may be advanced further into the bone. Should this be contemplated, accurate pre-operative measurements must be made of the intact tibia to assess the size of the nail to be cut. Alternatively, it is possible to keep a set of different lengths of nails of the commonly used diameters appropriately cut so that the surgeon may select the nail in the normal way during the operation. In reality it is probably easiest to keep a sterile hacksaw in theatre to cut the nail to the correct length during surgery.

Approximately 8 mm can be cut off the tip of the Grosse-Kempf tibial nail, but care should be taken not to transgress the lower screw hole. The shortened nail is introduced in the usual manner and the two distal screws inserted. Figure 8.5a and b shows an example of a shortened tibial nail. As the normal smooth conical tip of the nail has been removed, it is possible for the end of the nail to catch on the endosteal surface of the medullary canal. If this occurs, the surgeon should not attempt to hammer it down the canal as the tibia may fracture. Instead the canal should be reamed up a further 0.5 or 1 mm to facilitate nail insertion.

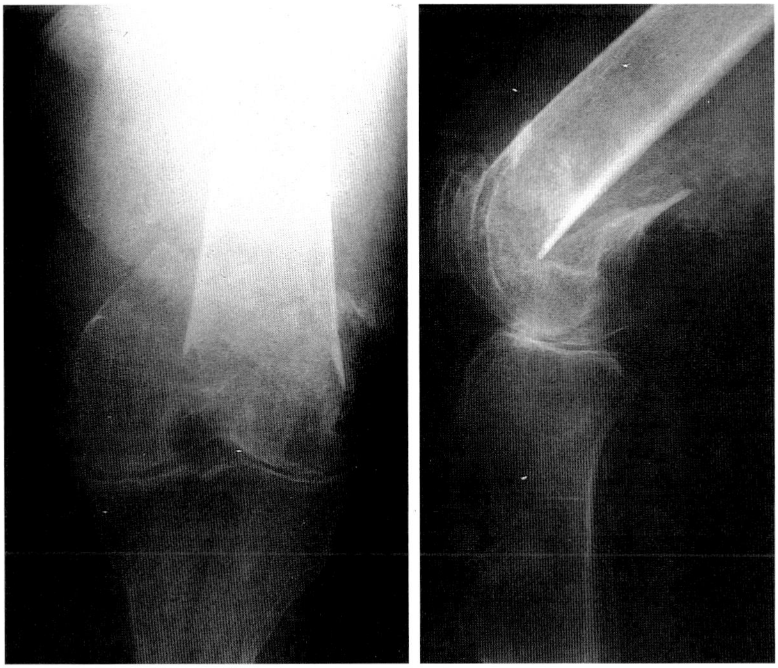

Figure 8.1

A supracondylar femoral fracture in a 79-year-old woman. This fracture is too low for the use of a locking nail.

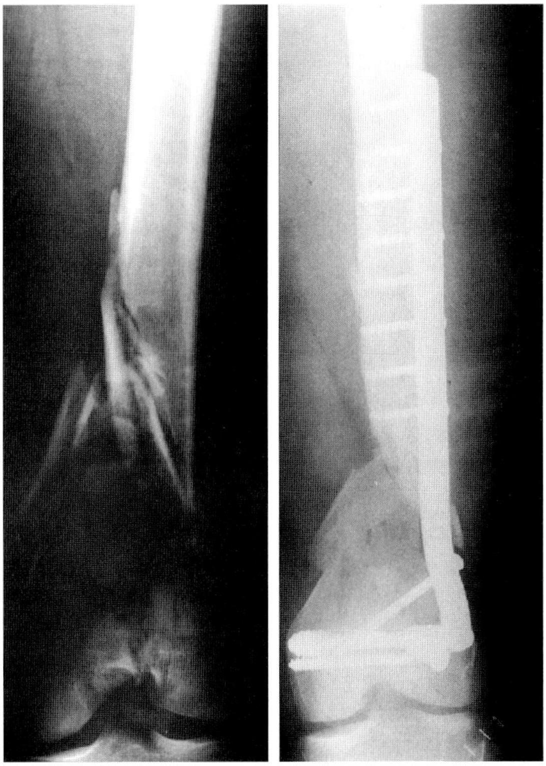

Figure 8.2

A Gustilo Type IIIb open comminuted intercondylar fracture. This was treated with a supracondylar compression screw and side-plate. The fracture healed without infection or the need for cortico-cancellous bone grafting.

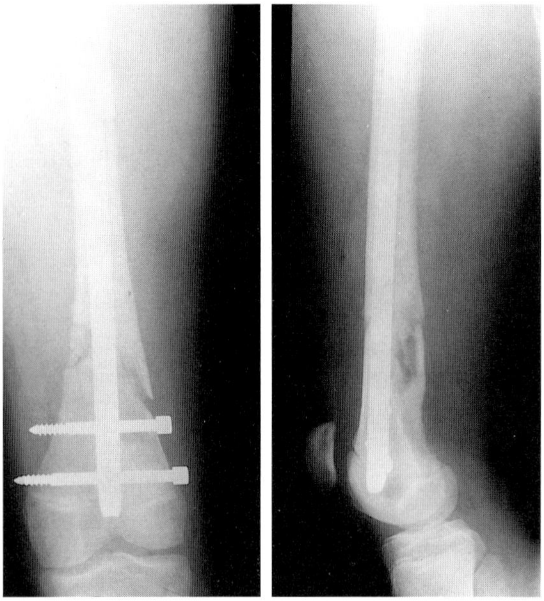

Figure 8.3

A closed distal femoral diaphyseal fracture. This fracture is well treated with a locking intramedullary nail but care must be taken in the placement of the transfixion pin as if this is placed posteriorly in the distal femur it may obstruct the passage of the nail.

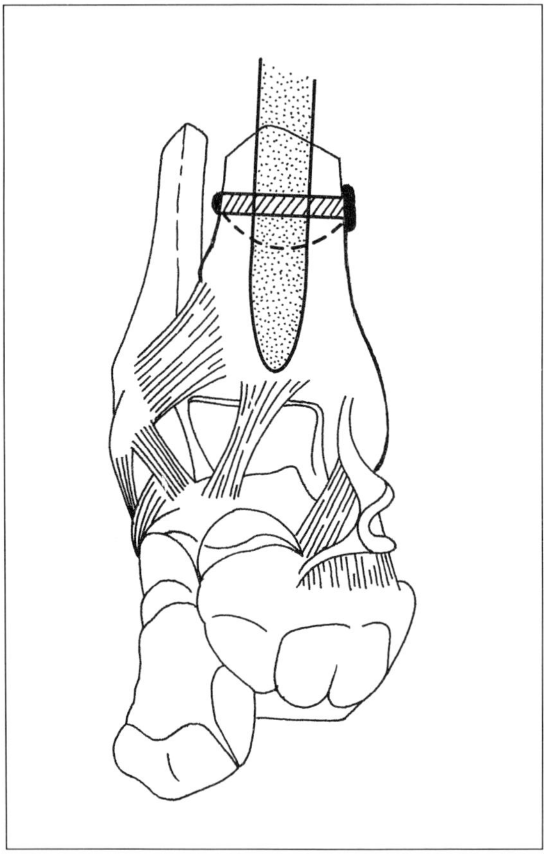

Figure 8.4

A diagram of the lower end of the tibia and ankle seen from the front. Distal tibial fractures can be stabilized by placing the nail into the metaphyseal bone and using one distal cross-screw. The strong ligamentous capsular attachments in the area prevent significant movement in the sagittal plane. Two cross-screws are only required if the bone is osteoporotic.

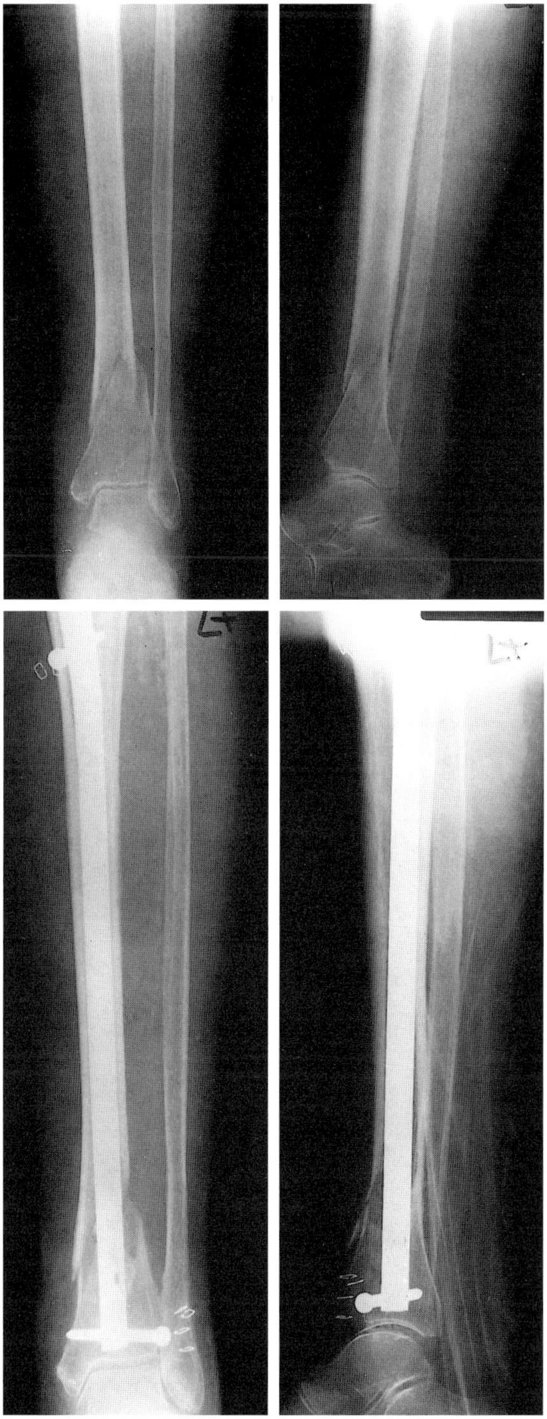

Figure 8.5

a Closed distal tibial fracture in a 63-year-old woman.

b The fracture has been stabilized with a statically locked tibial nail. The nail was cut short distally and one distal cross-screw was used. Fracture position was maintained until union.

CHAPTER 9 NAILING OF COMMINUTED FRACTURES

Closed locking nails provide the best solution to the problem of treatment of comminuted femoral or tibial diaphyseal fractures. As with the treatment of proximal or distal fractures, comminuted fractures that have an intra-articular extension are not usually suitable for nailing, although a combination of techniques can be used. Comminuted intra-articular distal femoral and proximal tibial fractures are more appropriately treated by other forms of internal fixation (see Figure 8.2). Intra-articular distal tibial fractures may be treated by either internal fixation or external fixation using the principle of ligamentotaxis. Closed external fixation is recommended for comminuted extra-articular proximal diaphyseal tibial fractures where insufficient stability will be gained in the proximal fragment (Figure 9.1a and b).

Comminuted diaphyseal fractures are usually relatively easy to nail. Often the isthmus is destroyed and only the proximal and distal fragments require to be reamed. Under these circumstances, the proximal and distal fragments should not be reamed to take an over-large nail but a nail of a size suitable for the patient should be chosen. Stability will be gained by the use of a static lock with the insertion of both proximal and distal cross-screws (Figure 9.2).

Reduction of comminuted fractures can usually be achieved by axial traction and guide wire placement is straightforward. The comminuted area should not be reamed as this may damage soft tissue in the area. Instead the reamers should be pushed through the comminuted area and only the proximal and distal fragments reamed. The nail and cross-screws are introduced in the usual way.

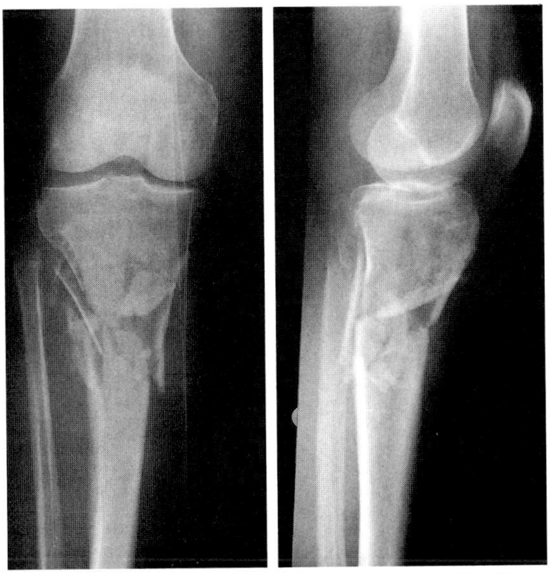

Figure 9.1

a A closed comminuted extra-articular proximal tibial fracture. This fracture is inappropriate for intramedullary nailing.

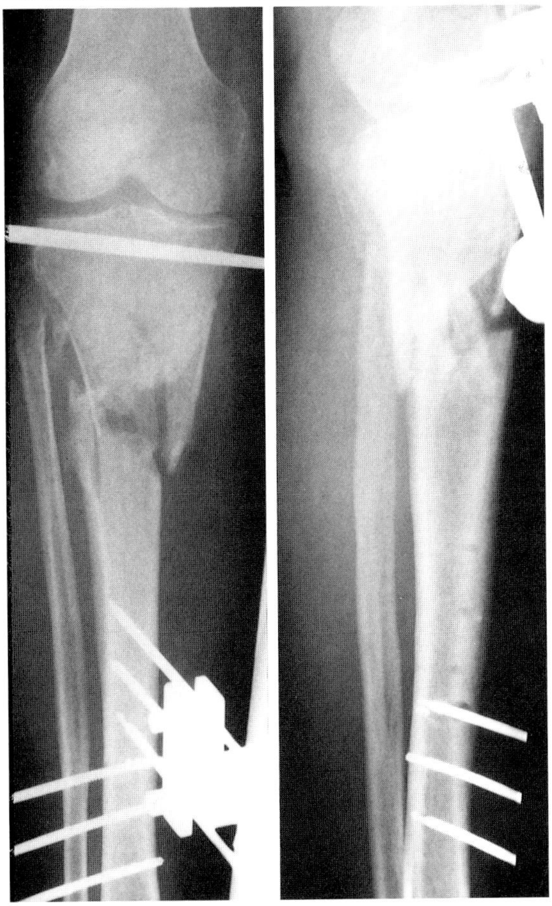

b Proximal extra-articular tibial fractures that are inappropriate for intramedullary nailing are well treated by external skeletal fixation. This method of treatment permits joint movement and allows for maintenance of fracture position.

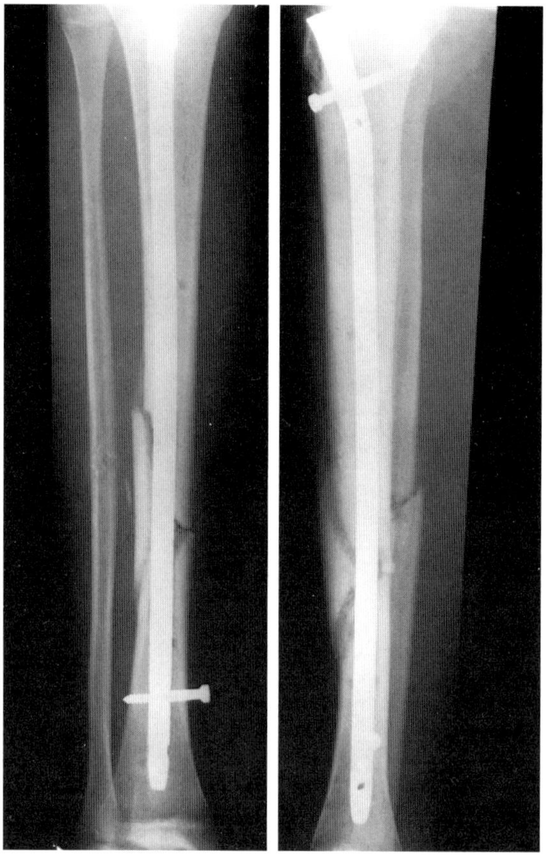

Figure 9.2

In comminuted tibial fractures, stability is gained by the use of a static lock. A static lock should be used regardless of the degree of comminution.

CHAPTER 10 NAILING OF SEGMENTAL FRACTURES

Many surgeons approach the nailing of segmental fractures with some trepidation because of the possibility of the segment spinning during reaming and therefore becoming avascular. In fact this is rare because of the considerable muscle, fascial and ligamentous connections of the femoral and tibial diaphyses. The major muscle attachments of the femur are shown in Figure 10.1. It can be seen that the wide insertions of the vastus intermedius, vastus medialis, vastus lateralis and the adductors along with the intermuscular septa will discourage a segment from spinning. In the tibia, the wide origins of tibialis anterior, tibialis posterior, flexor digitorum longus and soleus as well as the presence of the interosseous membrane also discourage segment spinning. Theoretically a loose segment in the distal quarter of the tibia could spin as there are few muscle or ligamentous attachments in this area, but distal quarter tibial diaphyseal segments are extremely rare and this is unlikely to be a problem that the surgeon will encounter.

It is obvious that the tendency of a segment to spin will depend on its length, the amount of adjacent soft-tissue destruction and the torque applied by the reamers. Longer segments, as shown in Figure 10.2, rarely spin as their soft-tissue attachments are extensive. However, care should be taken when a short segment is encountered (Figure 10.3) as spinning may occur. If the surgeon is concerned that a short segment might spin, he or she should immobilize the segment. In the tibia, this can be done by closed manual pressure or by the percutaneous application of sharp bone-holding forceps to the segment. This is preferable to opening the tibial fracture. In the closed femoral fracture it is impossible to hold the segment by external means. If the surgeon is concerned about the segment spinning, the thigh should be opened and the segment stabilized with bone-holding forceps. This was undertaken in the fracture shown in Figure 10.3. Such short segments are in fact unusual as in general the shorter the segment, the greater the chance that it will itself be fractured. Many resemble the broken segment seen in Figure 10.4. These are treated as comminuted fractures using the technique described in Chapter 9.

Open fractures provide the situation where segments have the greatest tendency to spin on reaming. This is because the severity of injury associated with Gustilo Type III fractures means that there is considerable soft-tissue damage. The use of locking nails in the management of open fractures is discussed in Chapter 11, but if a reamed nail is to be used to transfix a segment in a Gustilo Type III fracture, great care must be taken that the associated soft-tissue injury does not in fact allow the segment to spin. It is recommended that bone-holding forceps are used to stabilize such segments.

One further method of minimizing the risk of segment spinning is to use a smaller nail than would normally be used for that particular fracture. The use of a smaller nail means that less reaming is required and the torque generated within the segment will be less. However the surgeon should not use a nail of a size inappropriate for the patient.

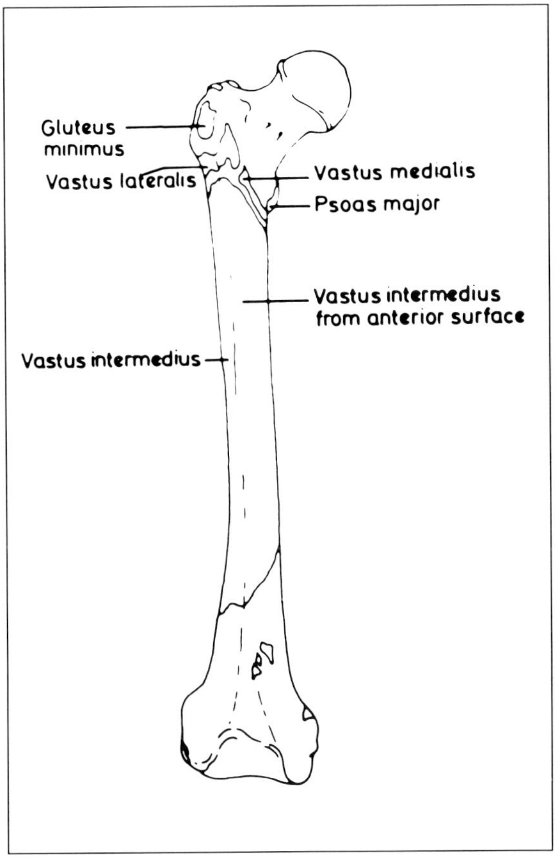

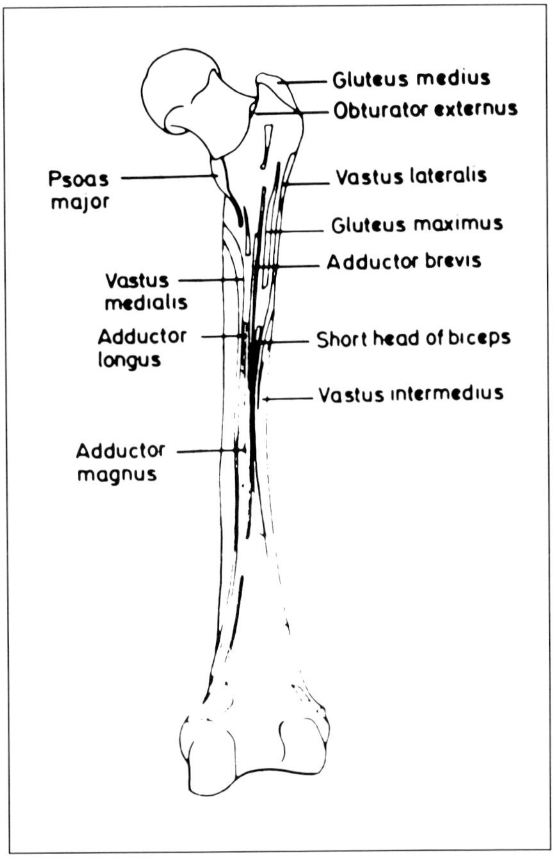

Figure 10.1

a Anterior aspect of the femur. The considerable origin of vastus intermedius stabilizes a separate diaphyseal segment.

b Posterior aspect of the femur. The extensive origins of vastus medialis and vastus lateralis and the extensive insertions of the adductor muscles in particular also help to stabilize loose bone segments and prevent their spinning during reaming.

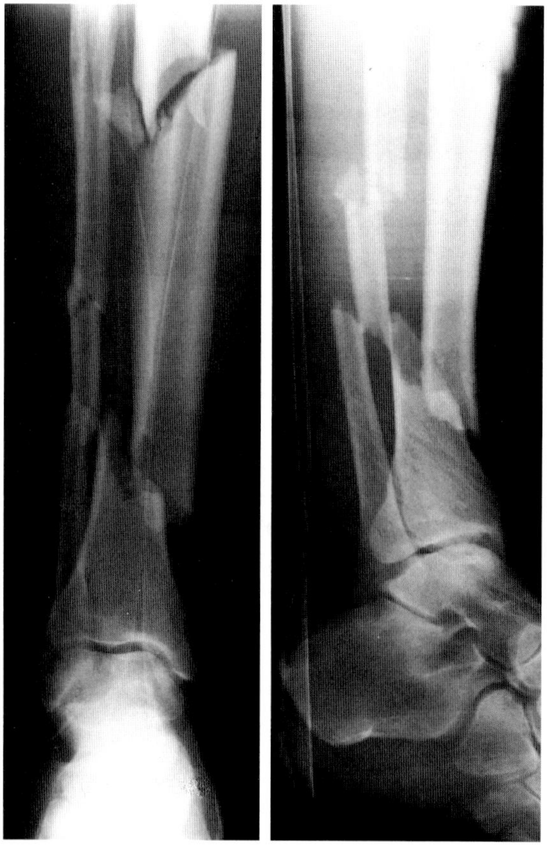

Figure 10.2

A long intact tibial segment. The extensive muscle attachment minimizes the risk of spinning a segment of this length.

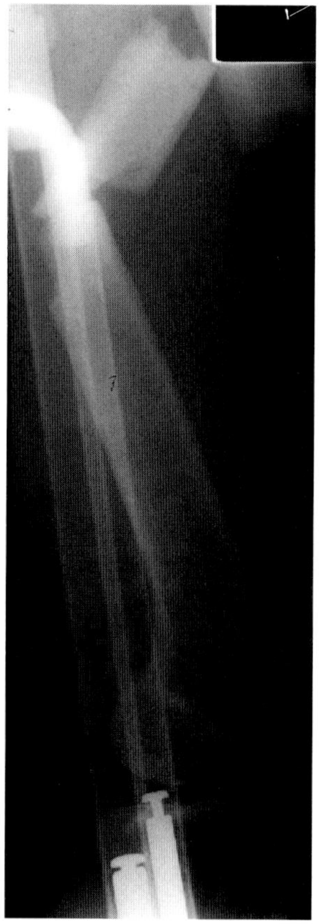

Figure 10.3

A short intact femoral segment in a closed fracture. The risk of this length of segment spinning is much higher and, if avascularity is to be avoided, this segment should be held with bone-holding forceps.

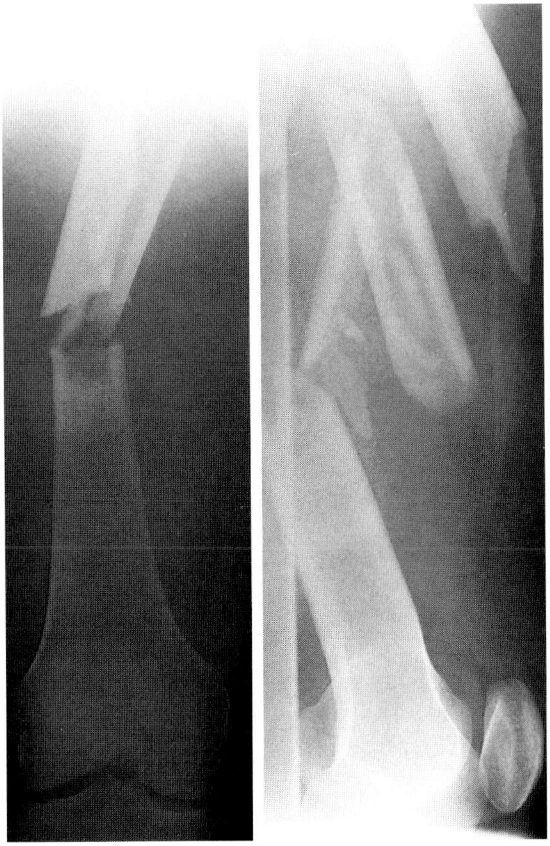

Figure 10.4

Many segments are themselves fractured. Such fractures are treated as comminuted fractures and a static lock should be used. Comparison of this fracture with the one shown in Figure 2.14 shows the advantages of locked nailing. If an unlocked nail is used an open operation is required.

CHAPTER 11 NAILING OF OPEN FRACTURES

The use of both reamed and unreamed intramedullary nails in the treatment of open fractures is controversial. A number of surgeons over the years have used reamed nails for all femoral and tibial fractures, including those associated with severe soft-tissue loss or damage. However, others find this practice unacceptable, believing that the use of reamed nails will damage an already compromised medullary circulation. This argument remains unproven, although it seems likely that in major open fractures the medullary blood supply will already have been considerably compromised by the force of the injury.

It is extremely important to assess the state of the soft tissues adequately if intramedullary nailing is contemplated in an open fracture. To do this it is essential to use a good open fracture grading system. In this book the system suggested by Gustilo and Anderson in 1976, and modified later by Gustilo et al in 1984, will be used. This system divides open wounds into three types based on the amount of bone and soft-tissue damage, with the Type III wounds being subdivided into a further three subtypes, again based on the extent of soft-tissue damage.

Type I	Wound less than 1 cm in length and clean
Type II	Wound longer than 1 cm with moderate contamination and/or muscle damage
Type III	Wound longer than 5 cm with severe contamination and/or severe muscle damage Any fracture occurring in a farmyard environment Any fracture which is segmental and displaced or due to a high-velocity gun shot or shotgun wound
Type IIIa	As Type III but with good bone and soft-tissue cover and limited periosteal stripping
Type IIIb	As Type III but with considerable exposed bone due to periosteal stripping
Type IIIc	As Type III but with a major vascular injury requiring repair

Open femoral fractures are much less common than open tibial fractures and tend to be associated with a more favourable prognosis. Most fracture surgeons will nail Gustilo Type I and II open femoral fractures and many find nailing acceptable in Type III fractures, although others prefer external skeletal fixation. The prognosis for open tibial fractures is worse and many surgeons prefer external skeletal fixation to intramedullary nailing. External skeletal fixation in severe open fractures is, however, associated with a relatively high incidence of mal-union (Court-Brown, Wheelwright, Christie et al, 1990) and in the author's centre intramedullary nailing has become the established method of treatment in Type III open tibial fractures. It has been found to be associated with a relatively low incidence of mal-union and joint stiffness compared with external fixation.

Primary treatment of open fractures

It has become a cliché to state that the most important component of open-fracture management is the initial wound excision or debridement, but it is undoubtedly true. In recent years, surgeons have unfortunately become more interested in the mechanical rather than the biological aspects of open-fracture management. Thus arguments have raged about the appropriate use of plates, external fixation devices and intramedullary nails, but there has been little discussion about the adequacy of wound toilet.

Initial wound management involves a thorough wound toilet with removal of all devitalized and dubious tissue. Different soft tissues have a different resistance to trauma. Skin is very resistant to damage and frequently only a small amount need be resected, although care must be taken when dealing with a degloved area of skin. Under these circumstances, the skin should be resected until dermal bleeding is encountered. All dead and devitalized muscle must be removed. It may be very difficult to assess at the first wound toilet procedure just how much muscle or fat is devitalized and therefore it is important to return a patient with an open fracture to the operating theatre 36 to 48 hours after the initial wound toilet to carry out a second wound toilet procedure to re-examine the soft tissues.

Unfortunately many surgeons return large pieces of avascular bone to the fracture site in the belief that the maintenance of bone structure is important. It is actually much more important to discard all avascular or potentially avascular bone to minimize the risk of post-traumatic osteomyelitis. There are a number of bone-grafting techniques available which will allow the surgeon to rebuild areas of large bone loss. The surgeon should also carefully assess the condition of any muscle that it attached to a large bone fragment. The fact that muscle is attached to the fragment may not necessarily mean that the fragment has an adequate blood supply. Should the muscle itself be traumatized the bone fragment should be removed.

Soft-tissue wounds associated with open fractures should never be closed. Small open wounds will heal by secondary intent and larger wounds can either be skin grafted or closed with a full-thickness flap at a later date. There is no doubt that modern plastic surgery techniques involving the early use of muscle flaps, myocutaneous flaps, osseous myocutaneous flaps and free vascularized flaps have revolutionized the treatment of severe open fractures (Cierny et al, 1983). It is usually unwise to perform flap cover primarily but once the wound has been re-examined, 36 to 48 hours after the initial injury, flap cover can easily be performed at that time or shortly thereafter. There is mounting evidence that the prognosis for an open fracture is greatly improved if adequate soft-tissue cover is achieved within one week of injury.

X-ray scans of an open fracture taken after wound excision has been performed frequently show pieces of bone which are significantly displaced from their correct position (Figure 11.1). These pieces of bone are usually devitalized and should be removed even if this necessitates re-exploring the limb. Failure to do this may result in post-traumatic osteomyelitis. Open fractures should be treated with a broad spectrum prophylactic antibiotic. This is usually a second-generation cephalosporin, although in fractures associated with considerable muscle damage it is wise to add benzyl penicillin. Studies in the USA

(Gustilo et al, 1984) and in the UK (Court-Brown, Wheelwright, Christie et al, 1990) have suggested that there has been a major increase in the incidence of Gram-negative sepsis in Gustilo Type III tibial fractures and it is probably wise to use a third-generation cephalosporin for these fractures.

Type I fractures

Many authors have stated that Type I open long bone diaphyseal fractures have the same prognosis as the equivalent closed fracture regardless of how they are treated. Such a fracture is shown in Figure 11.2. If nailing is to be undertaken, the basic principles outlined in Chapters 4 and 5 should be followed. After positioning, skin preparation and draping of the patient the open wound should be thoroughly excised and the bone ends cleaned. Nailing can then be undertaken as for a closed fracture with the wound being left open. In Edinburgh, the results of intramedullary nailing of Type I open fractures for both the femur and the tibia are the same as for closed fractures (Christie et al, 1988; Court-Brown, Christie, McQueen, 1990).

Type II fractures

Type II fractures are associated with some soft-tissue damage and a thorough wound excision is mandatory; an example is shown in Figure 11.3. Again nailing can be undertaken in the manner described in Chapters 4 and 5 with the wound being closed either secondarily or by plastic surgery techniques at a later date.

Type III fractures

Type III fractures are associated with a poorer prognosis regardless of their method of treatment. Work in Edinburgh (Court-Brown, Wheelwright, Christie et al, 1990) has shown that the rise in morbidity occurs with the Type IIIb fracture where there is extensive soft-tissue damage including periosteal stripping. The same study showed that Type IIIa fractures treated with external skeletal fixation have a 5 per cent incidence of deep infection, whereas Type IIIb fractures are associated with a 37 per cent incidence of deep infection.

If a Type III fracture is to be nailed, the patient should be placed on the fracture table in the position described in Chapters 4 and 5. Care should be taken that the limb is not overstretched as the loss of soft-tissue integrity associated with a Type III fracture may facilitate an unintentional limb lengthening. After the wound excision has been performed, the bone is nailed in the usual way. The soft tissues should be inspected at 36 to 48 hours after the initial operation and further wound excision performed if necessary. If the wound is clean, a full-thickness flap or split-skin graft can be used depending on the circumstances. Figure 11.4 shows a Type IIIa fracture in a multiply injured patient which was primarily nailed. A gastrocnemius muscle flap with an overlying split-skin graft was used to close the wound at 36 hours (Figure 11.5) and the fracture healed without bone grafting in 27 weeks (Figure 11.6). Nailing of Type III open fractures is usually straightforward as fracture reduction and nail placement is often easier than in a closed fracture.

Bone loss

There are a number of ways to treat bone loss, including vascularized bone grafts (Figure 11.7) and bone transport. If these techniques are to be used the surgeon must employ external skeletal fixation. Intramedullary nailing may be used to stabilize a bone with a missing segment provided the patient is prepared to accept cortico-cancellous bone-grafting procedures. Figure

11.8a and b illustrates the importance of good soft-tissue cover in the management of a Type IIIb tibial fracture with extensive bone loss. Good stability was obtained following nailing and a latissimus dorsi free flap was successfully used to gain skin closure.

The use that can be made of extensive cortico-cancellous bone grafting in the management of major bone defects in nailed fractures is shown in Figure 11.9. This is a Type IIIb tibial fracture (Figure 11.9a) with considerable bone loss following wound toilet (Figure 11.9b). After two bone grafting procedures the patient was walking without pain or walking aids (Figure 11.9c).

It is not intended to advocate the general use of locking nails for such fractures, although specialized units will continue to use these techniques in certain cases. External skeletal fixation and vascularized bone grafts have a proven place in the management of bone loss and bone transport techniques are currently being investigated to assess their use in the management of these difficult fractures.

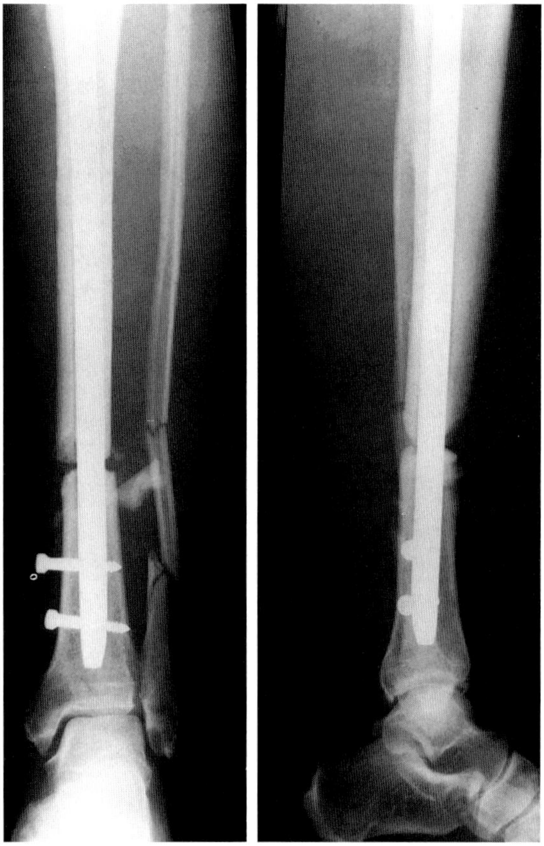

Figure 11.1

Type IIIa open tibial fracture after wound debridement and intramedullary nailing. A loose bone fragment is seen lying between the tibia and fibula. It is likely that the bone fragment is devitalized and it should be removed.

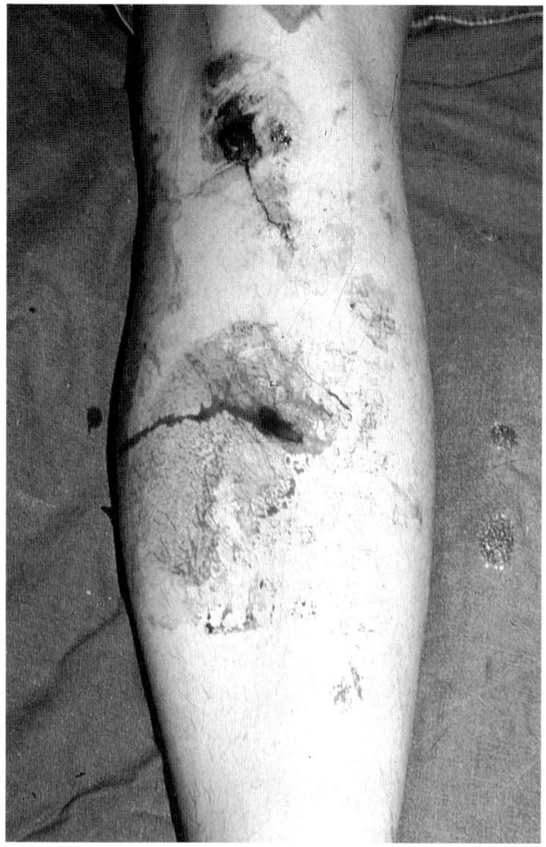

Figure 11.2

Gustilo Type I open tibial fracture. This was sustained in a soccer tackle. Such fractures are not associated with significant contamination and should have the same prognosis as closed fractures regardless of the method of management.

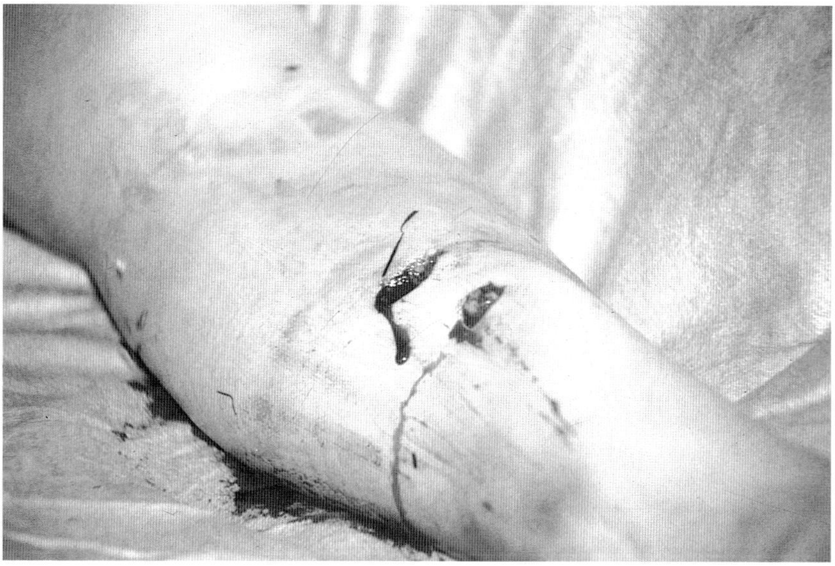

Figure 11.3

A Type II midshaft tibial fracture in a multiply injured patient who had jumped 150 ft. Such fractures are associated with a degree of soft-tissue damage and usually some contamination.

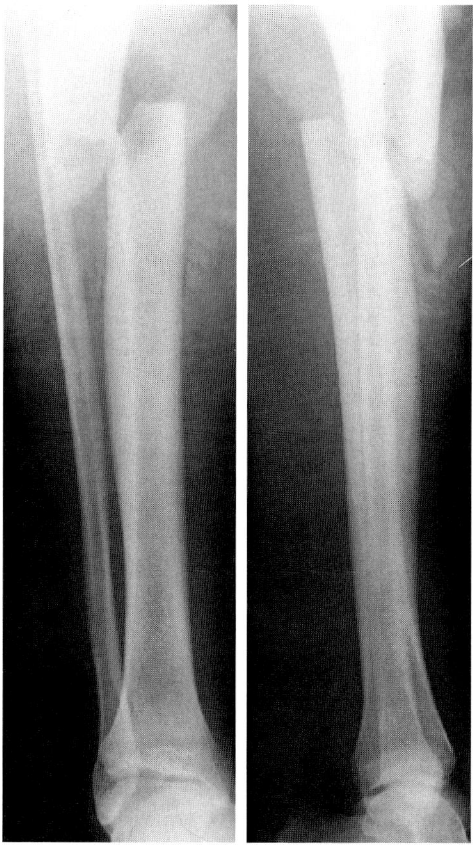

Figure 11.4

a A Type IIIa proximal tibial fracture in a 17-year-old male who had multiple injuries.

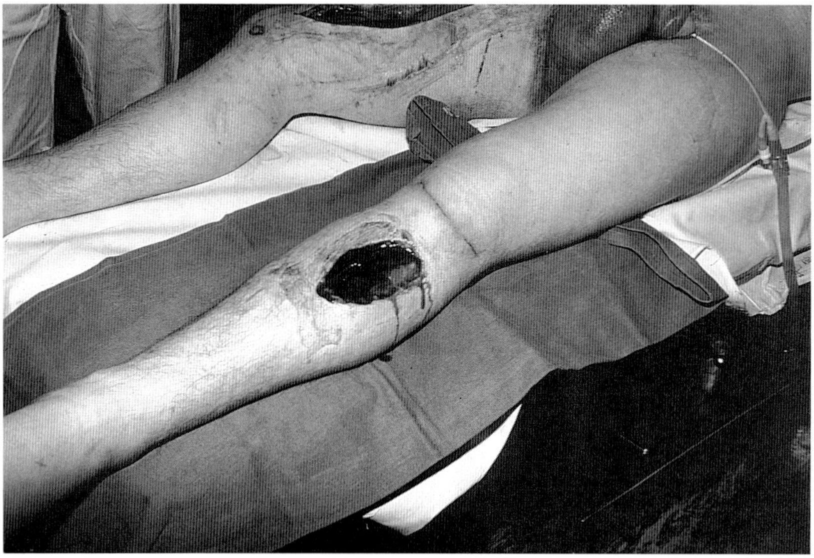

Figure 11.4 *continued*

b The fracture was treated with a primary proximal dynamically locked intramedullary nail after thorough wound toilet was performed.

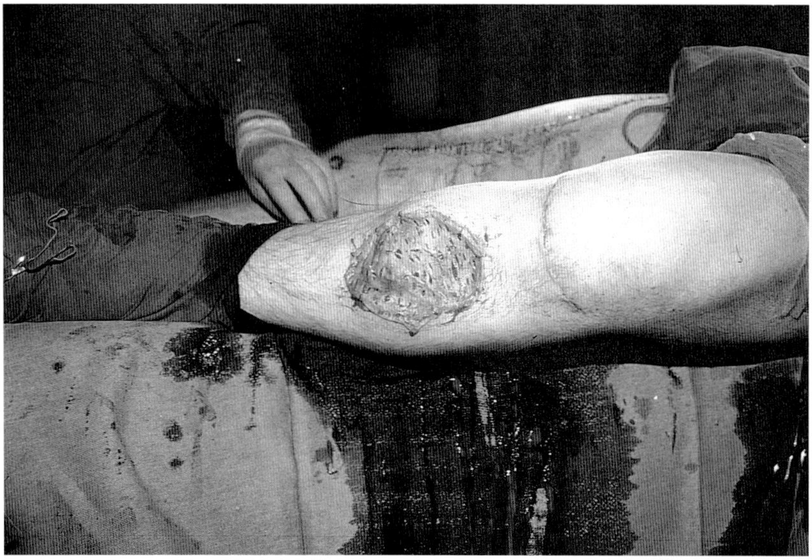

Figure 11.5

After 36 hours, a further wound toilet was performed and a gastrocnemius flap and split skin grafting used to close the defect. No further orthopaedic or plastic surgery procedures were required.

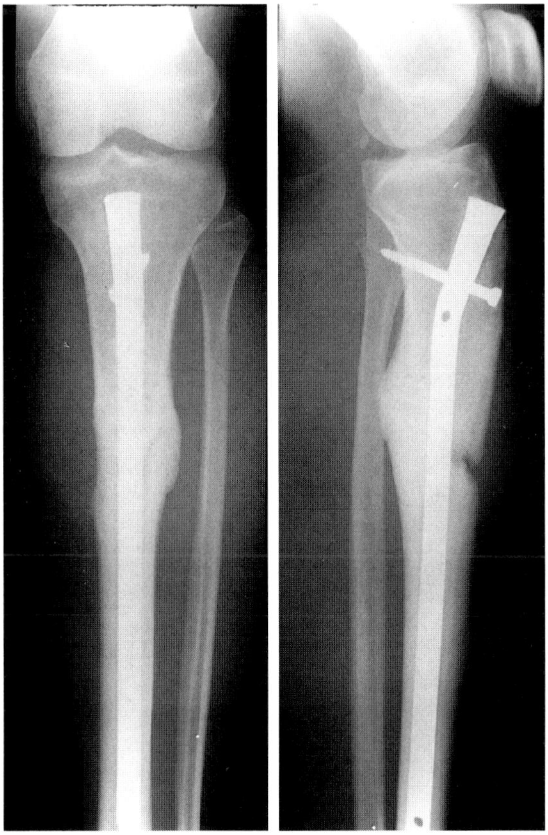

Figure 11.6

After 27 weeks the fracture was clinically and radiologically united. The patient had full function in his knee, ankle and subtalar joints.

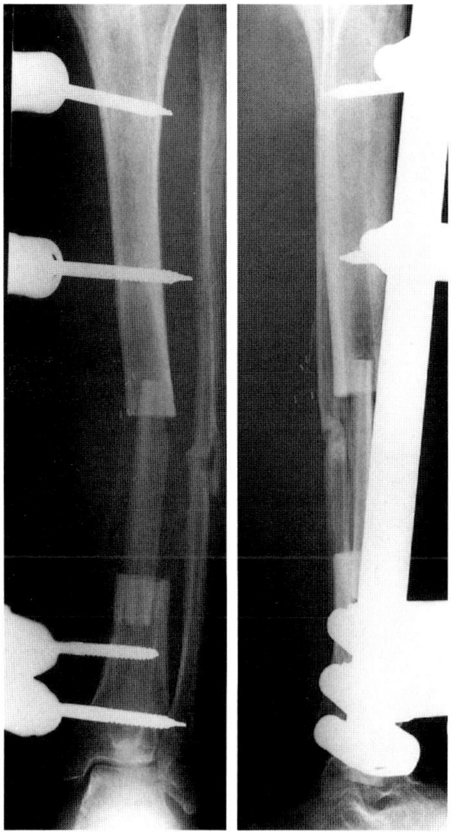

Figure 11.7

Vascularized fibular graft used to treat a non-union in a Type II open tibial fracture. Clearly intramedullary nailing is impossible if this procedure is used and this fracture has been held with an Oxford external fixator.

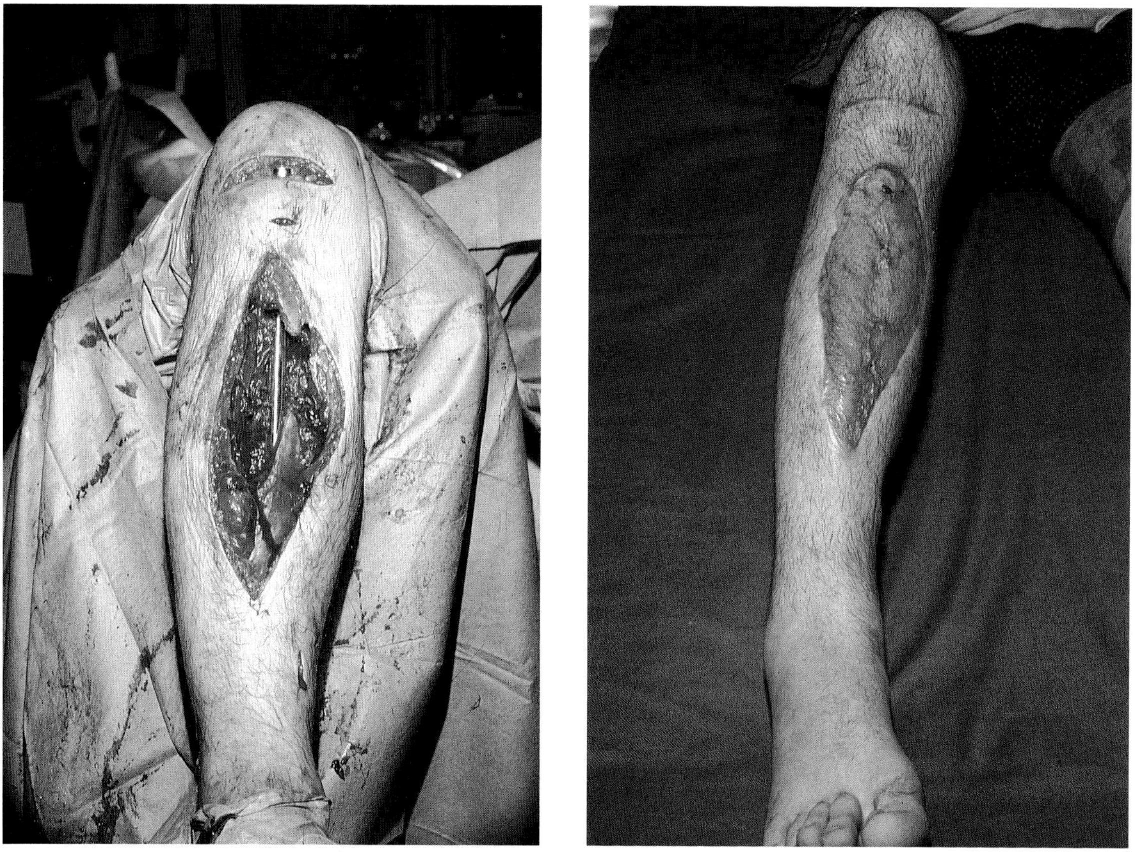

Figure 11.8

a A Type IIIb tibial fracture associated with considerable bone and soft-tissue loss. The fracture was nailed on the day of admission after a thorough wound toilet.

b After 3 days the wound was covered with a latissimus dorsi free flap. Four weeks later, the soft tissues are in a satisfactory condition and there is no evidence of sepsis. Cortico-cancellous bone grafting was carried out after 3 weeks using a posterolateral approach.

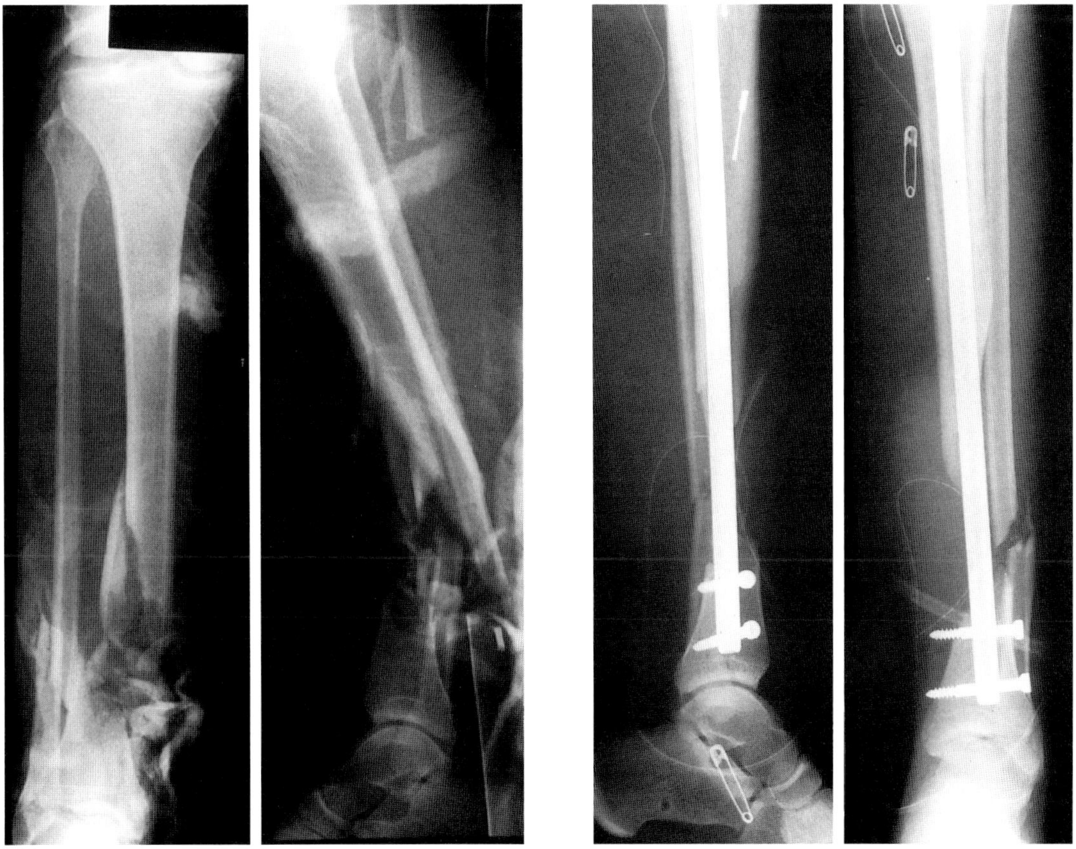

Figure 11.9

a A Type IIIb open distal tibial fracture.

b All devitalized bone was removed and the skin defect was covered with a latissimus dorsi free flap.

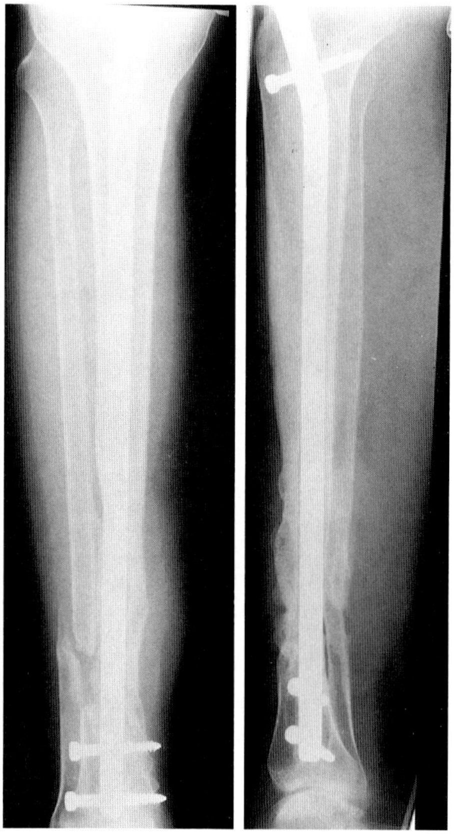

Figure 11.9 *continued*

c Following restoration of the soft-tissue envelope, two cortico-cancellous bone grafting operations were performed and union obtained. This X-ray scan was taken 15 months after the accident.

CHAPTER 12 MANAGEMENT OF NON-UNIONS

Non-unions can be either hypertrophic (Figure 12.1a) or atrophic (Figure 12.2a). Hypertrophic non-unions often occur after non-operative management of diaphyseal fractures and are probably related to the particular biomechanical environment imposed by that form of management. Atrophic non-unions are commonly associated with avascularity at a fracture site or the presence of infection. They are more often seen in Gustilo Type II and III open fractures and in closed fractures associated with significant soft-tissue damage. Open plating of femoral or tibial diaphyseal fractures may also be associated with atrophic non-union if the surgeon strips too much soft tissue from the bone to facilitate access.

Hypertrophic non-union can be successfully treated by altering the biomechanical environment of the fracture. Good results have been obtained with closed external fixation, plating and intramedullary nailing. There is no requirement for bone grafting and the hypertrophic non-union site should not be taken down unless one is dealing with a mal-aligned non-union which requires angular or rotational correction. There are a number of theoretical advantages in using locking intramedullary nails in the treatment of hypertrophic non-unions. The closed nature of the operation leads to a very low incidence of infection and axial loading at the fracture site is simply gained by the patient walking on the limb postoperatively. In addition, if the limb has been immobilized on traction or in a cast for a prolonged period the bone may be osteoporotic and bone screws and external fixation pins may gain a poor hold. Intramedullary nailing is particularly useful under these circumstances. There are, however, a number of circumstances where closed intramedullary nailing of hypertrophic non-unions may be difficult and may not be the treatment of choice. These are mainly related to any mal-alignment that persists following the initial treatment.

Atrophic non-unions do not generally unite without bone grafting. If intramedullary nailing is to be used to stabilize an atrophic non-union a cortico-cancellous bone graft may be required. The reamings produced during the nailing procedure may also act as a bone graft, although their role in the treatment of atrophic non-unions requires further research.

Intramedullary nailing of non-unions following conservative management

Many orthopaedic surgeons continue to use non-operative techniques for the management of femoral and tibial fractures, despite the considerable problems associated with their use. Surgeons will therefore encounter non-unions that follow femoral traction or tibial casting. Both these treatments are associated with a high incidence of mal-alignment and closed intramedullary nailing may be difficult or impossible to perform.

Hypertrophic non-unions that occur following conservative management may present with angular or rotational deformity or with a degree of overlap. The mal-position is impossible to correct by closed manipulation because of the presence of pseudarthrosis tissue in and around the fracture site. Thus only non-unions that are aligned or have an acceptable rotatory mal-alignment are suitable for closed intramedullary nailing. The problem is illustrated in Figure 12.3. If an intramedullary nail is hammered into an angulated non-union, the non-union will not straighten and cortical damage in the lower fragment is inevitable. Cortical overlap may also prevent the surgeon from using intramedullary nailing as even if a guide wire can be passed down the medullary canal into the distal fragment, the reamers may get stuck on the cortex and the nail, if hammered home, cause considerable cortical damage. This problem is illustrated in Figure 12.4. Rotationally mal-aligned femora and tibiae can be nailed if they are not associated with angular or overlap deformities. If the surgeon feels that the degree of rotation is unacceptable the non-union must be taken down to permit correction.

If there is sufficient mal-alignment to prevent intramedullary nailing, but insufficient deformity to necessitate taking down the non-union, another stabilization method must be chosen: either closed external fixation or open plating is suitable (Figure 12.1b).

Nailing of non-unions following plating

No major problems should be encountered in the use of intramedullary nailing to treat a non-union associated with the use of bone plates. Plate removal and closed nailing can be performed at the same operation provided there is no infection, but the surgeon should close the incision required for plate removal before nailing so that the medullary reamings remain at the fracture site.

Non-unions following plating are usually atrophic and occur because of poor plating technique, the surgeon having denuded a large area of bone of its blood supply. Such a non-union is shown in Figure 12.2a. This shows the X-ray scan of a closed tibial fracture which was plated. It was clear after 8 weeks that union was not proceeding and an open cortico-cancellous grafting operation was performed. Despite this, union had not occurred at 20 weeks and closed nailing was performed after plate removal. Good contact between the nail and the endosteal surface of the cortex was obtained and no cross-screws were used. A partial fibulectomy was performed and cortico-cancellous graft applied around the fracture site (Figure 12.2b). Full weight bearing was encouraged and the fracture was clinically and radiologically united after a further 16 weeks (Figure 12.2c).

Nailing following external fixation

The use of intramedullary nailing following previous external fixation is straightforward if the non-union is properly aligned. Although emphasis is always placed on the problems associated with pin-tract sepsis, the major problem of external fixation is actually mal-alignment with subsequent mal-union, this usually occurring because the surgeon is confused about when to remove the fixator. If an external fixator is removed before adequate callus has formed, mal-alignment and subsequent mal-union can occur. Since mal-alignment is the main problem following both conservative management and external fixation, the surgeon should take the same precautions in assessing externally fixed non-unions for intramedullary nailing as previously described for non-unions following conservative management. The mal-alignments shown in Figure 12.3 may occur after external fixation, and an open operation to take down the non-union may be required if secondary intramedullary nailing is to be performed.

If the externally fixed non-union is aligned nailing is straightforward and the only two problems that the surgeon may encounter are penetration of the non-union site with the reamers and possible infection from nailing across infected pin tracts. This latter problem is dealt with in more detail in Chapter 18.

Nailing of non-unions following previous nailing

Non-unions of closed and Gustilo Type I open tibial and femoral fractures are very rare after primary intramedullary nailing with a locked reamed nail occurring in about 1.5 per cent of such fractures. When they occur they are easily treated by further nailing – a process known as exchange nailing. This procedure is described in more detail in Chapter 17 but in essence it involves reaming the tibia a further 1 or 2 mm and inserting a larger nail. An example of this is shown in Figure 12.5. This is a high-velocity, technically segmental closed tibial fracture which was nailed primarily. The distal fracture was undisplaced and associated with little soft-tissue damage and distal cross-screws were not used, although they should have been inserted because of the comminution associated with the proximal fracture. The distal fracture healed but after 26 weeks the proximal fracture remained ununited (Figure 12.5b). Nine weeks after exchange nailing there was clinical and radiological union (Figure 12.5c).

It is obvious that there should be few difficulties encountered in nailing a non-union resulting from the use of a locked reamed nail. If the non-union follows the use of an unlocked unreamed nail, such as an Ender nail or Rush pin, then the exact operative procedure will depend on the appearance of the fracture. Such nails are not only rotationally unstable but they cannot maintain length in comminuted fractures. There may therefore be alignment problems such as are encountered in conservatively managed or externally fixed fractures and the appropriate action must be taken.

Technical problems of nailing non-unions

The techniques employed for nailing aligned non-unions are essentially those used in the nailing of fresh fractures and are described in Chapters 4 and 5. There are however a number of alterations in the surgical technique of which the surgeon must be aware.

The most important alteration of technique concerns the penetration of the plug of callus and fibrous tissue that exists within the medullary canal of all non-unions that are not primarily nailed using a large diameter nail. A typical non-union following external fixation and a period of cast immobilization is shown in Figure 12.6. Initially the fracture was treated by a Hoffmann frame and alignment was excellent. The frame was removed at 8 weeks and a slight valgus mal-alignment occurred. The lateral X-ray scan also shows a recurvatum deformity. By 16 weeks non-union was apparent radiologically and clinically and closed nailing was undertaken (Figure 12.6b). The valgus mal-alignment persists although the recurvatum has improved. After a further 10 weeks union was apparent clinically and radiologically (Figure 12.6c).

Image-intensifier views taken during the nailing procedure shown in Figure 12.6b show the method of penetrating the plug of non-union tissue at the fracture site. It is impossible to pierce this tissue with a guide wire or a power reamer. The only way to gain entry to the distal fracture fragment is by using progressively larger hand reamers. In Chapters 4 and 5 the use of hand reamers to breech the proximal metaphysis was described. In non-unions these should be passed distally through the non-union site. The nature of the tissue within the medullary canal at the non-union means that it may require considerable force to penetrate it. Once the first reamer is through progressively larger reamers are used until a 9 mm hand reamer can be passed across the non-union site. It is worthwhile keeping a set of Küntscher hand reamers in the operating theatre as these reamers are invaluable for penetrating non-union tissue. Occasionally, the use of more than one hand reamer may be necessary to penetrate the non-union adequately (Figure 12.7). Once the hole in the non-union site is 9 mm in diameter standard power reamers can be used to enlarge the defect until an appropriately sized nail can be inserted (Figure 12.8). There may be a considerable amount of fibrous tissue brought up on the initial reamer. Successive reamers will produce less fibrous tissue and more bone. Reaming should continue until all fibrous tissue at the fracture site is removed (Figure 12.9). Use of this technique at the author's centre has resulted in no hypertrophic non-union requiring bone grafting.

Open nailing of non-unions

Non-unions may be opened for two reasons. Both hypertrophic and atrophic non-unions may be so mal-aligned that the non-union must be taken down so that the fracture may be adequately aligned. The other reason for opening atrophic non-unions is to bone graft them using cortico-cancellous grafting techniques. It is, of course, theoretically possible to bone graft atrophic non-unions using the medullary reamings, but little information is as yet available on which atrophic non-unions might be suitable for this procedure.

An example of the need to take down a non-union to realign the fracture is shown in Figure 12.10a. This is the antero-posterior X-ray scan of a tibial non-union of 9 months' duration in a 23-year-old patient with juvenile osteoporosis. The state of the cortical bone negates the use of plates or external fixation. Open intramedullary nailing and grafting were undertaken. Two proximal and distal screws were used because of the osteoporotic nature of the bone (Figure 12.10b). Four months after fixation, union was proceeding and it can be seen that the nail has held the non-union securely (Figure 12.10c). A further example of the use of nailing is shown in Figure 12.11. A 48-year-old lady presented with tibial non-union following initial conservative management. This had been subsequently treated by plating and cortico-cancellous grafting, but the plate had broken after 18 months (Figure 12.11a). It is obvious that the non-union cannot be nailed using closed techniques and the fracture was taken down, realigned, nailed and grafted. A proximal dynamic lock (Figure 12.11b) allows early weight bearing and axial loading and after 9 months there was clinical union, although radiologically some of the fracture line can be seen (Figure 12.11c).

When taking down a non-union it is always tempting to release the soft tissues around the fracture to the extent that reaming of the proximal fragment can be undertaken in a retrograde direction from the fracture site. Ideally this practice should be discouraged as if it is carried out the degree of soft-tissue damage may deleteriously affect fracture union. Once the non-union has been taken down and the fracture site realigned nailing should be undertaken in the manner described in Chapters 4 and 5.

As with all good rules, this one may sometimes be broken and the surgeon may occasionally have to practise retrograde reaming. Figure 12.12a shows a difficult non-union of 6 years' duration where the patient had not taken weight for 5 years. A number of bone-grafting procedures had been undertaken including a sliding cortical graft. After taking down the non-union and resecting the avascular bone ends, it proved impossible to pass the hand reamer in a prograde manner down to the fracture site. Accordingly retrograde reaming was used to establish a nail passage. Predictably union was slow but an X-ray scan at 9 months (Figure 12.12b) shows it to be proceeding and at this time the patient was walking and pain-free for the first time in 5 years.

Infected non-union

The basic principles in the treatment of infected non-unions are the establishment of adequate bone stability and the eradication of bone infection. This is achieved with surgical bone debridement to remove dead or devitalized bone in combination with adequate antibiotic administration. Nowadays most surgeons would advocate the use of external skeletal fixation to provide the necessary bone stabilization to treat this problem. However, it is possible to use a locked intramedullary nail to achieve bone stability and a number of workers have made use of this method.

Klemm (1986) has described a technique for the treatment of infected non-unions with a locking intramedullary nail. Following removal of the existing metal implants, a statically locked intramedullary nail is used to stabilize the non-union. A continuous irrigation system is then set up (Figure 12.13). Initially fluid is introduced around the non-union site through a tube placed into the upper opening of the nail. A perforated tube placed close to the non-union collects the outflow. After 4 weeks the inflow and outflow tubes are cut close to the skin and secured with safety pins and both are used as outflow tracks. X-ray scans are then taken monthly until healing is seen, at which time the nail and tubes are removed and the medullary canal reamed to remove any infected material, in the manner described in Chapter 22. If infection persists, further irrigation is used or gentamycin-impregnated PMMA beads are introduced. According to Klemm, cancellous bone grafting is not required. Klemm has used this technique to achieve an 89.5 per cent union rate after infected femoral non-union, with 70 per cent union in the treatment of infected tibial non-unions. The infection could not be eradicated in 6 per cent of femora and 12.5 per cent of tibiae.

Despite these results, external skeleton fixation is probably the method of choice in the initial management of an infected non-union. Once the infection has been controlled by adequate surgical debridement and the use of either local or systemic antibiotics, the external fixation device can be removed and an intramedullary nail substituted in the manner described in Chapter 18.

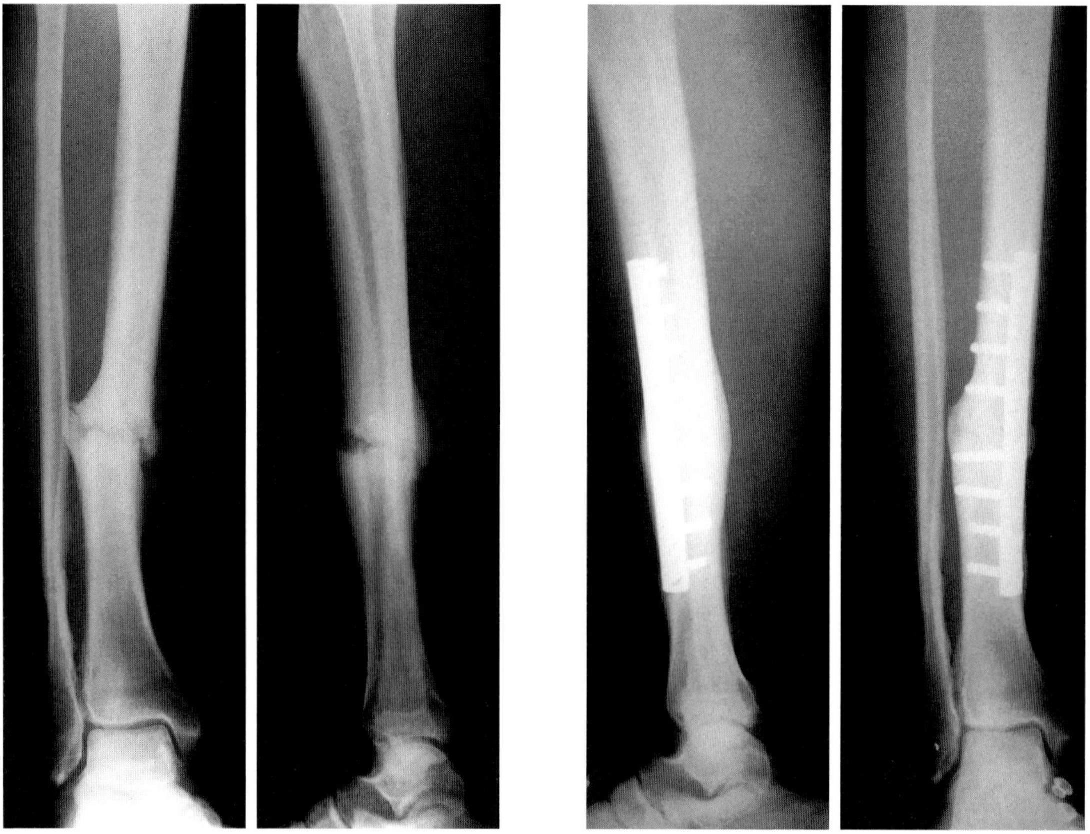

Figure 12.1

a Hypertrophic non-union of the tibia following treatment in a cast. It is clear that an attempt has been made to unite the fracture but the fracture line is still evident. An intramedullary nail could not be used to treat this non-union because of the varus deformity and slight overlap that are present.

b Rather than take down the non-union, it was elected to use a dynamic compression plate and the fracture has gone on to unite without cortico-cancellous bone grafting within 16 weeks.

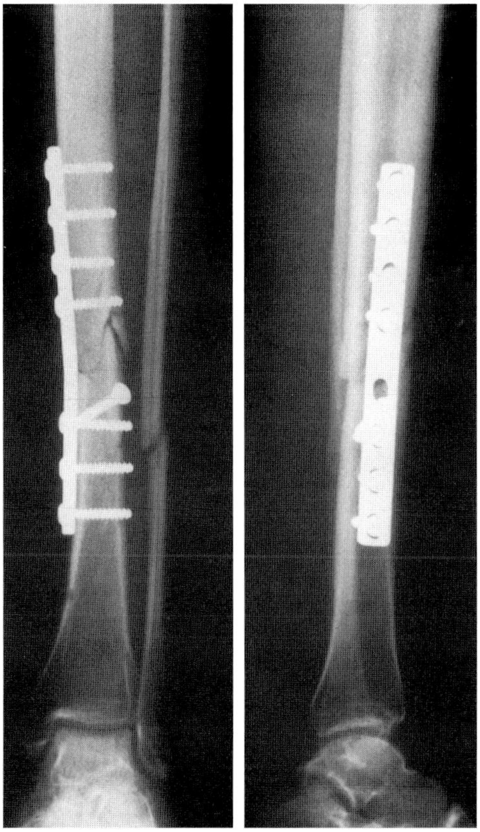

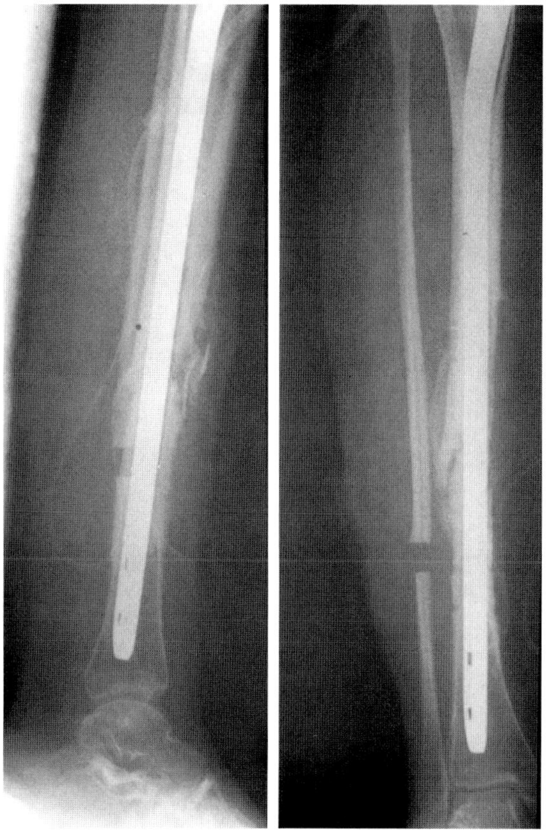

Figure 12.2

a Dynamic compression plate used to treat a closed tibial fracture in an 18-year-old woman. Despite cortico-cancellous bone grafting, non-union is evident at 20 weeks.

b Intramedullary nailing was straightforward. Cross-screws were not used because of the relative stability of the non-union. The fibula had healed and, to permit axial movement of the fracture site, a partial fibulectomy was performed.

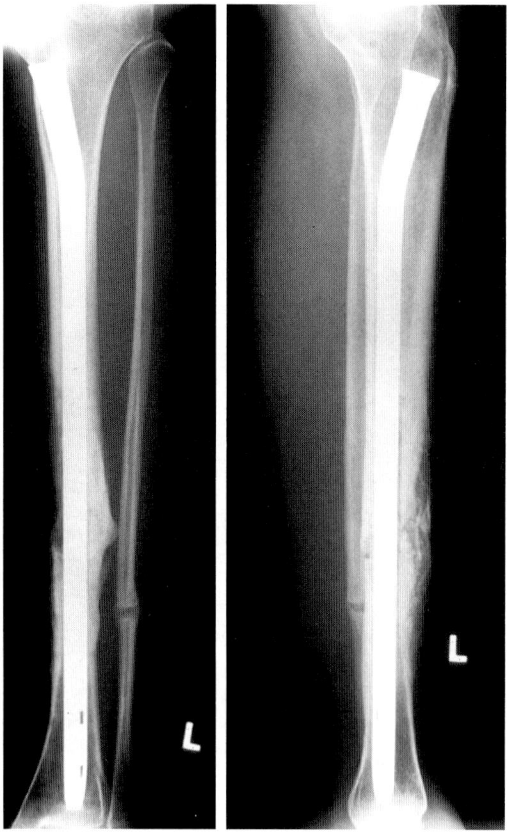

Figure 12.2 *continued*

c The fracture was clinically and radiologically united after 16 weeks, although the patient had regained full function before that time.

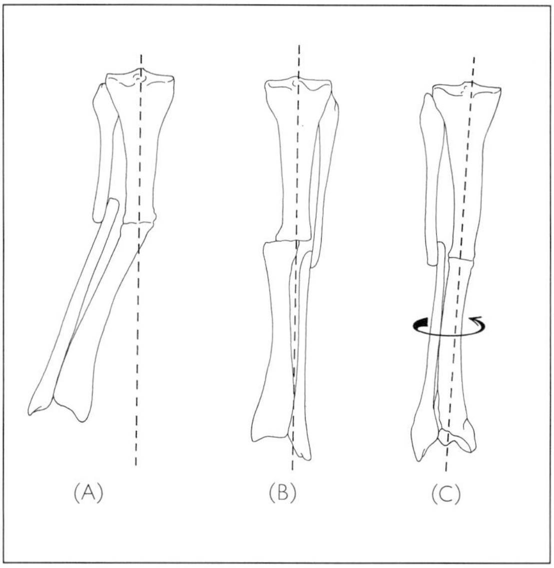

Figure 12.3

Femoral or tibial mal-alignment may be angular (left), rotatory (right) or there may be overlap (centre). If closed nailing is attempted in the presence of an angular deformity, there may be cortical damage to the lower fragment. If the fracture is overlapped by a complete bone diameter, it will be impossible to insert a nail into the lower fragment. A partial overlap may also render the fracture un-nailable as there may be cortical damage from the reamers or the nail. A rotatory mal-alignment does not prevent intramedullary nailing but, if the degree of rotation is unacceptable, the surgeon may have to take down the non-union and realign it prior to nailing.

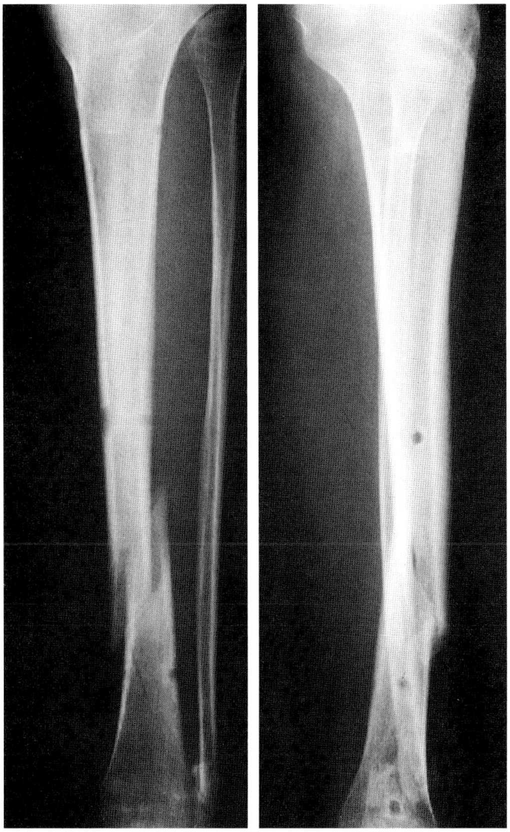

Figure 12.4

An example of bone overlap which would prevent closed nailing. This is a relatively common deformity following the closed management of a distal tibial oblique or spiral fracture. If the deformity cannot be reduced by closed means, an open procedure must be undertaken. In this case, the non-union was still mobile after 12 weeks of external fixation and closed reduction and intramedullary nailing were carried out.

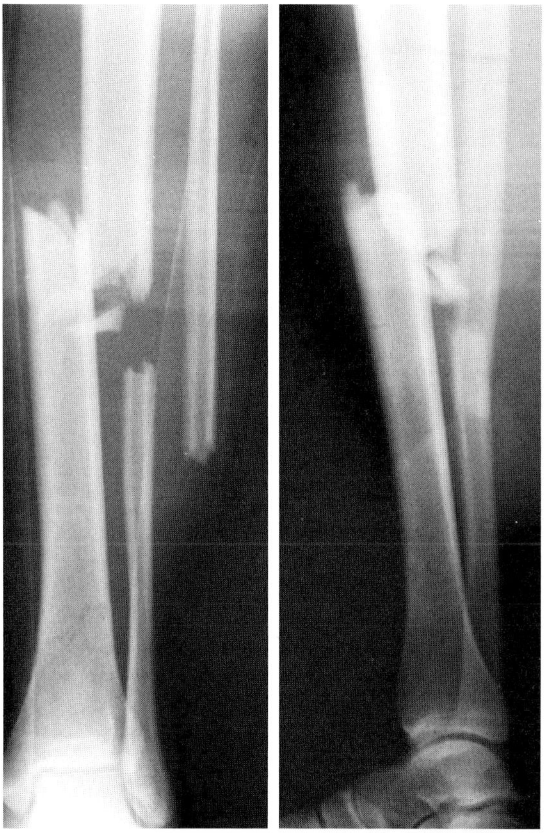

Figure 12.5

a Technically segmental closed tibial fracture occurring in a 19-year-old female. The upper fracture line is comminuted and the lower fracture line is undisplaced and almost certainly is not associated with significant adjacent soft-tissue damage.

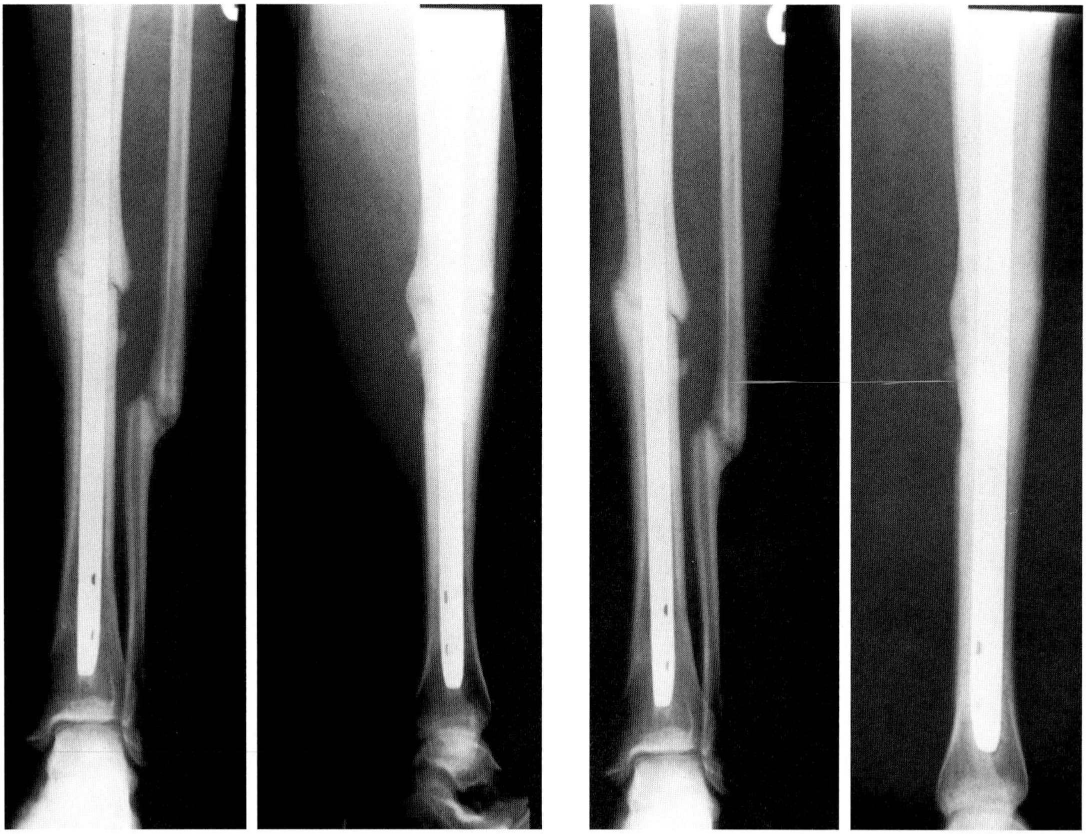

Figure 12.5 *continued*

b A static lock should have been used because of the presence of comminution at the proximal fracture. After 26 weeks, it was apparent that the lower fracture had healed but that there was a hypertrophic non-union at the upper fracture.

c Exchange nailing was undertaken and within 9 weeks there was clinical and radiological union. Cortico-cancellous bone grafting was not required.

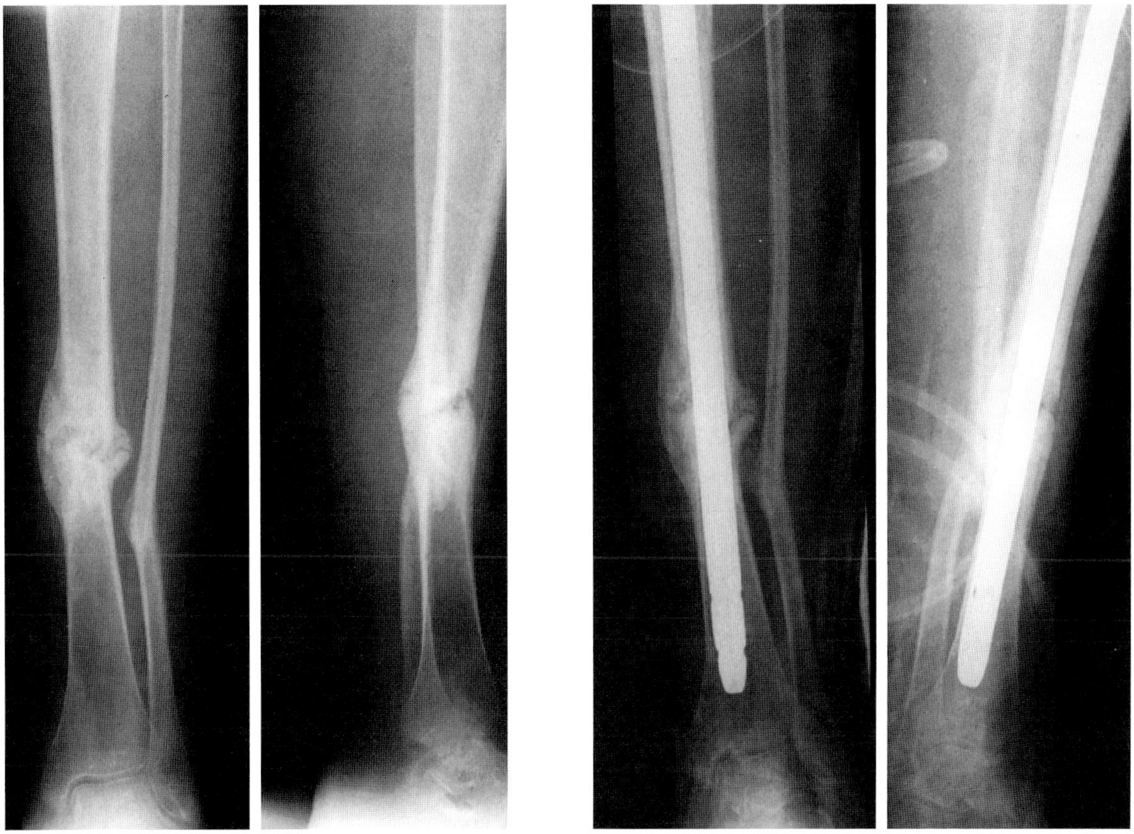

Figure 12.6

a Hypertrophic non-union in a closed tibial fracture following a period of external fixation with a Hoffmann frame. There are valgus and recurvatum deformities. Neither deformity is bad enough to prevent intramedullary nailing.

b Intramedullary nailing has improved the recurvatum deformity although the valgus deformity persists.

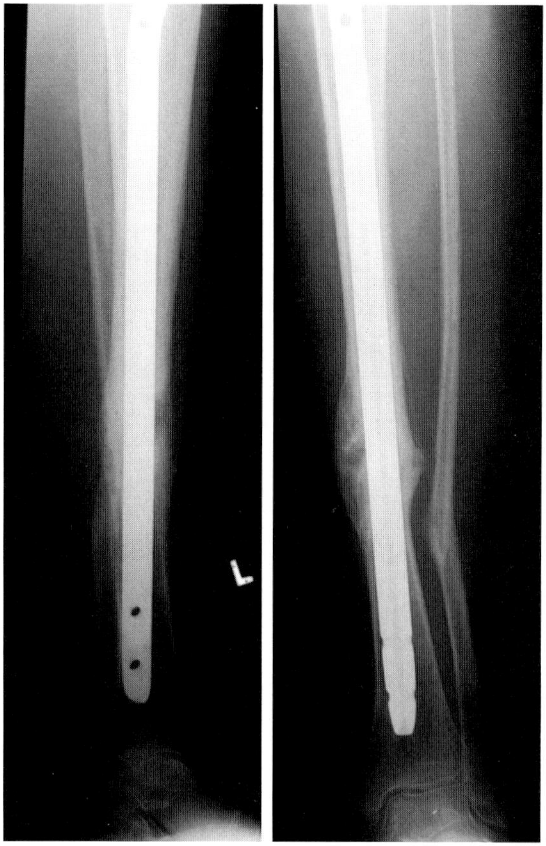

Figure 12.6 *continued*

c After 10 weeks, union was apparent clinically and radiologically.

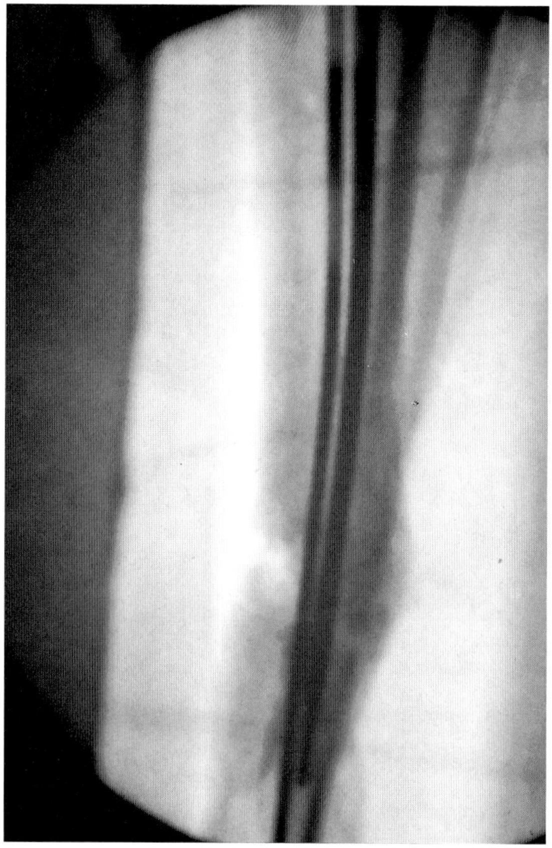

Figure 12.7

The penetration of intramedullary non-union tissue can only be undertaken with hand reamers. Usually it is sufficient to increase sequentially the size of the hand reamers until power reamers can be used. In this fracture, two hand reamers had to be inserted into the medullary canal to permit the clearance of enough tissue to allow for the introduction of power reamers.

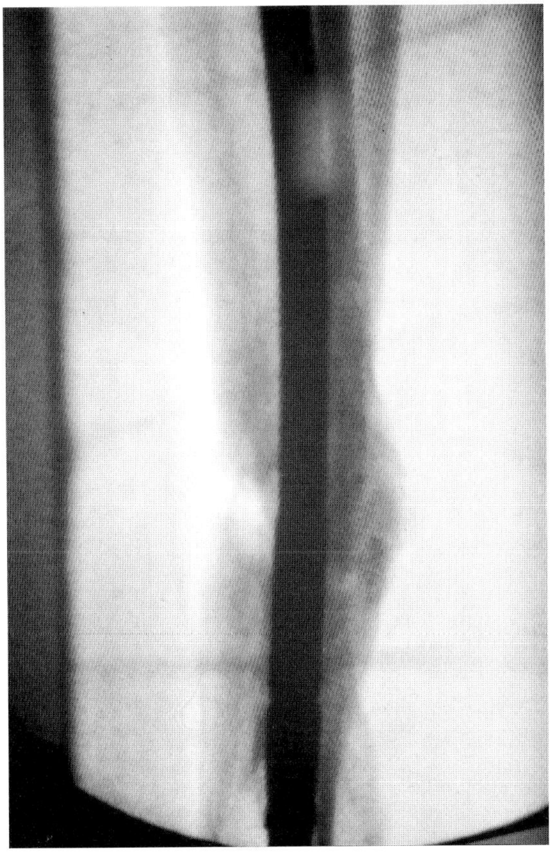

Figure 12.8

Once the non-union tissue has been breached, increasingly larger power reamers can be used in the standard way. It is interesting to note that the recurvatum deformity still persists but was corrected once the nail was inserted (Figure 12.6b).

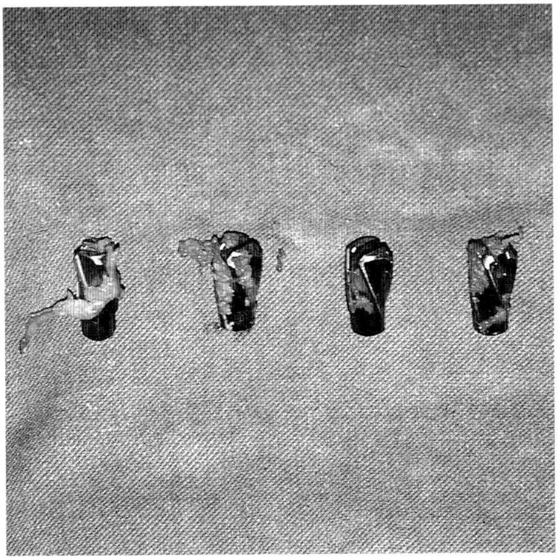

Figure 12.9

As progressively larger reamers are used, the amount of fibrous tissue decreases and the amount of bone seen on the reamers increases. The first reamer (extreme left) has removed the fibrous tissue at the non-union site. Subsequent reamers remove more bone until the last reamer shows only healthy medullary bone. A nail can then be inserted.

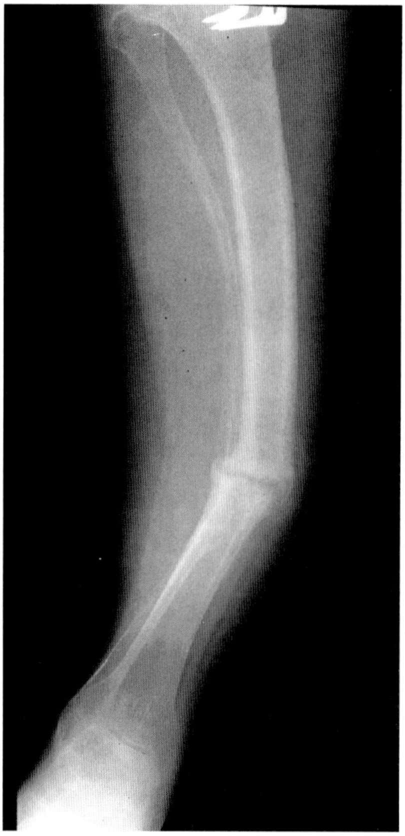

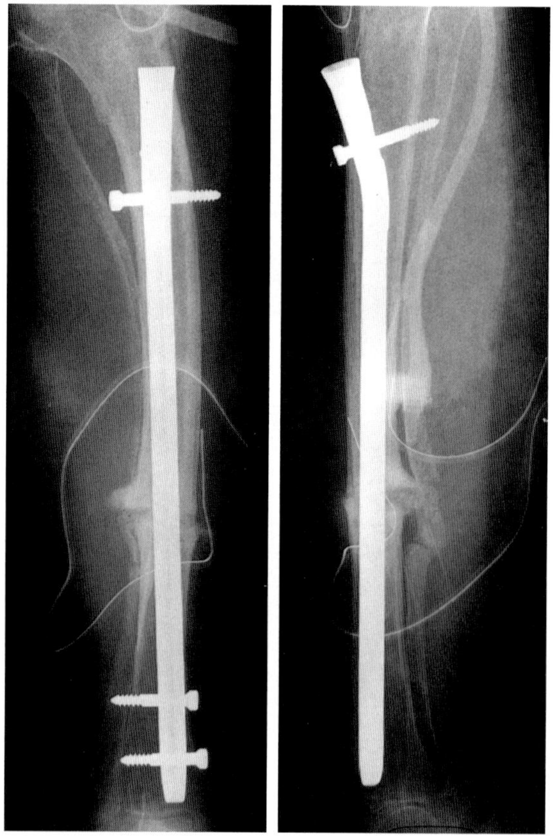

Figure 12.10

a An angulated non-union in a tibial fracture in a patient with juvenile osteoporosis. This fracture had been treated conservatively. The consistency of the bone precludes the use of external fixation pins and bone screws.

b Open nailing was performed. Obviously there is still an angular deformity in the tibia but no further correction could easily be obtained. Cortico-cancellous bone grafting was used.

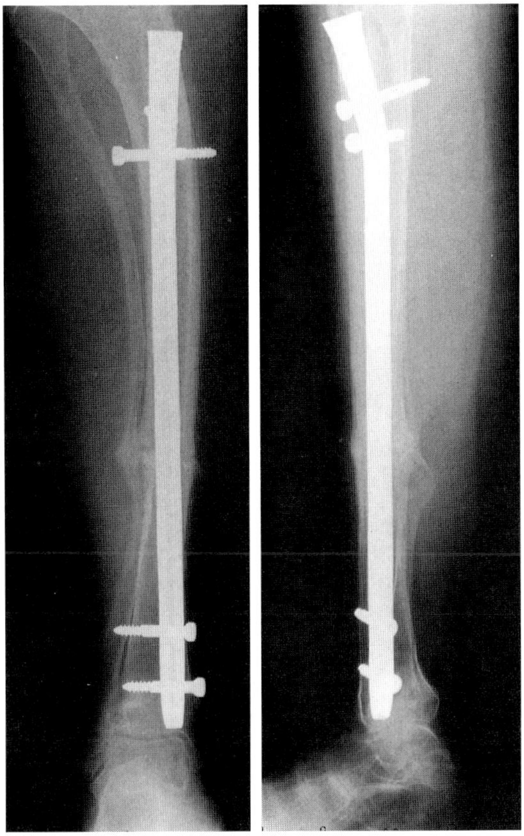

c Four months after nailing it is apparent that the fracture position has been maintained and that union is proceeding.

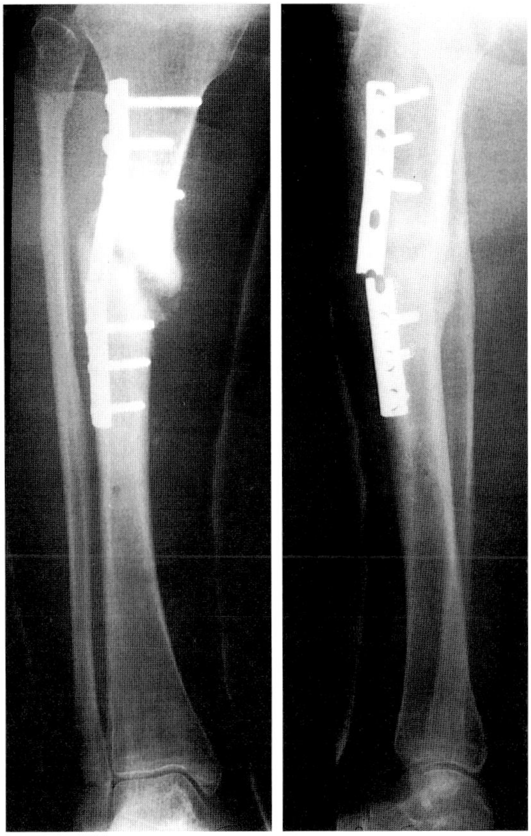

Figure 12.11

a Non-union of a proximal tibial fracture following conservative management. Immobilization with a dynamic compression plate had then been undertaken but 18 months after this operation the plate had broken.

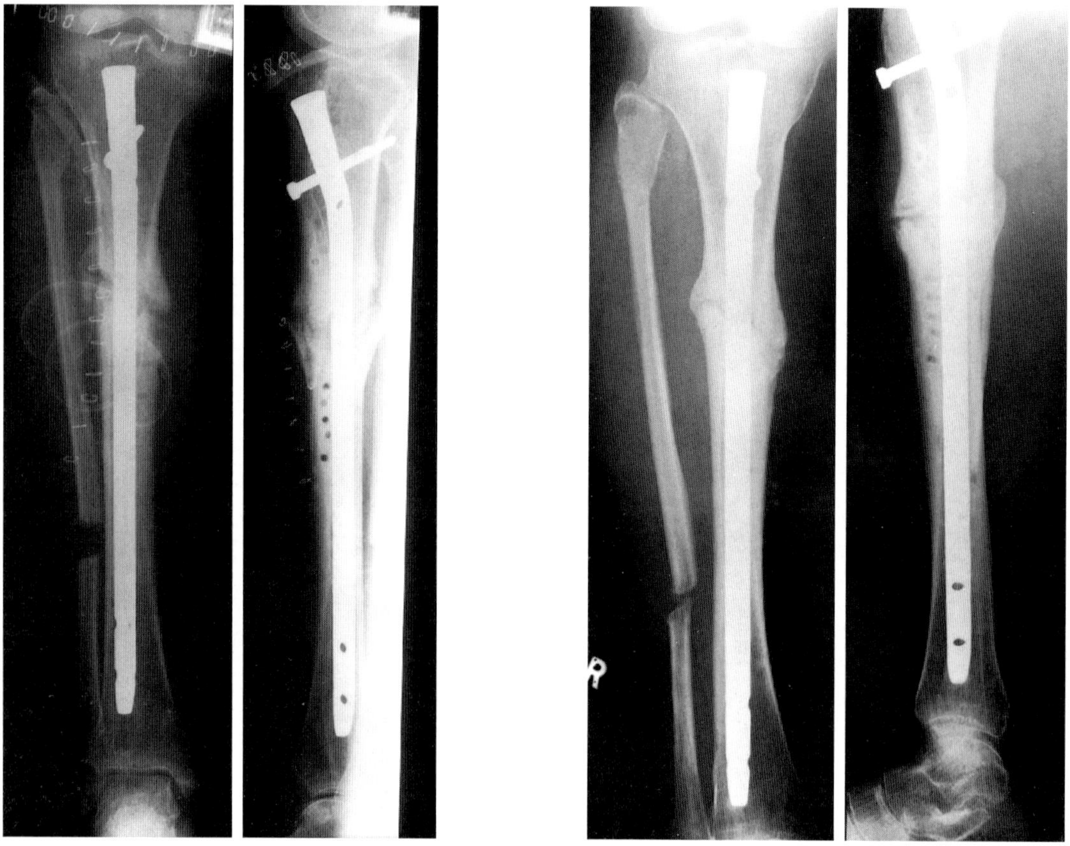

Figure 12.11 *continued*

b The non-union had to be opened to remove the plate and to straighten the tibia. It was realigned and nailed using a proximal dynamic lock. Axial tibial movement was encouraged by means of a lower partial fibulectomy.

c Clinically the patient was united after 9 months and it can be seen that the fracture position has been maintained. It is obvious that the fracture has closed as the nail is closer to the distal subchondral plate and the fibulectomy is partially closed.

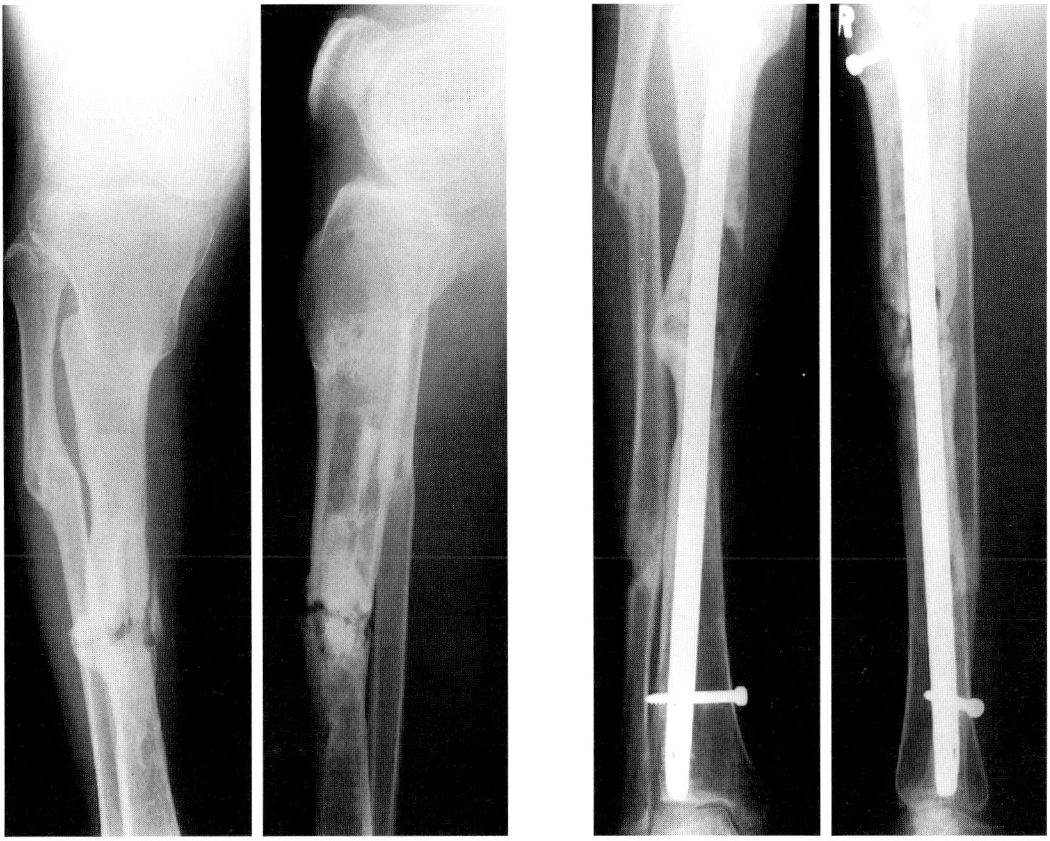

Figure 12.12

a Non-union of a tibia in an old closed segmental fracture. This fracture was initially treated conservatively and subsequently a number of bone-grafting operations were used to encourage union. The proximal fracture has healed with some overlap and a slight varus angulation.

b Following intramedullary nailing and bone grafting, union is proceeding. The patient was fully mobile and pain-free.

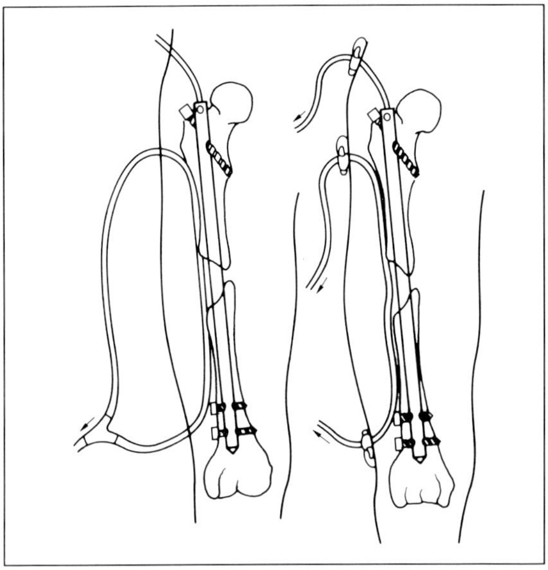

Figure 12.13

Klemm's method for treating infected non-unions with a statically locked intramedullary nail. Initially fluid is passed down the nail to exit through the non-union site. After 4 weeks, the inflow tube is removed and all tubes are used as outflow tubes (Klemm, 1986).

CHAPTER 13 MANAGEMENT OF MAL-UNIONS

Many mal-unions can be stabilized by the use of an intramedullary nail introduced following a corrective osteotomy. The nail is usually inserted by a closed technique, although the surgeon must decide about the advisability of carrying a closed or open osteotomy. Closed osteotomy is a procedure that requires specialist equipment in the form of intermedullary saws that will osteotomize the endosteal surface of the cortex working outwards to the periosteal surface. This procedure has the merit of preserving some of the blood supply to the bone, but is more time-consuming and difficult than open osteotomy.

If an open osteotomy is chosen, the surgeon has the option of closing the incision through which the osteotomy was performed and then nailing the fracture. This ensures that the reamings stay around the fracture site to act as a bone graft. If this is done, the need for cortico-cancellous bone grafting may be avoided. Such a fracture is shown in Figure 13.1. This shows the antero-posterior and lateral X-ray scans of a distal tibia and fibula fracture initially treated conservatively. At 10 weeks, the fracture is healing in significant varus despite several changes of cast. The distal nature of the fracture means that internal fixation is difficult unless a locking nail is used.

The leg is set up in the same manner as for a fresh fracture and the tibia is osteotomized through an appropriate incision. It is recommended that a fibular osteotomy or partial fibulectomy be performed if a tibial mal-union is to be correctly realigned. After osteotomy and wound closure, the tibia was nailed in the usual manner using a cut-down nail because of the distal position of the mal-union. After 14 weeks, the fracture was clinically and radiologically united (Figure 13.1b).

The extent to which the reamings can be used to graft a bone defect is not well defined in the literature, but there is no doubt that a number of mal-unions require open osteotomy and cortico-cancellous bone grafting to achieve a healed realigned fracture. An example is shown in Figure 13.2. Nailing in this situation is relatively straightforward and can be done on the nailing table using a mid-lateral approach to the femur and an anterior approach to the tibial diaphysis.

Kempf et al (1986) described one-stage lengthening of the femur using a Grosse-Kempf intramedullary nail. They stressed that this is a difficult surgical procedure and requires meticulous pre-operative planning and surgical technique. The desired length of nail should be calculated from pre-operative X-ray scans.

The operation starts with the patient in the prone position so the posterior iliac bone graft can be harvested. The patient is then placed supine and a distal femoral pin inserted. The patient is positioned on the fracture table with the knee and hip flexed to take the tension off the sciatic and femoral nerves. A standard approach as described in Chapter 4 is then made to the proximal femur and the medullary canal is reamed to 2 mm greater than the diameter of the nail to be used. This is more than for conventional fracture management, but ensures easy nail insertion and allows for sliding of the distal bone fragment around the nail during the lengthening procedure.

A second skin incision is then made unless a proximal osteotomy is to be undertaken, in which case use can be made of the proximal incision. After the femur is exposed a Z-shaped osteotomy is made (Figure 13.3) and distraction applied through the femoral pin and a femoral distractor. While lengthening is undertaken tight structures such as aponeuroses, fascia and septa are released. A nail is inserted and cortico-cancellous graft placed in the defect. After insertion of the proximal and distal cross-screws one or two 3.5 mm compression screws are placed at the osteotomy site to increase contact of the vertical arms of the Z-shaped osteotomy (Figure 13.3).

Kempf et al (1986) report a considerable morbidity with the technique and state that up to 4 cm length can be achieved. They recommend an external fixation technique if more length is required. The authors also describe femoral and tibial shortening by removal of a cylindrical fragment from the distal femur or tibia. Up to 4.5 cm can be removed from the femur and between 2.5 and 3.0 cm from the tibia. The femoral osteotomy is fixed with a distal dynamic locked nail and the tibia with a statically locked nail.

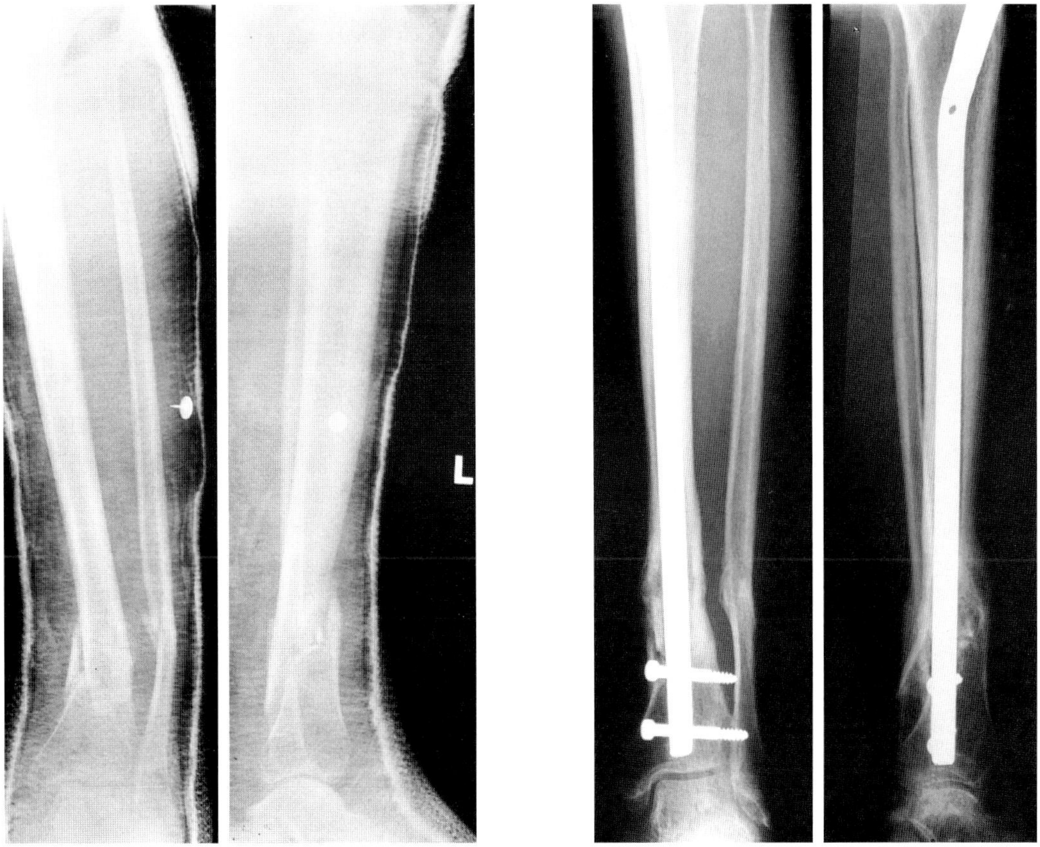

Figure 13.1

a Varus mal-alignment in a distal tibial fracture treated by cast immobilization.

b The osteotomy was performed at 10 weeks and held with a distal dynamically locked intramedullary nail. Weight bearing was allowed when tolerated and the fracture healed at 14 weeks. Full ankle and subtalar movements were regained.

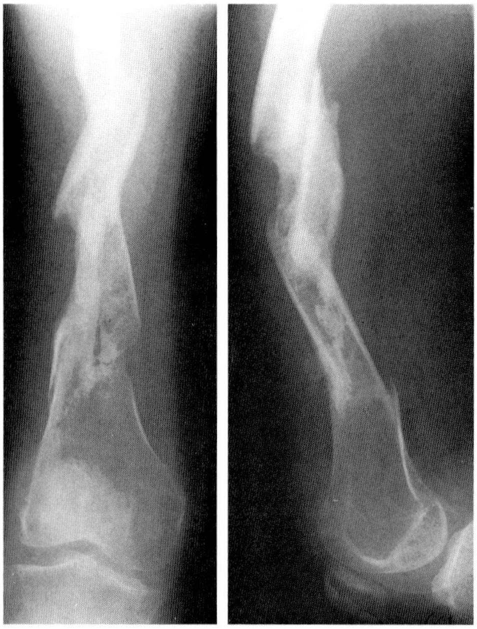

Figure 13.2

a Significant femoral antecurvatum in a 23-year-old man following the conservative management of a Type III open femoral fracture. The patient found the bow in his thigh troublesome.

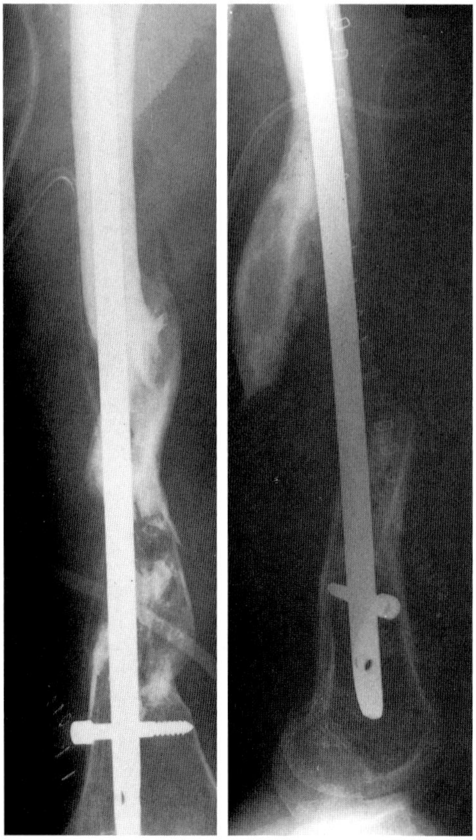

b A closed osteotomy is clearly impossible. An open osteotomy was performed and good correction achieved. Cortico-cancellous bone graft was used to fill the considerable defect.

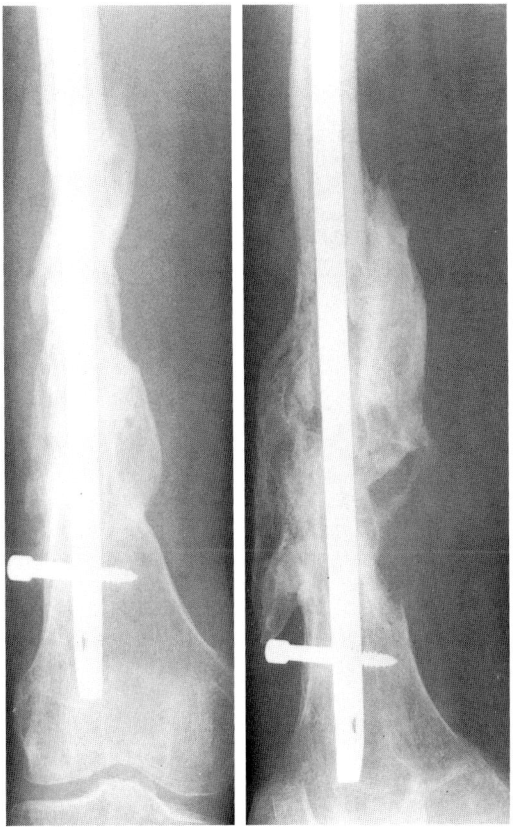

c The osteotomy healed well and good alignment was achieved. The patient was able to take weight on the leg 8 weeks after the realignment procedure.

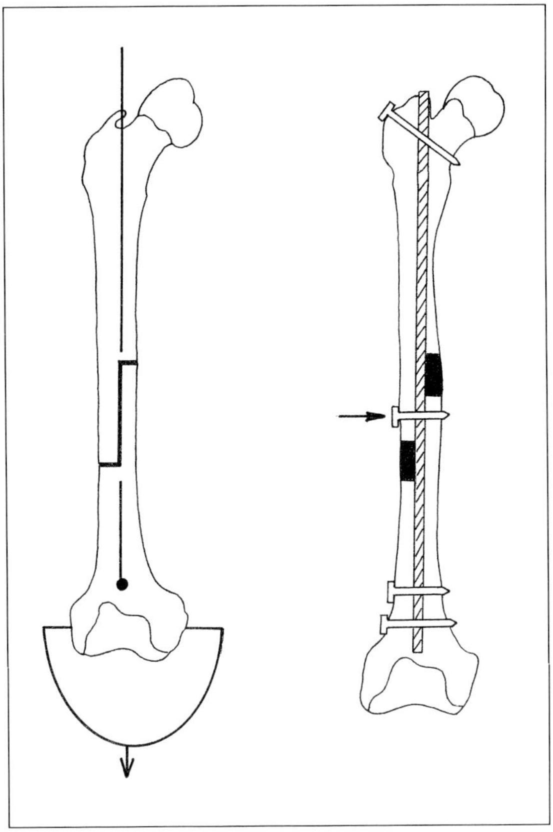

Figure 13.3

A Z-shaped osteotomy is made in the middle third of the femur and distraction applied. Kempf and his co-workers suggest the use of a statically locked intramedullary nail with interfragmentary screw fixation of the arms of the osteotomy to facilitate union. The defects in the femur are packed with bone graft (Kempf et al, 1986).

CHAPTER 14
POSTOPERATIVE MANAGEMENT

Immediately following surgery, the lower femoral, upper tibial or calcaneal transfixion pins are removed and dressings are applied to the leg. Dressing swabs are applied to the pin sites and the various wounds and bandages used to keep them in position. No plaster immobilization is required following femoral or tibial nailing.

Weight bearing is essentially dictated by the patient. When lower limb fractures are treated conservatively, surgeons attempt to predict the stability of the fractures and thereby what will happen to them on weight bearing. The use of an intramedullary nail means that all fractures are stabilized and weight bearing is mainly dependent on the degree of discomfort suffered by the patient. In over 500 femoral and tibial nailings in Edinburgh no nail has bent following normal weight bearing and only two cross-screws have broken, neither breakage causing fracture displacement. Thus it can be seen that it is safe for patients to take weight on femoral and tibial fractures stabilized with locking nails.

Usually patients with stable fracture configurations such as transverse or short oblique fractures are fully weight bearing soon after surgery. Patients with extensively comminuted fractures may need about 6 weeks before weight bearing after a tibial fracture or longer after extensive femoral fractures. Postoperatively, patients should be encouraged to mobilize as soon as possible with the use of whatever walking aids are required.

Approximately 40 per cent of patients with closed or Gustilo Type I open tibial fractures as their only injury manage immediate weight bearing, although most require the use of a walking aid (Court-Brown, Christie, McQueen, 1990). Three weeks postoperatively, approximately 60 per cent of patients are weight bearing with over 90 per cent weight bearing after 6 weeks. The remaining 10 per cent take longer, these consisting mainly of the severe, high-velocity closed fractures where there is considerable subcutaneous soft-tissue damage.

Weight bearing in Type II and III open fractures tends to be dictated by the requirement for plastic surgery and the presence of any other injuries. Following satisfactory split-skin grafting or flap-cover, mobilization can be commenced. Most of these patients have significant comminution and weight bearing is delayed for several weeks. However, as with the closed fracture, it should be encouraged as soon as the patient can tolerate it.

Weight bearing following the treatment of hypertrophic non-unions is usually straightforward as the non-union site is stable and does not give rise to significant discomfort. Immediate postoperative weight bearing should be encouraged.

If a non-union or mal-union has to be taken down to realign the femur or tibia and is subsequently bone grafted, the situation is similar to that seen in a comminuted fresh fracture. Weight bearing can be allowed when the patient finds it tolerable, but is usually delayed for several weeks.

Joint mobilization

The stability of the femur and tibia following closed nailing means that passive and active mobilization of the joints can be started at an early stage. Following femoral nailing, passive movement of the hip and knee can be instituted within 24 hours. The same regime can be commenced for the knee, ankle and subtalar joints following tibial nailing. Continuous passive mobilization is not particularly useful following tibial nailing, but is indicated following nailing of distal femoral fractures. The other situation where continuous passive movement is of benefit in helping to regain joint movement is where there are multiple injuries or other significant injuries in the same limb. It is particularly useful where there are ipsilateral femoral and tibial diaphyseal fractures. If continuous passive movement is employed, it should be used until the patient regains active use of the muscles and can take over joint movement.

In a population of closed and Type I open tibial fractures, where joint movement could reasonably be expected to be normal after treatment, 55 per cent had full movement in knee, ankle and subtalar joints by 3 months, 89 per cent by 6 months and 93 per cent by one year (Court-Brown, Christie, McQueen, 1990). A number of the remaining patients had other injuries to the leg which reduced the likelihood of regaining full joint movement.

CHAPTER 15 SCREW REMOVAL AND DYNAMIZATION

Cross-screws are removed for two principal reasons: either the patient finds them uncomfortable or the surgeon wishes to dynamize the fracture. Dynamization is the term given to the conversion of a static lock to a dynamic lock, and this is carried out to increase axial loading at the fracture site and thereby at least theoretically improve the chances of fracture healing.

Dynamization is performed between 6 and 8 weeks after the initial nailing procedure. It is usually carried out because of a paucity of signs of union at that time. Either the proximal or distal screws can be removed, the surgeon usually selecting the screw or screws which are positioned in the shorter fragment. Selection of the shorter bone fragment for screw removal means that there will be less contact between the nail and the endosteal surface of the cortex to interfere with axial movement. There is little doubt that dynamization does permit axial bone movement (Figure 15.1), but there is doubt as to the clinical relevance of the radiological findings.

Experience with dynamization in Edinburgh has led to the belief that it has little clinical relevance. Analysis of the figures for union time in closed and Type I open tibial fractures that were originally statically locked shows that those fractures that were subsequently dynamized did not have a higher rate of union or unite faster than those that were not. The dynamized group in fact had a somewhat longer time to union, although there were more high-velocity tibial fractures in this group than in the statically locked group (Court-Brown, Christie, McQueen, 1990). The overall clinical impression, however, is that dynamization does not accelerate bone union. The reason for this is fairly obvious when one considers that those fractures that are dynamized are those which show little evidence of healing at 6 to 8 weeks. These fractures are mostly high-velocity ones which take on average over 20 weeks to unite. If the surgeon merely waits, without dynamizing the fracture, union will occur.

If a fracture has been inadvertently lengthened during nailing, then conversion of a static to a dynamic lock may allow for correction of the length discrepancy. The surgeon should wait until the fracture regains a measure of stability before removing cross-screws under these circumstances. It is, of course, always better to prevent lengthening of a fracture by adherence to the correct nailing technique.

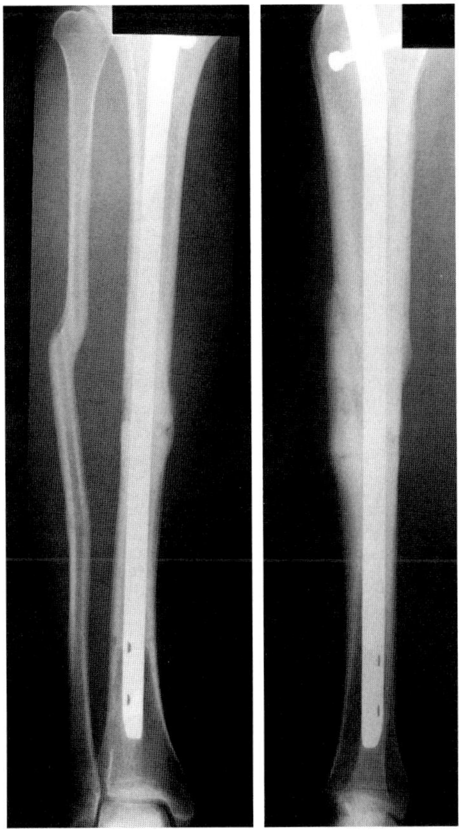

Figure 15.1

A closed fracture of the tibia and fibula. This fracture was dynamized at 8 weeks and subsequently went on to union. Evidence that axial loading has taken place can be seen at the proximal of the two distal screw holes. After weight bearing, the screw hole is clearly seen above the hole in the nail.

CHAPTER 16
PATHOLOGICAL FRACTURES

Most surgeons now accept that intramedullary nailing is the ideal treatment method for actual and incipient pathological fractures of the femoral or tibial diaphysis (Figure 16.1). The subtrochanteric area of the femur is a particularly common site for the deposition of metastases from lung, breast, renal and other tumours. Unfortunately, once the patient presents with femoral or tibial metastases, the prognosis is usually poor and systemic treatment only palliative. The treatment of most pathological fractures is therefore not aimed at curing the patient but at rendering the femur or tibia pain-free and stable enough to allow immediate weight bearing if the patient's general condition permits it.

It is always preferable to nail the femur or tibia before it actually fractures (Figure 16.2), but unfortunately it is all too common for the patient to be referred late and to present to the orthopaedic surgeon with a fracture. Nailing should be undertaken as soon as possible after admission, as the patients tend to be in poor physical condition and bed rest leads to major complications. The technique is the same as for the nailing of non-pathological fractures discussed in Chapters 4 and 5. However, the surgeon should be aware of the extent of the disease in the bone on which he is operating. Proximal disease such as shown in Figure 3.2 will interfere with the correct insertion of a proximal cross-screw and decrease the stability of fixation. Equivalent changes in the distal femur may persuade the surgeon that another fixation technique is preferable.

When pathological fractures are nailed, it is always wise to use a static lock, no matter what the actual configuration of the fracture is, as the disease may be more widespread than it appears radiologically and a dynamic lock may prove to confer insufficient stability to the fracture. The surgeon should also be careful when inserting the initial guide wire into the femur or tibia, as it is easy to push the guide wire out of the cortex in the areas where this has been largely replaced by tumour. If the surgeon does not notice this, he or she may end up reaming into the soft tissues and placing the nail incorrectly.

If the surgeon wishes to use bone cement as an ancillary fixation method, this can be introduced after the bone is reamed to the appropriate size. It is important that the surgeon is certain that the nail will pass down the bone into a good position, without any difficulty, before the cement is introduced into the medullary canal. It is therefore advisable to undertake a trial nailing before the cement is introduced. Failure to do this may result in the nail becoming stuck as the bone cement hardens. This is a serious complication that may necessitate the surgeon having to cut the nail at the greater trochanter. Clearly it is very difficult to remove such a nail without actually opening the limb and splitting the bone. A low-viscosity cement should be used and it should be introduced through a wide-bore cement syringe of the type used to introduce cement into the femoral shaft during hip arthroplasty. Usually two mixes (80 g) of cement are adequate. The nail must be introduced as soon as possible after the cement has been injected into the medullary canal. Postoperative mobilization should be encouraged as soon as possible in the manner described in Chapter 14. The nail is not removed.

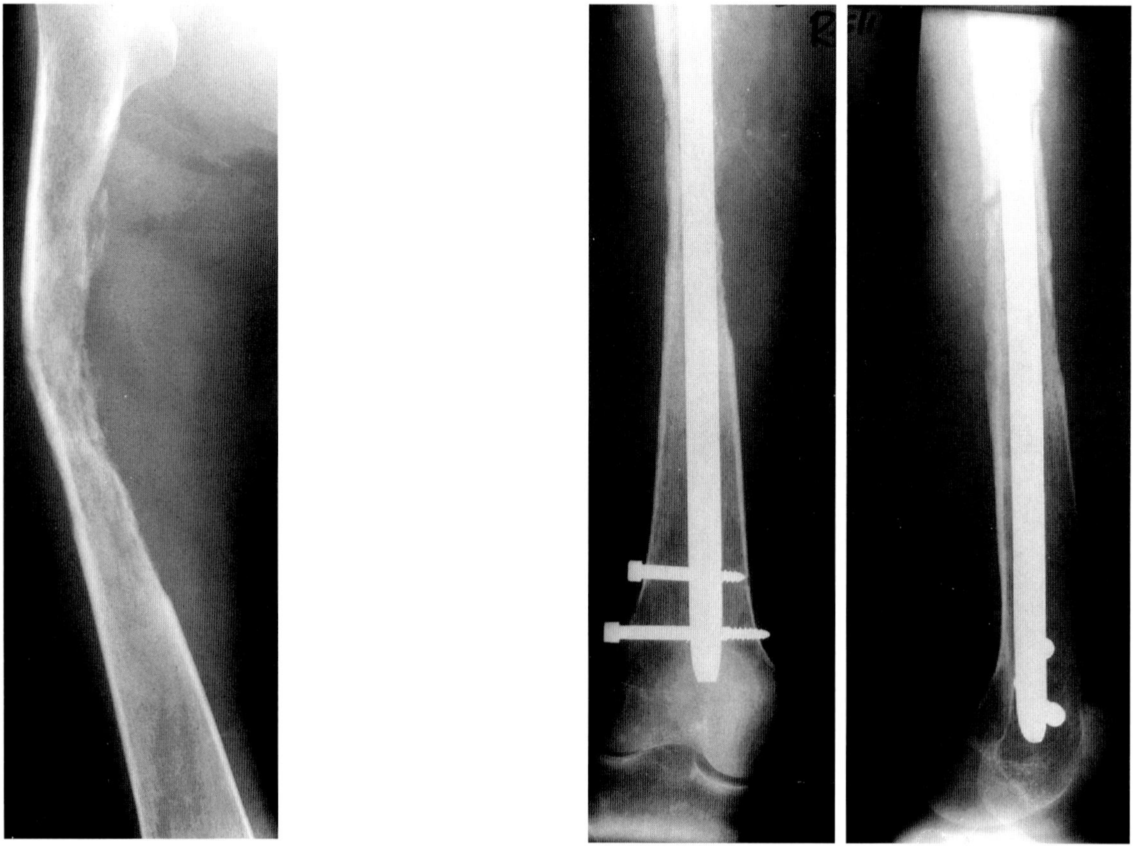

Figure 16.1

a An antero-posterior X-ray scan of a pathological fracture in the femoral diaphysis in a patient with known bronchogenic carcinoma. Intramedullary nailing represents the best method of treating such fractures. In view of the prognosis in patients who present with this type of problem, the nail need not be removed.

b A static lock should always be used and the fixation can be supplemented with the use of bone cement. In this particular case, it was felt that injection of bone cement down the femoral canal would merely result in its intrusion into the soft tissues.

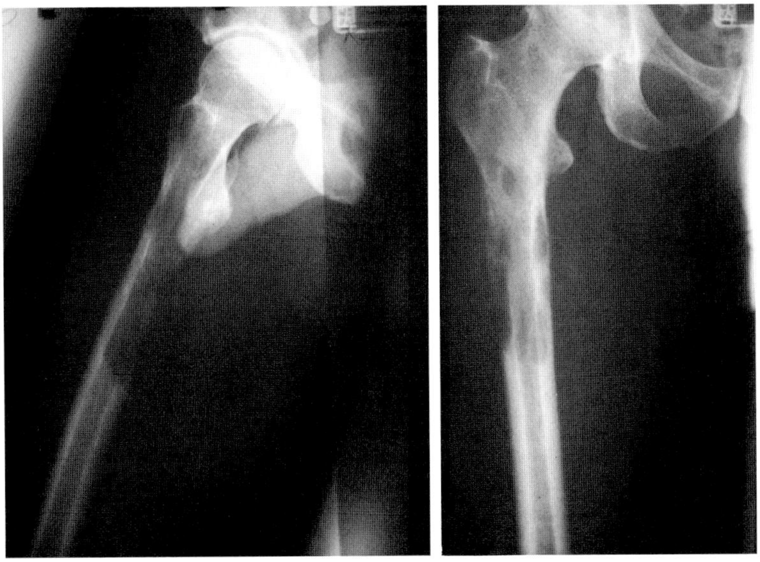

Figure 16.2

Subtrochanteric metastases in a patient with known bronchogenic carcinoma. Despite widespread involvement, the bone has not as yet fractured. Nailing is straightforward under these circumstances and ideally should be performed before the fracture actually occurs.

CHAPTER 17
EXCHANGE NAILING

Exchange nailing, or the substitution of one intramedullary nail for a larger second nail, is usually performed because of actual or incipient non-union in a previously nailed fracture. This has been discussed in Chapter 12. Non-unions are unusual in those closed or Type I open femoral and tibial fractures treated primarily by the use of a locking nail, comprising about 1.5 per cent of such fractures. The non-unions that do occur in these fractures are usually hypertrophic and unite after exchange nailing.

The principal use of exchange nailing is in the treatment of Type III tibial fractures. Such fractures are associated with a high incidence of non-union regardless of their method of treatment. Experience in Edinburgh has shown that exchange nailing of Type IIIa fractures results in the majority of such fractures uniting without the need for open bone grafting. The periosteal stripping associated with Type IIIb fractures ensures a low incidence of bone union without grafting. Exchange nailing has also been shown to be useful in treating Type IIIb fractures that are not associated with significant bone loss.

The procedure of exchange nailing is the same as that of primary nailing described in Chapters 4 and 5. After the patient is set up on the operating table, the cross-screws are removed and the lateral thigh or proximal tibial wound re-opened. The nail is extracted by the method described in Chapter 19 and a straight olive-tipped guide wire is then placed down to the distal end of the nail track. It is unnecessary to use an initial curved guide wire as reduction should not be a problem.

The initial nail should have been placed into a track reamed to 1 mm larger than the diameter of the nail. It is usually wise to start re-reaming the nail tract with a reamer the size of the primary nail, as this starts to remove the fibrous layer that exists between the nail and the endosteal surface of the cortex. As with primary nailing, the reamer size should be sequentially increased in 0.5 mm increments and usually the canal is reamed by a further 1 mm and a 1 mm larger nail inserted.

The surgeon must assess whether the fracture requires the use of the same number of cross-screws that were used initially. Usually the fracture is more stable and fewer cross-screws are required. More research is required to investigate just how often exchange nailing can be productively performed. It is assumed that exchange nailing promotes bone grafting of the fracture, but just how often this can be relied on to stimulate fracture healing remains unknown.

Figure 17.1 shows an example of exchange nailing. The serial X-ray scans are of a 36-year-old man who sustained a Type IIIa open tibial fracture (Figure 17.1a) which was primarily treated with a statically locked nail. After 18 weeks there was no sign of union (Figure 17.1b) and an exchange nailing was performed. After a further 16 weeks the non-union was hypertrophic but the patient remained symptomatic (Figure 17.1c). A second exchange nailing was performed and the fracture seen to be united after a further 14 weeks. The nail was then removed (Figure 17.1d). The patient required two operations to achieve fracture union, but avoided open bone grafting. He has been left with full movement of the knee, ankle and subtalar joints.

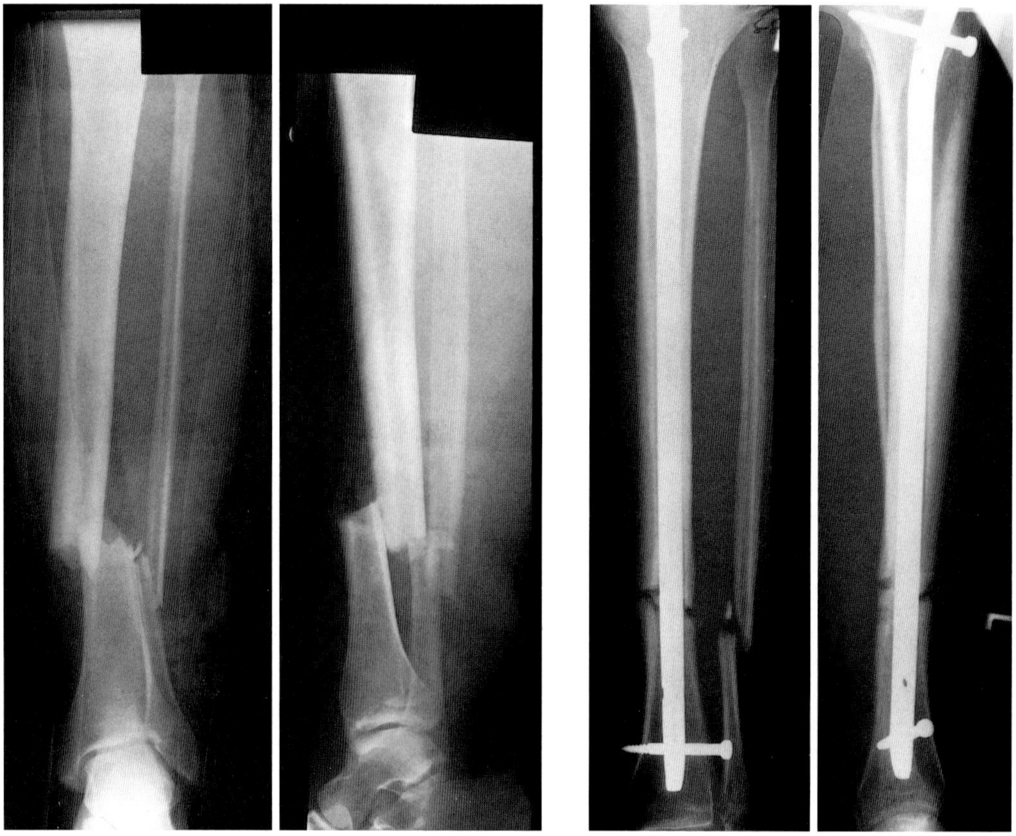

Figure 17.1

a A Gustilo Type IIIa open tibial fracture in a patient involved in a road-traffic accident. Intramedullary nailing was undertaken following thorough wound toilet. The open wound was closed with split skin graft after 36 hours.

b After 18 weeks there is an obvious atrophic non-union of the tibia and fibula. Exchange nailing was performed.

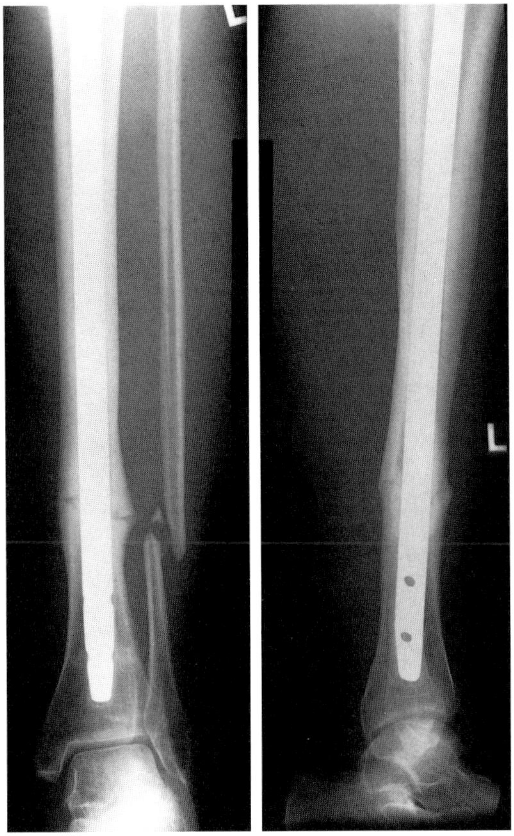

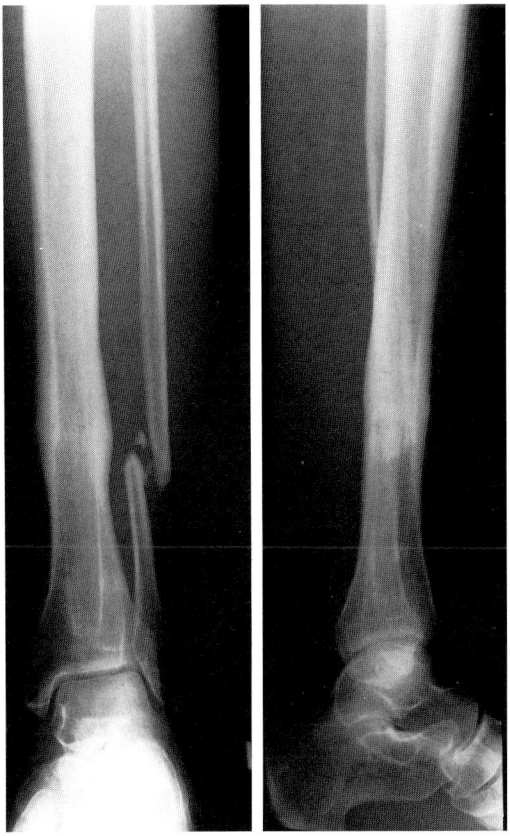

c Sixteen weeks after exchange nailing, the atrophic non-union has been converted to a hypertrophic non-union. The patient still complained of local discomfort.

d Fourteen weeks after the second exchange nailing, the fracture was clinically and radiologically united and the nail was removed. The use of the intramedullary nail has allowed the maintenance of full knee, ankle and subtalar movements.

CHAPTER 18 CONVERSION OF EXTERNAL FIXATION TO INTRAMEDULLARY NAILING

A recent study of intramedullary nailing of severe open tibial fractures that were primarily treated by external fixation suggests that pin-site infection is a contra-indication to later nailing (Maurer et al, 1989). In this study, 24 Gustilo Type II and III open tibial fractures were dealt with and it was shown that five of the seven patients who had pin-tract sepsis with external fixation subsequently developed infection around the intramedullary nail. In contrast, only one of the 17 patients who did not have initial pin-tract sepsis developed infection around the nail.

In Edinburgh, conversion of 20 externally fixed tibial fractures to locked reamed nails has tended to confirm the observation made by Maurer and his co-workers. Most of these patients had either closed or Type I open tibial fractures and none of this group of patients developed sepsis. In the more severe injuries there were two infections, one of which is covered in detail in Chapter 22. Both resolved with appropriate treatment but they suggest that conversion of external fixation to intramedullary nailing in severe open fractures may be associated with a high rate of sepsis, although this does not appear to be the case in closed or Type I open fractures. If the surgeon does wish to convert an externally fixed fracture to intramedullary nailing it is important that meticulous care should be taken of the pin tracts. Transfixion pins should be inserted using an optimal technique so that the risk of loosening and subsequent sepsis is lessened. The skin should not be allowed to impinge on the transfixion pins and the pin sites should be dressed carefully and checked for superficial sepsis on a routine basis.

In Edinburgh, immediate exchange from external fixation to an intramedullary nail has not been practised. If the surgeon makes the decision to change from external fixation to intramedullary nailing, the patient is admitted to the hospital and the external fixation device is removed under general anaesthesia. The stability of the fracture site is assessed and, if the surgeon feels that further fixation is required, a Steinmann pin is placed in the calcaneus and traction applied. The pin sites are then carefully cleaned and dressed and the patient is returned to the ward. Intramedullary nailing is not undertaken until all pin tracts have granulated. If the pin tracts are not infected, granulation is complete within 24 hours. The patient is then returned to the operating theatre at a convenient time and intramedullary nailing performed using the technique described in Chapters 4 and 5. Where pin-tract discharge persists, this is treated with systemic antibiotics and local measures until the discharge stops and granulation tissue is evident. Not until this has occurred is intramedullary nailing performed. If this method of delayed nailing is followed, it is associated with excellent results in closed and Type I fractures.

An example of successful conversion of external fixation to intramedullary nailing in a Type IIIa open tibial fracture is shown in Figure 18.1. The fracture (Figure 18.1a) was externally fixed using a Hoffmann frame (Figure 18.1b). After 12 weeks, there was little sign of union and a conversion to intramedullary nailing was performed using the method described above. The leg was placed on calcaneal traction for 48 hours, following which nailing was carried out and the calcaneal pin removed. The fracture was united after a further 9 weeks (Figure 18.1c).

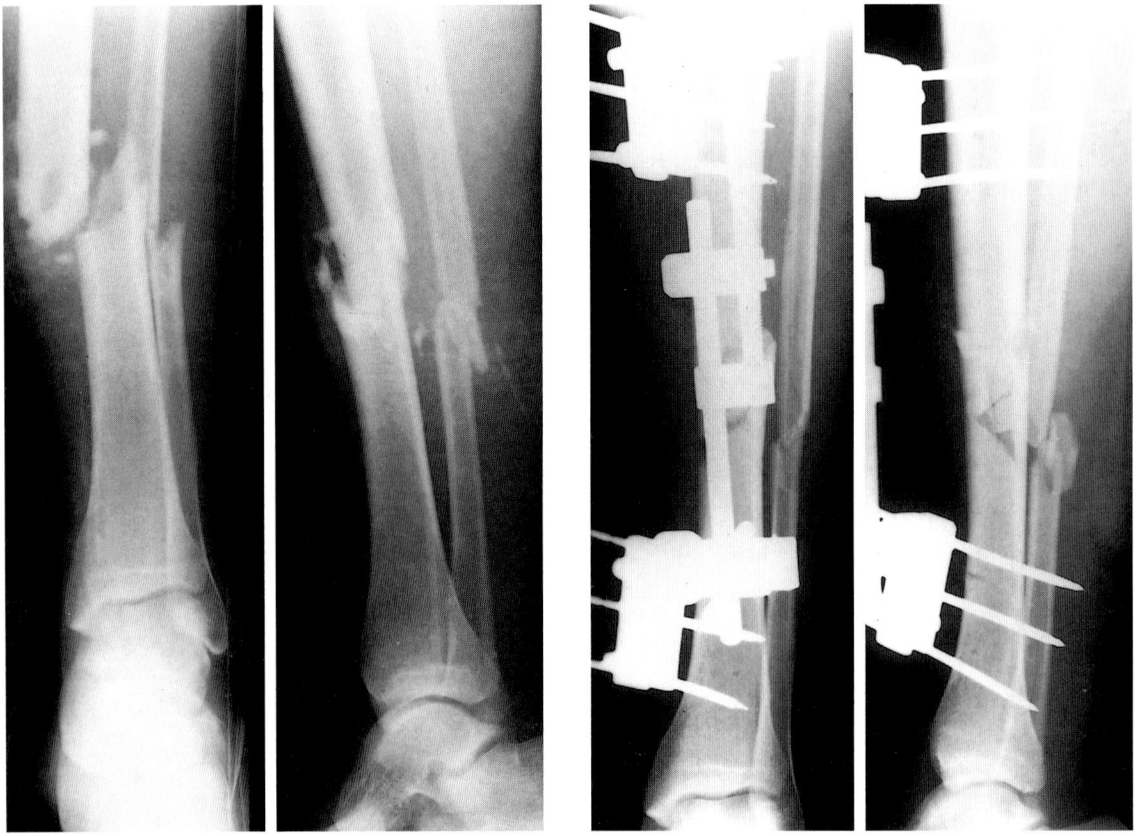

Figure 18.1

a Gustilo Type IIIa open tibial fracture in an 18-year-old male sustained in a road-traffic accident.

b After thorough wound toilet, a unilateral Hoffmann frame was applied with the fracture in excellent position. After 12 weeks it can be seen that there is little sign of union.

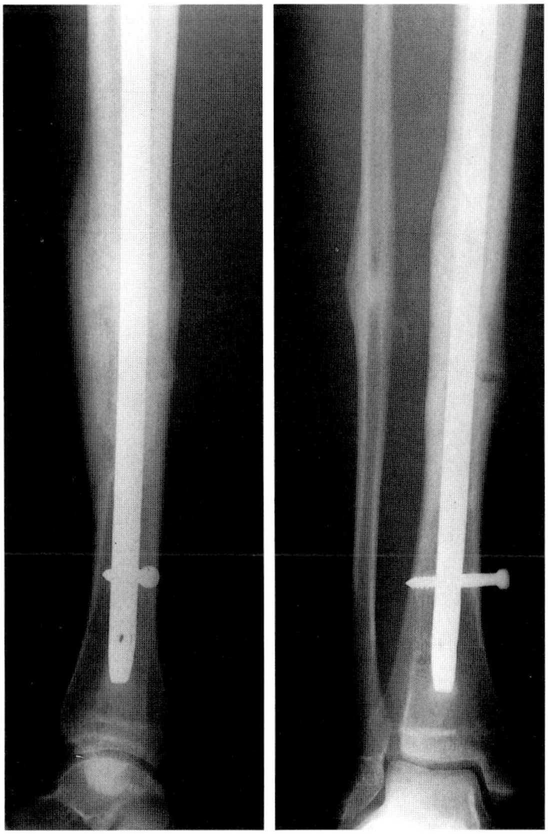

c A calcaneal pin was inserted and the leg placed on a Braun frame for 48 hours. Intramedullary nailing was then undertaken and the fracture healed without cortico-cancellous bone grafting after a further 9 weeks.

CHAPTER 19 NAIL REMOVAL

There are two basic methods employed for the removal of large diameter nails. The original Küntscher nail had a rectangular slot cut close to each end of the nail (see Figure 1.1). A hook (Figure 19.1) is passed into the slot and the nail is removed. This necessitates the proximal end of the nail being left slightly proud of the bone, to facilitate engagement of the hook into the nail slot. This type of system is also used in the Brooker-Wills locking nail.

In contrast, the Grosse-Kempf intramedullary nail has a screw thread inside the proximal end of the nail. An extractor is screwed into the nail and after the threads engage, the nail can be removed (Figure 19.1). This system allows the nail to be buried in the bone at the time of initial surgery. The screw system tends to be somewhat easier to use than the hook system, particularly if the nail is securely fixed within the bone and is difficult to remove. The improved grip provided by the screw thread under these circumstances facilitates nail extraction.

Femoral and tibial nail removal is very similar and the procedure will be discussed with reference to the tibia as this is a slightly more difficult procedure. The Grosse-Kempf intramedullary nail extractor is very similar to other nail extractors (Figure 19.2). The screw connector is initially screwed into the proximal end of the nail and then screwed on to a long steel rod on which a hammer can move in both directions.

The operation can be performed on a normal operating table. For femoral nail removal, the patient should lie in the lateral position and, for tibial nail removal, the patient is supine. Once the patient has been prepared and draped the knee is bent to facilitate tibial nail extraction. All cross-screws are removed by re-opening the small incisions through which they were inserted. Tibial cross-screws are usually easily found but the distal cross-screws in the femur may be difficult to locate because of the bulk of the overlying muscle. Once the screws have been located they should be unscrewed with the appropriate screwdriver. It is often useful to use an artery forcep to grip the neck of the screw to facilitate extraction. The incision through which the nail was inserted is then re-opened and the proximal end of the nail is located. This is usually straightforward with femoral nails, although a piece of bone may need to be removed from the proximal end of the nail (see Figure 23.17) to allow the insertion of the extractor. The proximal end of the tibial nail can be surprisingly hard to locate as it may be buried well into bone and filled with fibrous tissue. Once located, all soft tissue should be removed from the proximal end of the nail and any bone overhanging the posterior wall of the nail should be curetted away to allow the insertion of the extractor. It is always worth taking time to clear the proximal end of the tibial nail adequately as if this is not done it is impossible to insert the extractor easily.

The extractor should be screwed home into the proximal end of the nail and the extraction rod assembled with the hammer in situ (Figure 19.3). The hammer is struck upwards and the nail is removed (Figure 19.4). Care must be taken to move the operating light away from the operative field so that the extractor and the surgeon do not become contaminated during the procedure. There is always a considerable amount of tissue ingrowth into the nail (Figure 19.5) but this does not usually interfere with nail removal.

After removal of the nail the wounds should be closed and dressed. A suction drain should be placed in the thigh after femoral nail removal but it is not necessary to place one in the leg after tibial nail removal. Immediate weight bearing is allowed and no cases of re-fracture of either femur or tibia have occurred in the author's centre after nail removal.

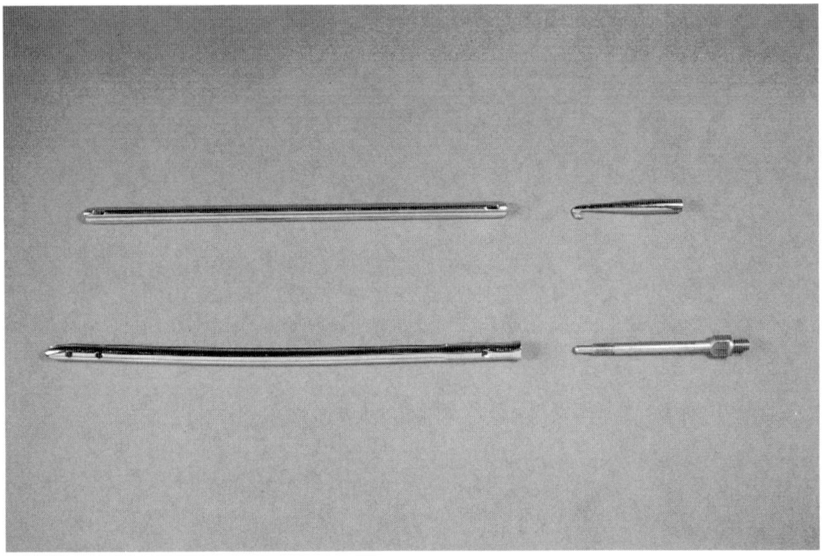

Figure 19.1

The Küntscher nail is extracted by the use of a hook inserted into the proximal slot in the nail. The Grosse-Kempf nail (lower in the picture) is removed by a threaded extractor.

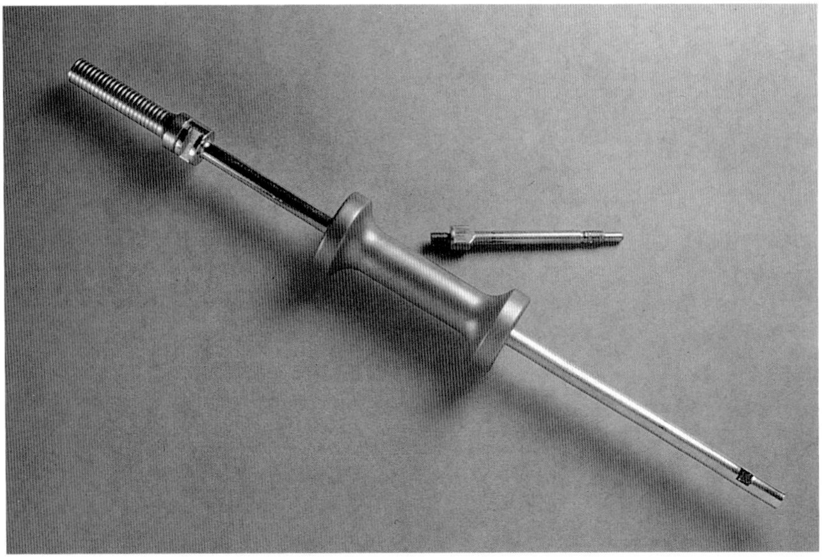

Figure 19.2

Most nail extractors are similar. The extraction hook or bolt is screwed into a long metal rod on which slides a hammer.

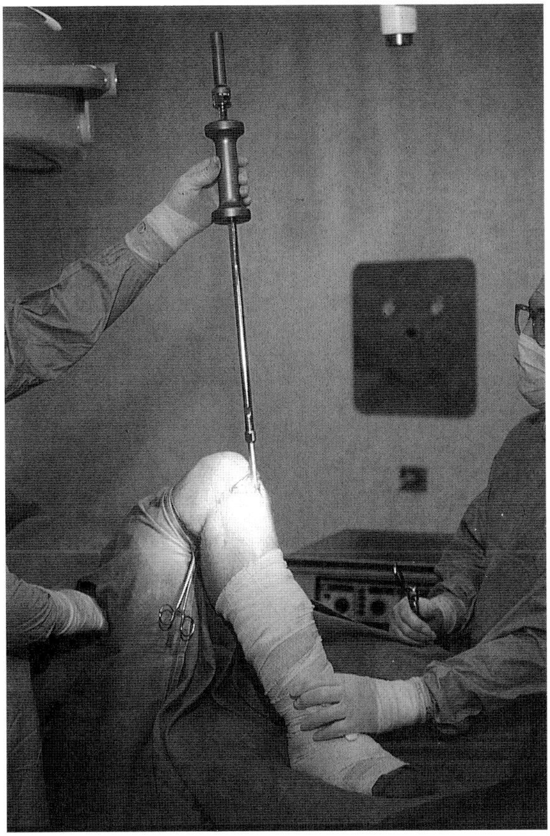

Figure 19.3

In this fracture, there were no cross-screws but if distal cross-screws are to be removed then the leg must be cleaned and draped to allow exposure between the lower femur and the ankle. After insertion of the extraction bolt, the extractor assembly is attached to the bolt. Care must be taken to remove the operating light from above the surgeon in case the surgeon's hands and the extraction assembly become contaminated.

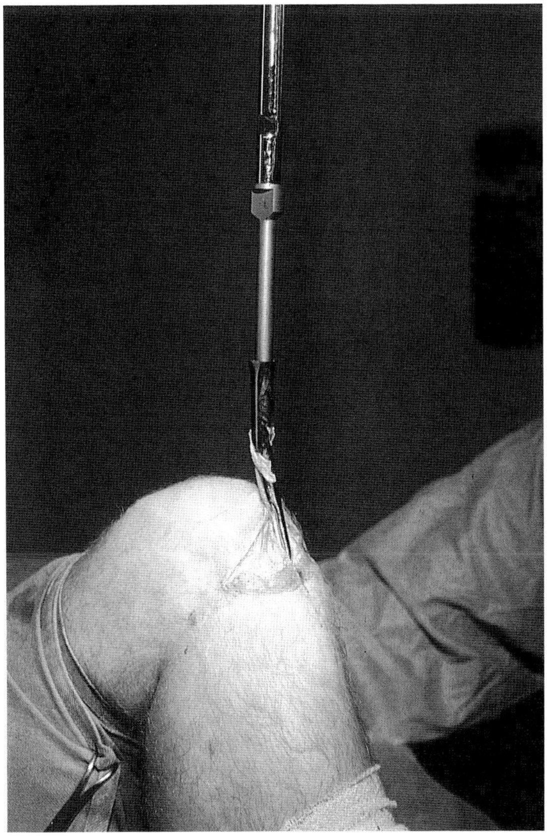

Figure 19.4

By striking the hammer upwards, it is possible to remove the nail fairly easily. Fibrous tissue is seen around the proximal nail.

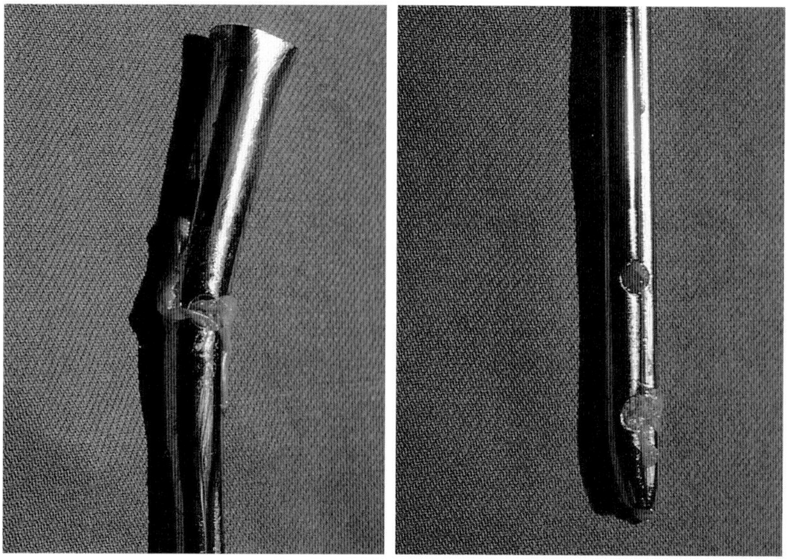

Figure 19.5

The proximal and distal screw holes contain a surprising amount of bone unless they have been used. This bone does not obstruct nail removal. There is a considerable amount of fibrous tissue within and around the nail on extraction (Figure 19.4), but there is no need to ream the fibrous tissue from the endosteal surface of the medullary canal unless bone has been previously infected.

CHAPTER 20
RECONSTRUCTION NAILS

With **Mr James Christie** *FRCS*
Consultant Orthopaedic Surgeon,
Royal Infirmary of Edinburgh

Although locking nails can be used to treat all diaphyseal and most metaphyseal femoral fractures, there are a number of fractures where their use is inappropriate. Conventional femoral locking nailing is contra-indicated when there is tumour involving the lesser trochanter (see Figure 3.2) or if there is a proximal femoral fracture such that the fracture is either partially or completely situated above the lesser trochanter (Figure 20.1). Such a fracture could of course be fixed with one of a number of hip screw systems, but the recent development of a reconstruction type of nail has given the surgeon a new treatment alternative.

Reconstruction nails are locking femoral nails that have the proximal holes drilled such that the proximal screws are placed within the femoral head and neck. The distal screws are the same as on the conventional locking nail. An example of such a nail is the Russell-Taylor reconstruction nail shown in Figure 20.2. A modification of the reconstruction nail is seen in the Gamma nail which has been designed for use in intertrochanteric fractures. In this nail, the femoral component has been shortened, although the overall principle remains the same (Figure 20.3).

A number of designs of reconstruction nail have been used in Edinburgh. An example of one of them is shown in Figure 20.4. They are inserted in a similar manner to the conventional locking femoral nail, with a jig being used to insert the proximal screws into the femoral neck. There are, however, a number of difficulties which the surgeon should be aware of when inserting reconstruction nails.

The procedure is difficult to keep entirely closed as the fracture line is often at or close to the point of insertion of the nail. If the fracture site is opened widely with unnecessary soft-tissue and bone-fragment mobilization, it may be difficult to get a good insertion point and to maintain the correct neck shaft angle. There is therefore a tendency for comminuted proximal fractures to go into slight varus at the time of fixation (Figure 20.4).

In very comminuted fractures, there may be no obvious starting point and the surgeon will merely insert the nail through the fragments in an appropriate position. Under these circumstances, the surgeon has to rely exclusively on the proximal screws for fixation in the proximal femur.

The combination of femoral neck and diaphyseal fracture will be encountered by the trauma surgeon from time to time. This can be treated by a combination of a conventional locking nail and cancellous bone screws, as shown in Figure 20.5, just as the combination of a femoral condylar fracture and a diaphyseal fracture can also be treated by combining the use of interfragmentary screws inserted either percutaneously or in an open operation, with an intramedullary nail (Figure 20.6). If this combination is used, care must be taken that the bone screws do not obstruct the passage of the nail. The reconstruction nail represents a good alternative to the use of an intramedullary nail and cancellous screws to stabilize femoral combined diaphyseal and neck fractures. In reality, the reconstruction nail differs little from the fixation shown in Figure 20.5, although it is perhaps a rather neater approach. As yet there is little documentation regarding the use of reconstruction nails but indications, advantages and disadvantages of these systems will emerge soon.

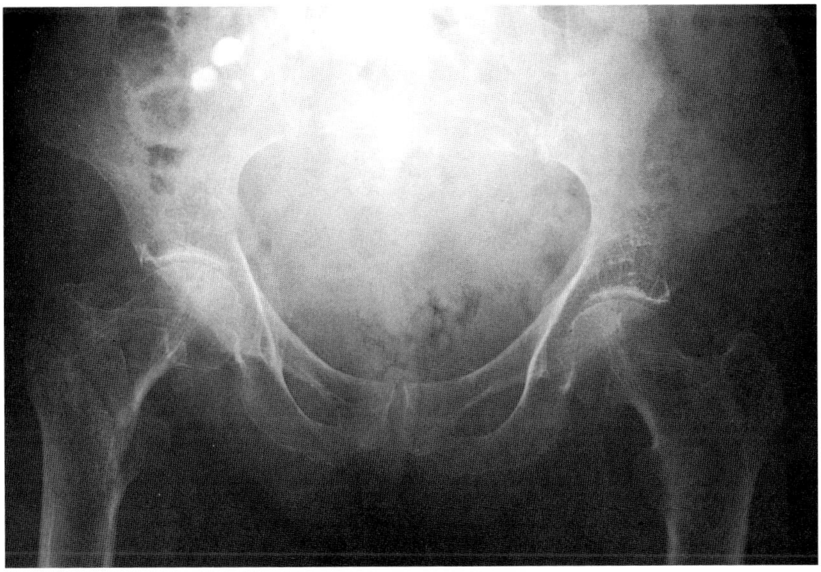

Figure 20.1

There is a high spiral fracture of the right proximal femur extending above the lesser trochanter. The use of a conventional locking nail would be inappropriate in this fracture as proximal stability would not be obtained.

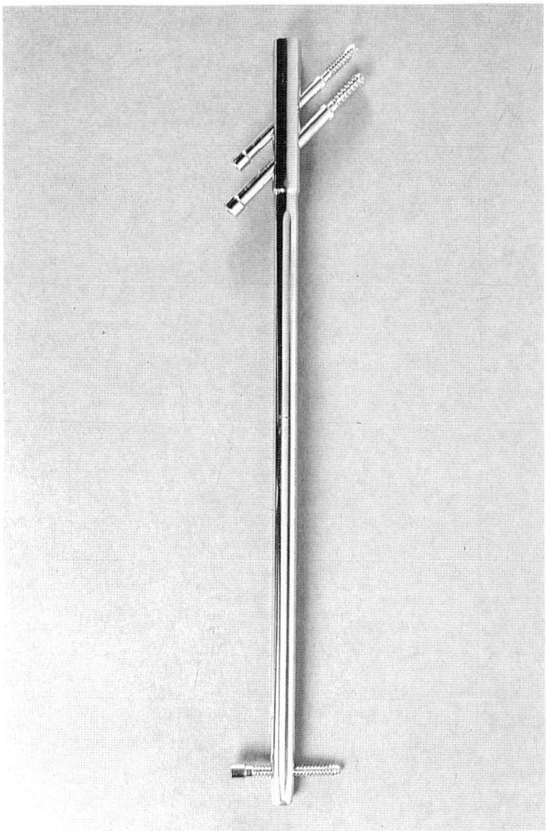

Figure 20.2

The Russell-Taylor femoral reconstruction nail. Two screws can be passed upwards and medially into the femoral head and neck. Distal cross-screws are used in the usual way.

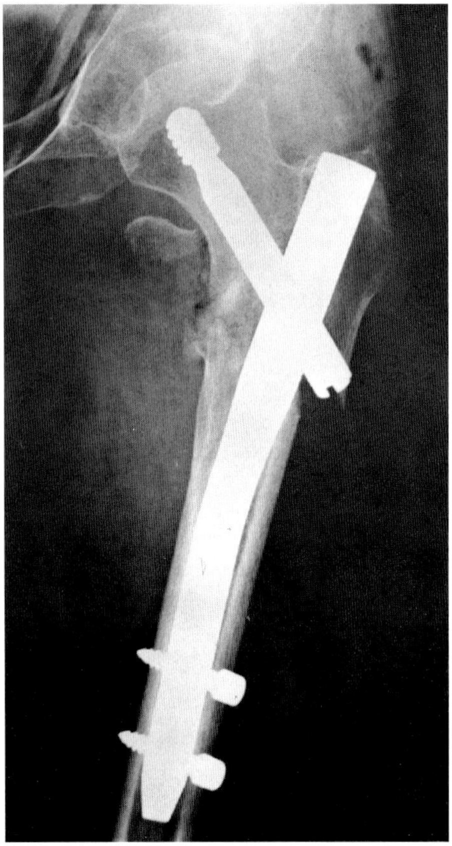

Figure 20.3

The Gamma nail. This is a shortened reconstruction nail used for intertrochanteric and high subtrochanteric fractures. The proximal side arm and the distal screws are inserted with a jig. (Photograph courtesy of Howmedica Ltd.)

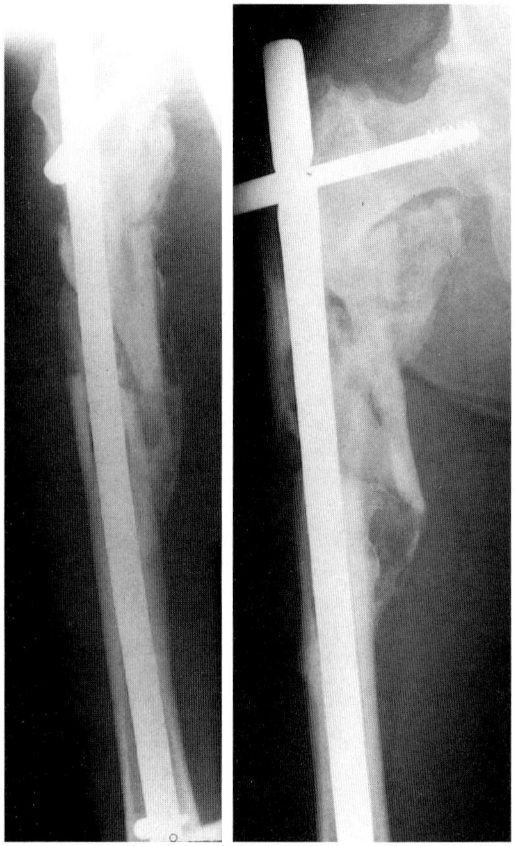

Figure 20.4

The use of a reconstruction nail to stabilize a high proximal femoral fracture. Good union has been obtained although a coxa vara is present.

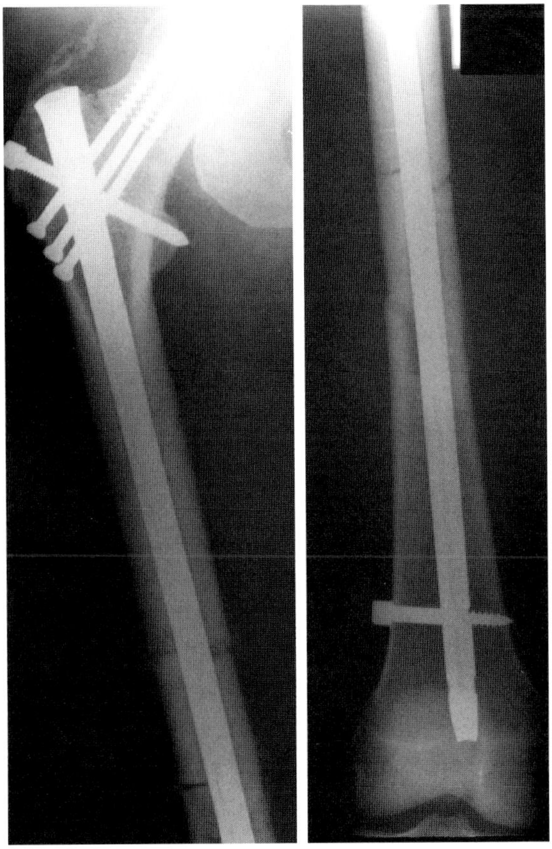

Figure 20.5

The combination of subcapital fracture and femoral diaphyseal fracture can be difficult to treat. If a hip screw system is used to treat the subcapital fracture an intramedullary nail cannot be used to treat the diaphyseal fracture. An alternative is shown here with the use of a locking femoral intramedullary nail to treat the diaphyseal fracture and cancellous bone screws to stabilize the subcapital fracture. Both fractures healed well.

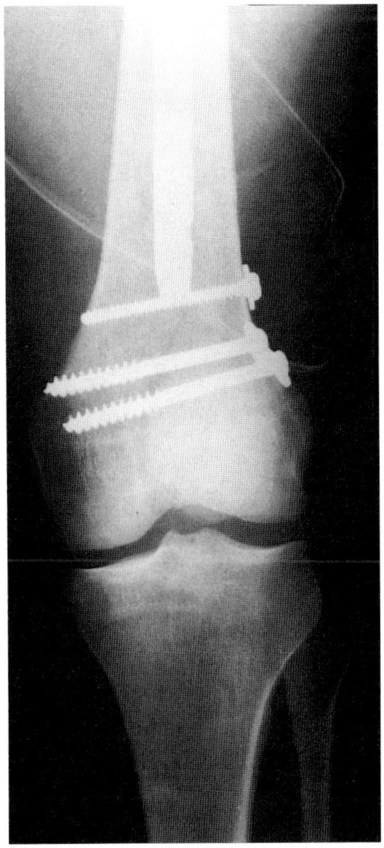

Figure 20.6

Closed intramedullary nailing can be used in association with other internal fixation techniques. Here a lateral condylar fracture has been internally fixed with three bone screws in an open procedure. Following this intramedullary nailing of the femoral diaphysis was undertaken. If a distal third femoral fracture is to be treated in this way the intramedullary nail must be passed far enough into the distal fragment to ensure fracture stability.

CHAPTER 21 COMPARTMENT SYNDROMES

With **Miss Margaret M McQueen** *FRCS Ed (Orth)*
Senior Lecturer/Consultant Orthopaedic Surgeon, Royal Infirmary of Edinburgh

One of the criticisms that has been levelled at intramedullary nailing is that it causes raised intracompartmental pressure and thereby increases the incidence of both compartment syndrome and the sequelae of raised compartment pressure, namely muscle tightening, claw toes and pes cavus. Some surgeons have suggested that these effects are ameliorated by delaying nailing for a few days to allow the soft-tissue swelling to diminish. There is, however, little evidence in the literature to confirm or refute this belief.

Compartment syndromes of the thigh following femoral fracture are very rare, few surgeons having experience of more than one or two cases. Schwartz et al (1989) undertook a retrospective review of over 6000 patients admitted to a centre in the USA and found 21 thigh compartment syndromes, of which 10 were associated with femoral fractures. The remaining 11 were associated with prolonged hypotension, a history of external compression of the thigh, the use of anti-shock trousers, coagulopathy or vascular injury. They emphasized the relationship between thigh compartment syndrome and multiple trauma.

In the author's centre, there have been four documented cases of thigh compartment syndrome associated with a femoral diaphyseal fracture in the last 8 years, giving an approximate incidence of 0.8 per cent. Unfortunately, none of these patients had compartment monitoring in position at the time of diagnosis or treatment.

Compartment syndrome following tibial fracture is more common. Court-Brown and McQueen (1987) estimated that there was a 1 per cent incidence of compartment syndrome in closed and Type I open tibial diaphyseal fractures treated by conservative management. Owen and Tsimboukis (1967) reported a 10 per cent incidence of the sequelae of raised compartment pressure following plaster treatment of tibial diaphyseal fractures.

Compartment pressure monitoring of the anterior compartment of the leg has been standard practice in the author's centre for 3 years and therefore considerable knowledge of the effect of intramedullary nailing on compartment pressures has been collected (McQueen et al, 1990). Monitoring of the anterior compartment only is open to criticism as theoretically there might be a low pressure in this compartment but a high pressure in, for example, the deep posterior compartment. We do not believe that under normal circumstances this is the case and monitoring of the anterior compartment seems to give a pressure reading representative of the leg as a whole.

Following the commencement of routine compartment monitoring, fasciotomy was initially performed on the traditional clinical grounds of pain on passive or active movement along with signs of paraesthesiae or impaired capillary circulation. However, as confidence in pressure monitoring grew, it became clear that if the need for fasciotomy was dictated exclusively by the pressure reading, the operation was performed 8 to 12 hours earlier and was not associated with significant complications. Compartment pressure monitoring is now relied on to dictate the need for fasciotomy, although it is not the absolute compartment pressure that is important but rather it is the relationship between compartment pressure and the diastolic blood pressure that dictates the need for fasciotomy. If the difference between the diastolic blood pressure and the compartment pressure falls below 30 mm mercury, a compartment syndrome should be considered.

Technique of pressure monitoring

The equipment required for pressure monitoring is straightforward and should be found in any anaesthetic department. The surgeon requires a slit catheter, a length of plastic manometer tubing connected to a pressure transducer, a pressure measuring device and a chart recorder.

After the patient has been prepared and draped, the slit catheter is inserted into the anterior compartment of the leg through a stab incision. The catheter is passed distally and the trochar withdrawn. Slit catheters are commercially available but can also be made easily from jugular central venous catheters, as shown in Figure 21.1.

After insertion of the slit catheter into the leg, a small quantity of normal saline is injected into the catheter to fill the dead space. A small-bore plastic manometer tube, pre-filled with normal saline, is then connected through a three-way tap to the slit catheter and a pressure monitor. It is important to check that there are no air bubbles in the system. The three-way tap is then connected to a pressure recorder. The pressure recorder is connected to a chart recorder to allow for a permanent trace to be made.

The system relies on an uninterrupted column of saline between the compartment and the pressure transducer. The height of the pressure monitor should be level with the end of the slit catheter as the hydrostatic pressure within the system will be altered by variation in this relationship. The height of the pressure monitor is best controlled by securing it to a drip stand after estimating its correct position (Figure 21.2). Before commencing pressure recording, the system should be set to zero by exposing the pressure monitor to atmospheric pressure. This is conveniently done by opening the three-way tap, adjacent to the pressure monitor, to the atmosphere.

Pressure monitoring of tibial fractures

The position that is used for closed nailing of the tibia shown in Figure 5.2 tends to increase compartment pressure for two main reasons. First, there is compression of the popliteal fossa and the upper calf muscles from the circular pad on which the leg rests. Second, the traction which is often required to reduce the fracture tends to increase the intracompartmental pressure.

Accordingly, when the surgeon starts to record the pressure in the anterior compartment it may well be high. A typical peroperative pressure trace is shown in Figure 21.3.

Pressure rises in response to interference with the tibia, particularly in response to instrumentation of the medullary canal. Figure 21.3 illustrates the temporary rise in pressure that accompanies intramedullary reaming and nailing. Surgeons should not be unduly concerned about the apparently high peroperative pressure levels as they will drop postoperatively. Postoperatively the slit catheter is left undisturbed and the plastic tube and pressure monitor are bandaged into the dressings, care being taken not to kink the tubing. The pressure recorder and chart recorder are transferred to the ward and the system is set up once again. The surgeon should take care to re-zero it prior to recording the postoperative pressures.

The usual postoperative findings are that the pressure falls to acceptable levels over the 24 to 36 hours after surgery. As the important relationship is between the compartment pressure and the diastolic blood pressure, the blood pressure should be taken every 2 hours and recorded on the pressure-monitoring record. A typical postoperative record is shown in Figure 21.4. If a compartment syndrome is going to occur, the pressure will continue to rise so that it is within 30 mm mercury of the diastolic blood pressure (Figure 21.5). This trend will only be reversed by fasciotomy which should be performed as soon as the surgeon is happy that the overall pressure trend is upwards. At the time that the record shown in Figure 21.5 was taken, the patient had no clinical signs suggestive of compartment syndrome but the diagnosis was undoubtedly confirmed at the time of fasciotomy (Figure 21.6). It is the experience of the author and co-workers that machine-recorded pressure increase is apparent several hours before the onset of clinical signs.

Results of compartment pressure monitoring

Over 100 patients have now had compartment pressure monitoring following tibial fractures in Edinburgh. The overall incidence of acute compartment syndrome is 2 per cent, which does not differ significantly from the 1 per cent reported by Court-Brown and McQueen (1987) following conservative management in the same centre. It is interesting to note that there was no significant difference in the pressures recorded between closed and open tibial fractures or between low- and high-energy fractures. In addition, there was no significant difference in the pressures recorded between fractures nailed within 24 hours of injury and those nailed after this time (McQueen et al, 1990). It would appear that intramedullary nailing transiently increases the compartment pressures during surgery but that postoperatively these fall to normal levels. Not only is there no increased incidence of compartment syndrome following closed intramedullary nailing, but delaying the nailing procedure does not alter the pressure.

Court-Brown and McQueen (1987) noted a relationship between compartment syndrome and fracture union with a significantly prolonged time to union in patients over 18 years of age who had had compartment syndrome. They felt that this was probably a vascular phenomenon. It is of interest that none of the patients who have had early decompression as a result of pressure monitoring has had union problems.

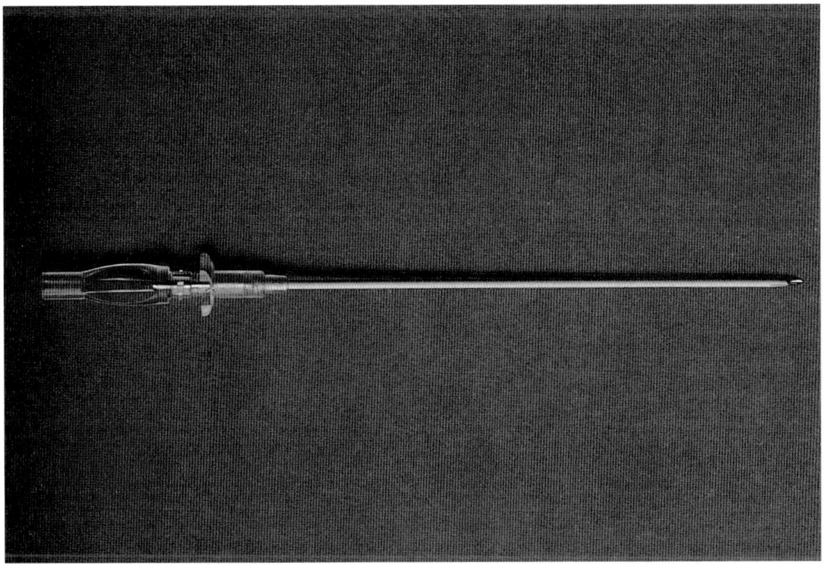

Figure 21.1

a A commercially available jugular central venous catheter. With modification, this is suitable for use as a slit catheter.

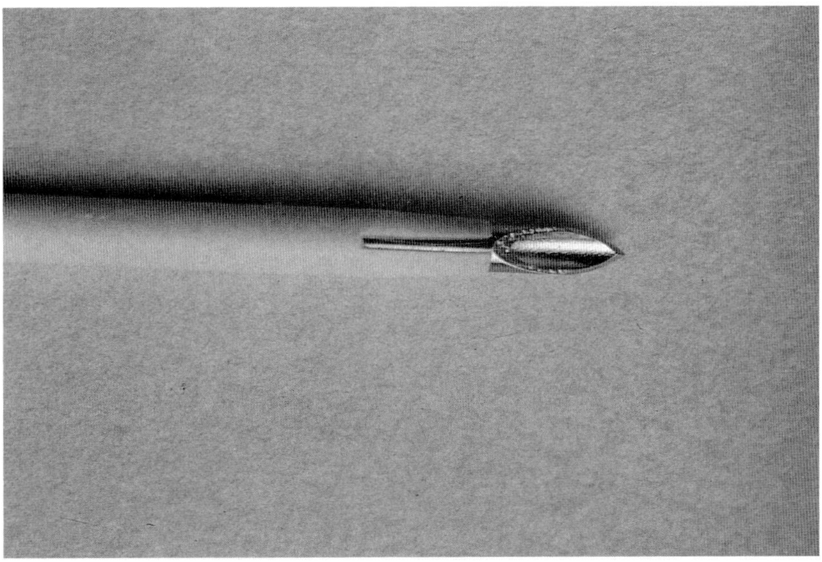

b The slit catheter is made by cutting two small slots out of the distal end of the catheter with a sharp scalpel blade. One slot is cut on each side of the catheter. The trochar should be left in the catheter while the slots are cut.

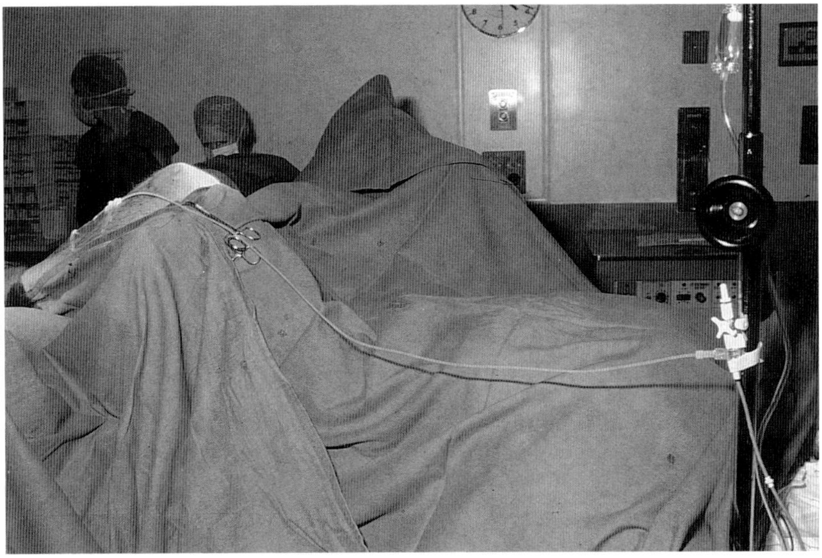

Figure 21.2

The pressure transducer should be at the same level as the distal end of the catheter. This is best achieved by securing the transducer and the attached three-way tap to a drip stand and then altering the height in relation to the slit catheter.

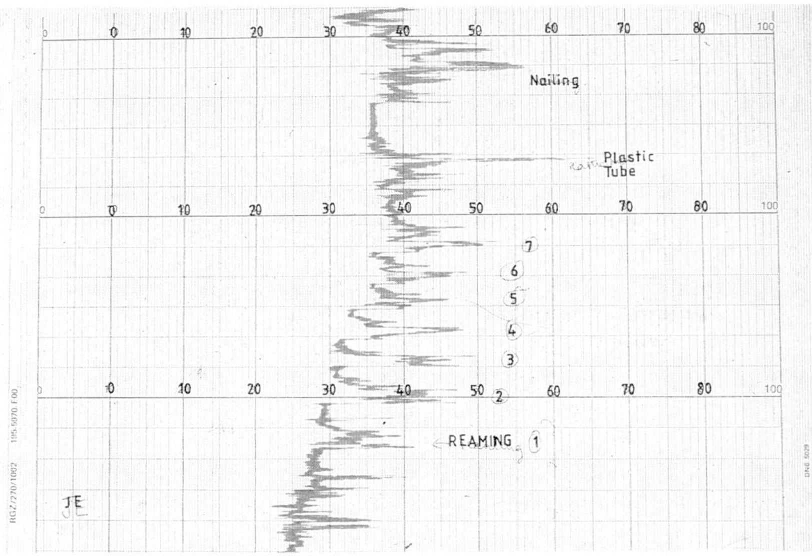

Figure 21.3

A typical per-operative pressure trace. The transient increases in the pressure during the insertion of seven different reamers, a plastic tube and the nail itself can all be seen. The overall trend is of a small increase in pressure during the procedure.

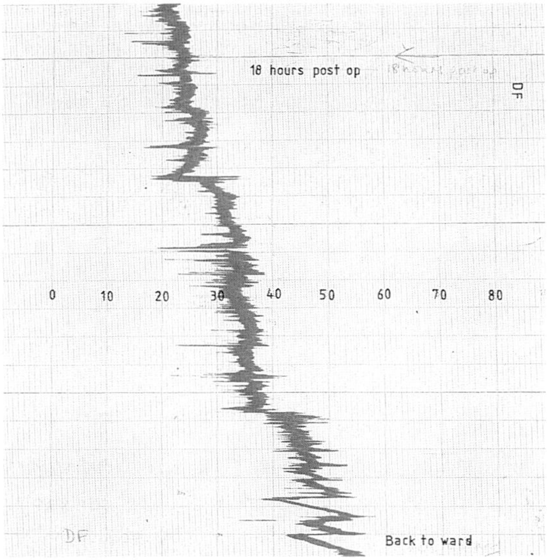

Figure 21.4

A typical postoperative pressure trace, showing a gradual lowering of the intracompartmental pressure after surgery. Eighteen hours after surgery, the pressure has fallen to about 25 mm of mercury.

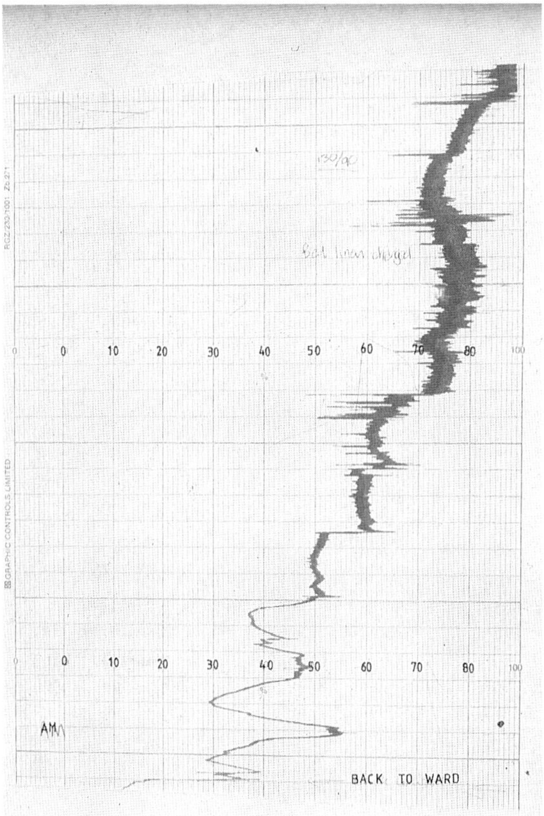

Figure 21.5

A pressure trace from a patient developing a compartment syndrome. At the time that the patient was returned to the ward, the pressure was approximately 45 mm of mercury but rose to approximately 80 mm. At that time, the blood pressure was recorded as 130/90. The patient did not have the characteristic symptoms of a compartment syndrome.

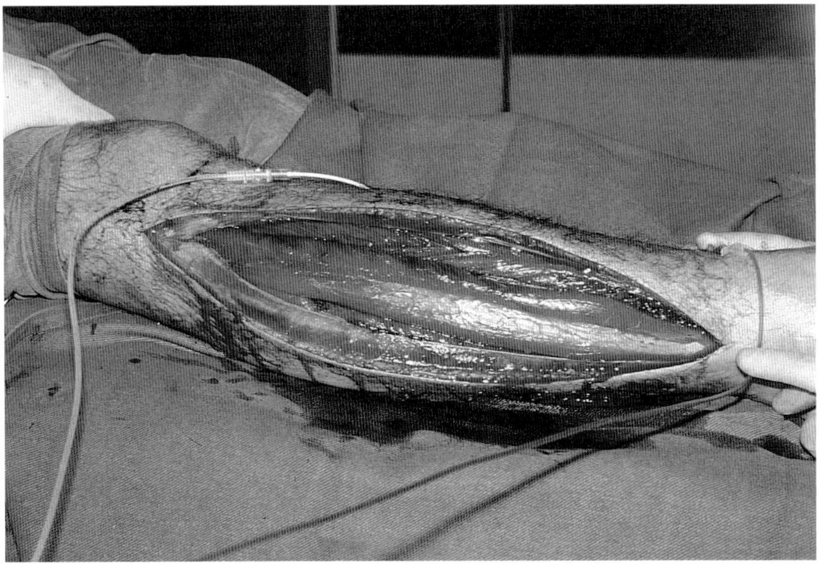

Figure 21.6

Fasciotomy confirmed the compartment pressure results shown in Figure 21.5. A two-incision approach was used. The upper catheter is in the anterior compartment and the lower in the deep posterior compartment. It is interesting to note that after decompression of the anterior compartment pressure in the deep posterior compartment fell from 70 mm to 35 mm of mercury.

CHAPTER 22 INFECTION

Any operative treatment used for the management of closed femoral or tibial fractures must have a low incidence of infection or it should be abandoned. What constitutes an acceptable incidence of infection is open to debate. If a surgeon selects an operative treatment method then sooner or later deep infection will occur and he or she should know how to deal with the problem.

The incidence of superficial infection following closed nailing of closed femoral and tibial diaphyseal fractures is 1.4 per cent and 2.6 per cent respectively. Superficial wound infection in the thigh following femoral nailing has not proved to be a problem. All such cases have responded to local treatment and the use of antibiotics and none has been complicated by bone infection. Superficial infection of the proximal tibial wound following tibial nailing is potentially more serious. The proximity of the skin wound to the underlying nail entry point means that there is a risk of bone infection following superficial infection. The author has seen two such cases. If superficial infection occurs it is preferable to treat the patient as an in-patient with appropriate local treatment and antibiotics.

The incidence of deep infection following closed nailing of closed and Type I open femoral fractures in the author's centre is 0.5 per cent. The incidence of deep infection following closed nailing of closed and Type I open tibial fractures is 1.5 per cent. These figures are comparable to other series (Winquist et al, 1984; Klemm and Borner, 1986). All nailing procedures of closed or Type I open fractures of the femur or tibia are covered by the routine prophylactic administration of a second-generation cephalosporin. A three-dose regime is currently used with the initial dose given at the time of anaesthetic induction and the two subsequent doses administered after a further 6 and 12 hours.

The incidence of deep infection following the use of a locking nail in Type III open femoral fractures is currently 5 per cent and is comparable to the incidence that occurs with other treatment methods. The centre's policy of using locking nails to treat Type III open tibial fractures was introduced because of the observation that the use of external skeletal fixation was associated with a deep infection rate of 5 per cent in the Type IIIa open tibial fractures and 37 per cent in the Type IIIb open fractures. The overall incidence of infection in Type III fractures following external fixation was 17.6 per cent (Court-Brown, Wheelwright, Christie et al, 1990). This figure is comparable to other series of externally fixed fractures (Chan et al, 1984) and plated fractures (Clifford et al, 1988). It was also observed that the externally fixed Type III fractures had a high incidence of mal-union. It was assumed that nailing would more or less abolish the problems of mal-union and muscle penetration by transfixion pins and it was felt that, even if the infection rates were the same, this would constitute a more successful treatment method for these difficult fractures. The subjective impression is that the incidence of infection is no higher than that seen with external fixation, but research into this continues.

If infection does occur it is important that it be treated correctly. Many surgeons resort to conservative management when faced with an infected fracture. This, however, is the wrong approach and it is vital that the stability of the fracture is maintained if infection occurs. The surgeon could substitute external fixation for the intramedullary nail but there is in fact no need to do so. The presence of infection does not necessarily mean that healing will not occur. This is particularly true when infection occurs in a closed fracture, as shown in Figure 22.1. A 23-year-old man sustained a closed tibial fracture while playing football (Figure 22.1a). This was treated by a distal dynamically-locked nail (Figure 22.1b). After 6 weeks the patient presented with increasing pain, swelling and erythema at the fracture site. X-ray scans showed signs of bone infection (Figure 22.1c) and he was treated with in-patient bed rest and intravenous antibiotics. Despite the infection, the tibia had united by 14 weeks and the nail was removed after a further 8 weeks (Figure 22.1d). After a further 12 months there was no evidence of recurrent sepsis. At the time of nail removal it is important to ream out the pyogenic membrane from the medullary canal and if there has been a discharging sinus at any time this should be curetted at the time of nail removal. This treatment method has proved satisfactory for all closed and Type I open femoral and tibial infections that have been encountered following intramedullary nailing in the author's centre. All have healed without changing the treatment method and none has required open bone grafting.

In Type III open fractures, the same basic procedure is followed. Infection is more common but, if basic principles are adhered to, the incidence can be kept within acceptable limits. An example is shown in Figure 22.2. This shows a Type IIIa open tibial fracture which was initially treated by external fixation (Figure 22.2a). A gastrocnemius flap with a superficial skin graft was used to cover the skin defect at the second wound inspection after 36 hours (Figure 22.2b). After 12 weeks, there was no sign of bone union and instead of using open bone grafting it was elected to change to an intramedullary nail (Figure 22.2c). The exchange between external fixation and intramedullary nailing was carried out as described in Chapter 17, but the patient developed bone infection with a discharging sinus that was not related to a previous external fixation pin tract. The nail was not removed and the fracture was clinically and radiologically united at 27 weeks (Figure 22.2d). At this time, the nail was removed and the medullary canal reamed until no fibrous tissue was apparent in the reamings. The sinus was curetted and the wound left open to granulate. All wounds healed and after two years there was no sign of recurrent infection (Figure 22.2e).

The incidence of infection in Type III open tibial fractures is related more to the skill with which the initial wound toilet is performed and to the adequacy of subsequent plastic surgery than to the type of internal or external fixation used by the orthopaedic surgeon. Results at the author's centre suggest that locking intramedullary nailing is a satisfactory method of treating all open femoral and tibial fractures provided there is expert management of the soft tissues and an appreciation of how to deal with any deep infection that does occur.

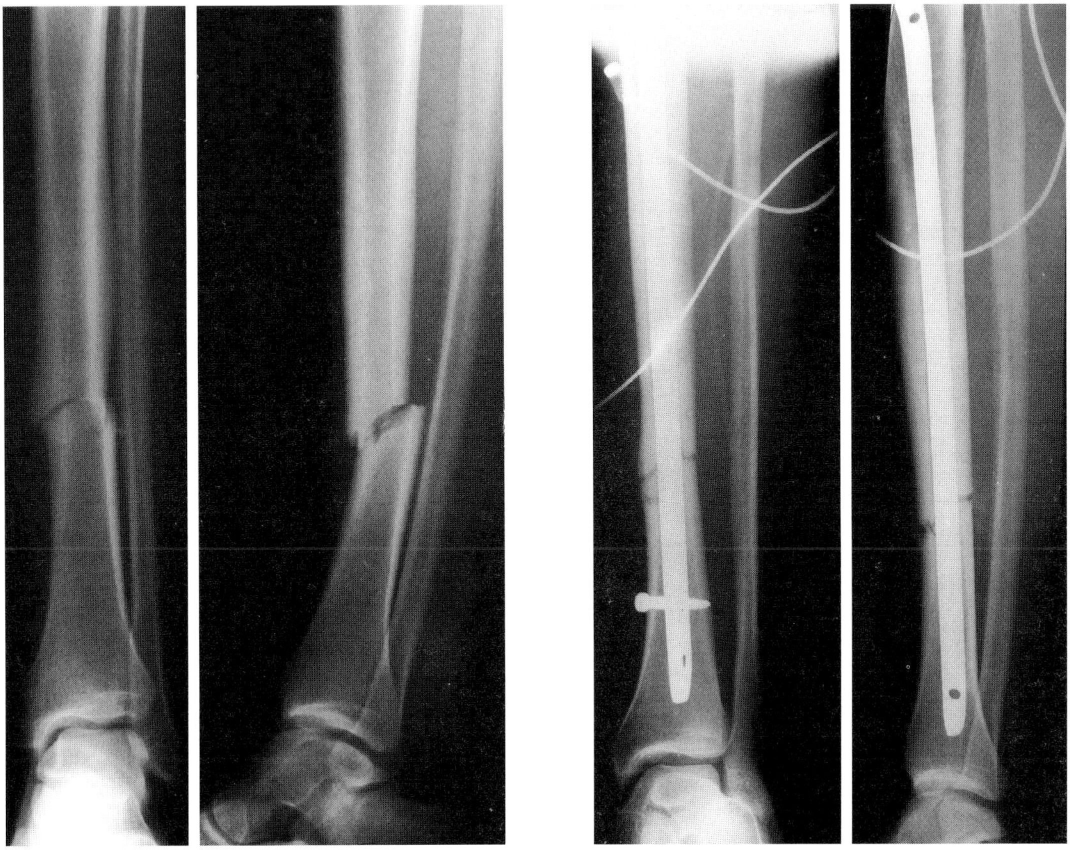

Figure 22.1

a A closed tibial fracture in a 23-year-old male. The fracture occurred as a result of a soccer tackle.

b The fracture was treated with the use of a dynamically locked intramedullary nail and postoperative recovery was uneventful.

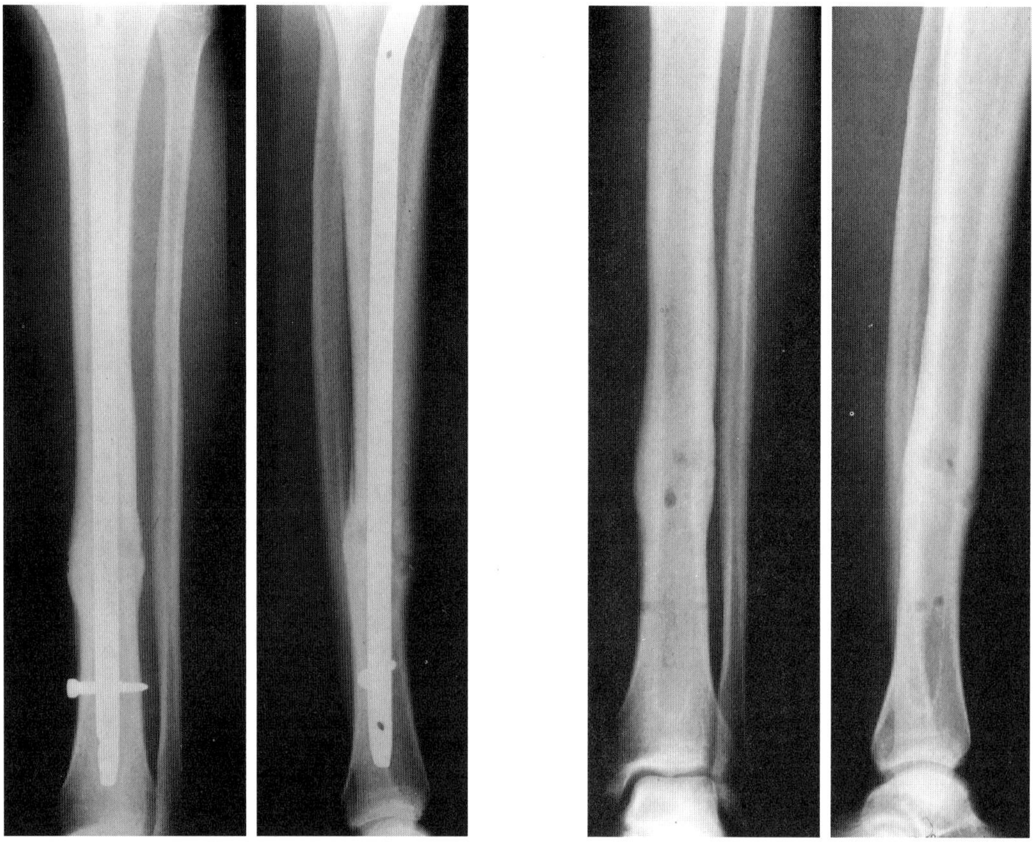

Figure 22.1 *continued*

c Six weeks after nailing, the fracture is clearly uniting but there is evidence of sepsis around the fracture site. There is a lucent area in the anterior cortex at the level of the fracture site as well as evidence of a posterior collection.

d The tibia had united by 14 weeks. Nail removal was carried out after 22 weeks, at which time the pyogenic membrane was reamed from the medullary canal. There has been no recurrence of the infection.

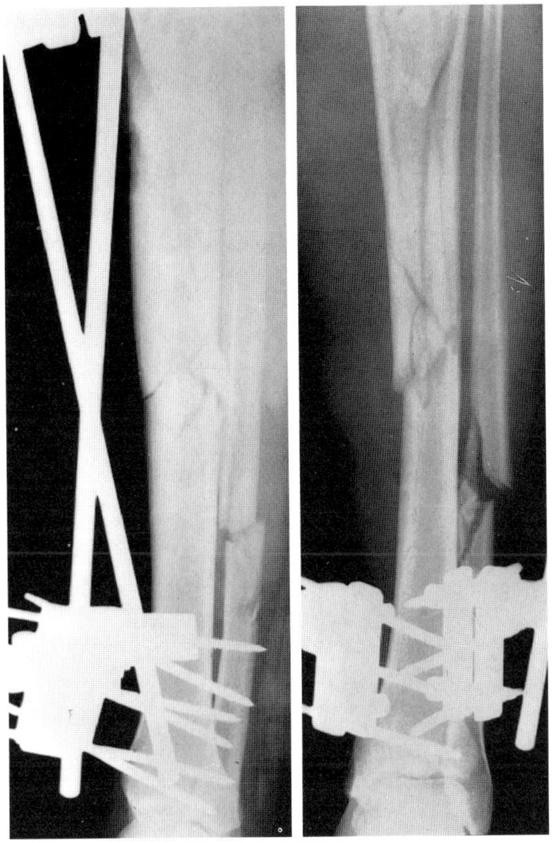

Figure 22.2

a Gustilo Type IIIa open tibial fracture in a 24-year-old male. This was initially treated by the application of a Hoffmann external fixation frame.

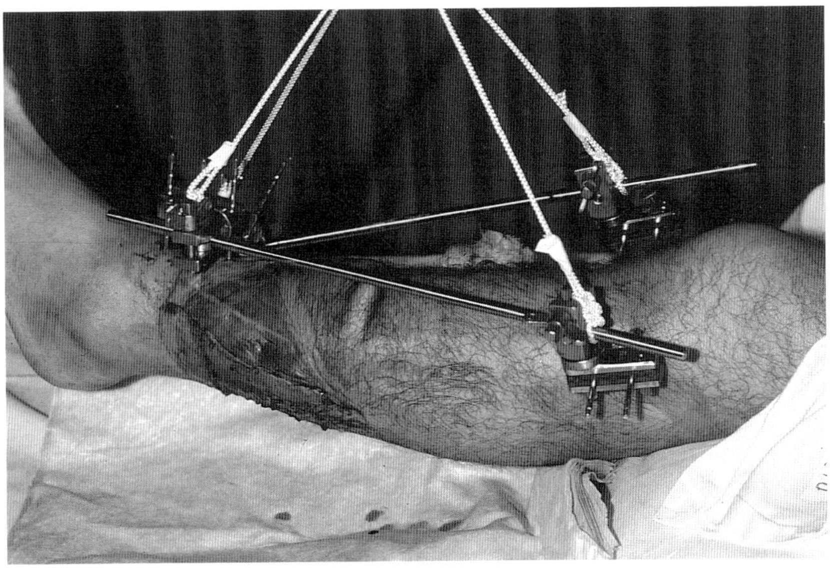

b Thirty-six hours after the initial surgery, a gastrocnemius flap with an overlying superficial split-skin graft was used to cover the skin defect.

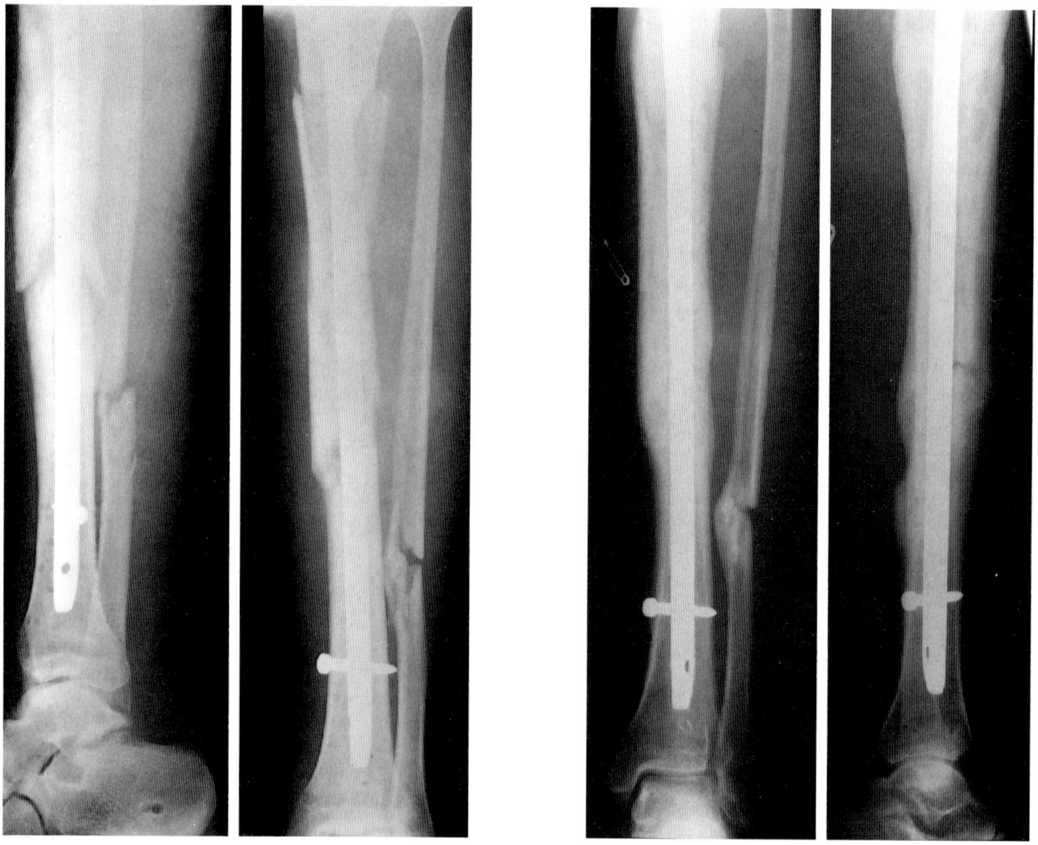

Figure 22.2 *continued*

c Twelve weeks after the accident, there was no sign of union in the tibia and it was elected to change from the Hoffmann fixator to a statically locked intramedullary nail.

d Three weeks after this operation, the patient developed a discharging sinus in the proximal third of the tibia. This was not related to a previous external fixation pin tract or to the cross-screws. As bone union appeared to be progressing, the nail was not removed and the fracture was clinically and radiologically united at 27 weeks. At this time, the proximal sinus was still discharging.

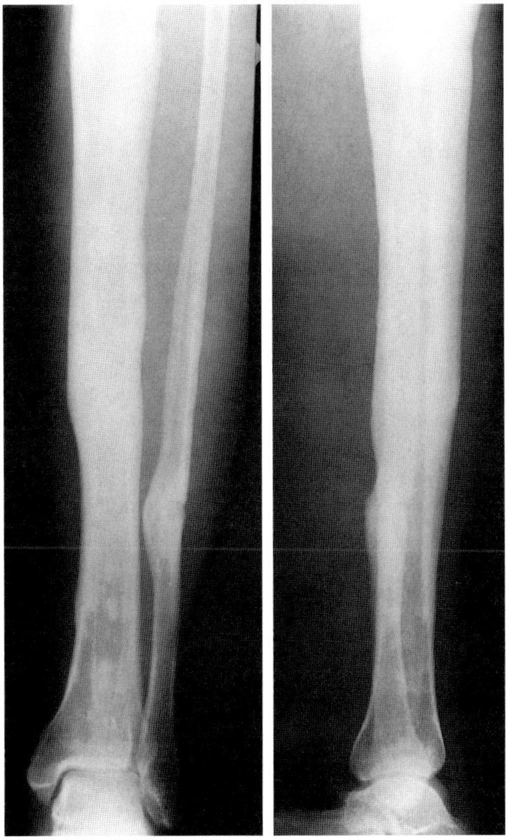

e The nail was removed and the medullary canal reamed. The sinus was opened and curetted free from granulation tissue. All wounds healed and there has been no subsequent evidence of sepsis.

CHAPTER 23 OTHER COMPLICATIONS

As with all surgical techniques, complications can occur during and following intramedullary nailing, although adherence to correct surgical practice will minimize the incidence and effect of any complications. Some of the complications are avoidable and are directly related to poor surgical technique. However, as all surgeons know, complications will occur despite experience. A number of complications apart from infection and compartment syndrome are common to both the femur and the tibia and will be dealt with together. Complications that are unique to the femur or the tibia will be discussed separately.

Non-union

The use of intramedullary nailing to treat non-unions is discussed in Chapter 12. The incidence of non-union following reamed locking nailing is very low, being between 1 and 1.5 per cent for both the femur and the tibia. Older series where small diameter Küntscher nails were used had a higher incidence of non-union. This is presumably related to the inability of the smaller nail to stabilize the fracture adequately and the relative lack of bone graft material gained from the endosteal surface of the cortex.

The incidence of non-union following locked reamed nailing can be reduced by:

- Not opening the fracture site
- Using a nail of adequate diameter: at least 11 mm in the tibia and 12 mm in the femur
- Adequate reaming of the intramedullary canal
- Proper use of cross-screws

Mal-union

This complication should be non-existent following the use of a correctly inserted locking intramedullary nail. Where mal-unions do occur following nailing they are produced by:

- Incorrect reduction of the fracture: usually a rotational mal-alignment of the femur
- Incorrect placement of the transfixion pin
- Incorrect guide wire placement
- Incorrect cross-screw insertion

Incorrect fracture reduction

Straight traction and the use of proper surgical technique as described in Chapters 4 and 5 should minimize the incidence of fracture mal-reduction. However, if a surgeon does not assess rotation correctly, the bone can be nailed with rotational mal-alignment. This in fact is rare in the tibia where alignment of the distal fragment is easily obtained by aligning the second toe with the patella. Femoral alignment is more difficult to obtain, particularly if there is considerable thigh swelling. The surgeon may detect a rotational mal-alignment by comparing the width of the cortices above and below the fracture site. This is illustrated in Figure 23.1. If this problem occurs the surgeon should remove the nail, correct the rotation and renail the femur.

Incorrect placement of transfixion pin

In femoral nailing, traction is applied through a distal femoral or upper tibial transfixion pin. In the tibia, the pin is placed in the calcaneum. It is important to align the pin at 90 degrees to the axis of the femur or tibia. Failure to do this may cause an incorrect angulation of the distal fracture fragment. This problem is accentuated in distal fractures, as in proximal fractures the passage of the nail down the medullary canal helps to align the fracture. Figure 23.2a shows a tibial fracture that was nailed badly for two reasons. First, the transfixion pin was inserted at about 20 degrees to the correct axis, causing the distal fragment to go into varus. Second, the surgeon leant on the tibia while carrying out the nailing procedure, causing a recurvatum deformity. The only possible treatment is renailing, and Figure 23.2b shows that a satisfactory result was eventually obtained.

Incorrect placement of the guide wire

The importance of centring the guide wire in the distal fragment of both femoral and tibial fractures has been emphasized. This is usually straightforward in proximal or middle third fractures, but becomes more difficult with distal fractures. Figure 23.3 illustrates the problems of a mal-position of the guide wire. The guide wire has been placed down the medial side of the distal femoral fragment and the result after nail insertion is a valgus mal-alignment. Renailing with correct fracture reduction was carried out.

Failure of cross-screw insertion

This is usually an iatrogenic failure to lock an unstable fracture statically. All spiral, segmental and comminuted fractures should be statically locked, regardless of the degree of comminution. The need for static locking is frequently obvious, but the surgeon must realize that the passage of a large intramedullary nail down a femur or tibia may displace a previously undisplaced fracture. Thus an apparently stable fracture may be converted into an unstable fracture by nailing. It is wise to lock any fracture statically if there is the slightest doubt about its stability.

Figure 23.4 shows a tibial fracture where the surgeon failed to appreciate the extent of the fracture. After nailing, it is obvious that the comminution was more extensive than was initially thought (Figure 23.4b). At this point, the patient should have been returned to the operating theatre and a proximal cross-screw inserted. Seven weeks after nailing, the fracture position has altered (Figure 23.4c). A cast was applied in a futile attempt to minimize further displacement but this was unsuccessful and the result was a mal-union (Figure 23.4d). This situation is easily avoided by the use of the correct cross-screws.

Nail failure

Nail failure may take two forms: the nail may either bend or break. These problems are usually associated with the use of a nail of too small a diameter or with a non-union where the nail has to take all the stresses that pass through the bone. The problems of using a narrow nail are illustrated in Figure 23.5a, where a small diameter nail has been used to stabilize a femoral fracture. The nail has bent and the patient presented at 6 months with a non-union. After a further 3 months, the nail broke at the fracture site (Figure 23.5b). This problem is commonly encountered when hand reamers have been used to prepare the medullary canal. It is impossible to do more than lightly curette the endosteal surface of the cortex with hand reamers and therefore a small nail is often inserted. The use of power reamers and correct reaming technique should abolish this problem.

Some early nails tended to fail at the junction between the solid proximal portion and the slotted distal portion 30–60 mm below the proximal end of the nail (Figure 23.6). This problem no longer exists as the design of nails has improved, but a surgeon may encounter an older nail which has broken at this location.

Nail bending

Although most nail bending follows submaximal loading of a small diameter intramedullary nail, the author has encountered one case of a bent Grosse-Kempf nail following a single incident where a bending stress was placed on the fracture site. This is illustrated in Figure 23.7. An 18-year-old man was playing football 6 weeks after his original closed tibial fracture was nailed. He slipped on the ball and bent his tibia and its nail.

The treatment of any bent nail is to remove it as soon as possible. This applies to both the nail that is bending under chronic submaximal loading and the acutely bent nail. Nails that are bent only a few degrees can be removed in the usual way as outlined in Chapter 19. However, it would be difficult to remove the nails shown in Figures 23.5 and 23.7 by conventional means. An attempt should be made to straighten such nails. This can usually be achieved by the surgeon bending the thigh or leg across his knee. This somewhat crude manoeuvre is usually successful in straightening the nail sufficiently so that it can be removed in the conventional way. This was successfully performed in this case.

The alternative to straightening the nail and then performing an exchange nailing is to wait until the nail breaks, as it will eventually. Since the nail will usually break at the non-union site it can then be extracted by either closed or open means. It is preferable to extract such a broken nail by closed means if possible. The proximal end can usually be removed easily by the use of an appropriate nail extractor. The distal end can be removed by the use of a long hook that can be used to engage the distal end of the nail. If this fails, an open removal should be performed, but as the non-union must be extensively taken down bone graft must be used to promote bone union.

Should a bent nail refuse to break, the surgeon may have to cut the nail to allow removal. This obviously is an open procedure and should be done with great care to avoid excessive soft-tissue damage. A small pad saw can be used to saw through the nail and the two pieces then extracted.

Cross-screw failure

Failure of the cross-screw can occur in two ways. Either the screw can break or it can back out of the bone and thereby lose function. Screw breakage is extremely rare and has occurred in only two patients in the author's centre in the last six years, giving an approximate incidence of 0.4 per cent. One case is shown in Figure 23.8. This was a Type IIIa tibial fracture which was primarily nailed. The distal screw broke at 6 weeks for no obvious reason. In neither case of screw breakage was the outcome apparently affected by the breakage.

Failure of the screw to retain its hold in the cortex is even rarer and there has been only one case of this in the author's centre, giving an approximate incidence of 0.2 per cent. This occurred in a 38-year-old mentally defective patient whose bones were extremely osteoporotic (Figure 22.9). There has been no other case of a screw backing out to the detriment of fracture position.

Cross-screw discomfort

The use of distal cross-screws in the femur is sometimes accompanied by discomfort. The subcutaneous position of much of the tibia however means that the proximal antero-posterior cross-screw and any medially introduced distal cross-screw can be associated with local discomfort, particularly if the screws are not fully inserted (Figure 23.10). Where a patient complains of pain over the head of a screw it should be removed if sufficient time has passed to stabilize the fracture. The screws can usually be removed under local anaesthetic on an out-patient basis.

Nail mal-position

In osteoporotic bone an incorrectly located intramedullary nail can penetrate the cortex; this is shown in Figure 23.11. This is an incorrectly located Grosse-Kempf nail in the femur of a patient who was osteoporotic. The nail was removed and correctly repositioned.

Callus formation

Fractures treated by closed intramedullary nailing tend to heal with abundant callus due to the preservation of movement at the fracture site and the stimulation of the extra-osseous blood supply. Figure 23.12 shows a situation where callus had formed which caused discomfort as the quadriceps moved over it. In this case, the callus mass was removed, although this is rarely required.

Broken drill bits

Drill bits may break when used to drill both the proximal and distal bone cortices opposite the holes in the interlocking nail. The common reason for this occurrence is the surgeon's attempt to rotate a bent drill bit. This usually occurs in three situations (Figure 23.13). If the entry point of the cross-screw is slightly off-centre compared with the hole in the nail the surgeon will be able to move the bit across the proximal cortex and through the hole in the nail, but will be forced to bend the drill bit to try to penetrate the distal cortex in the correct position. As soon as the bent bit is rotated within the nail it will break (Figure 23.13a).

A similar situation has been encountered with insertion of the proximal screw in both the tibia and the femur if the proximal jig is not secured tightly to the nail. Even if the jig is only standing off the nail by 1–2 mm, the alignment of the proximal hole will be incorrect and although the drill bit may pass through the proximal cortex and the hole in the nail, it will tend to bend and snap (Figure 23.13b).

Drill bits can also break in the proximal tibia if the drill bit hits the ascending slope of the posterior cortex when the surgeon is inserting a proximal screw. Unless the drill bit is very sharp, rather than pierce the posterior cortex, it can bend and travel along the cortex, which causes weakness and breakage (Figure 23.13c).

Broken drill bits have been left in to act as cross-screws, but this is not advisable. They should be removed. This is usually straightforward if one end is outside either the proximal or distal cortex. If it is not, the surgeon may choose to leave the drill bit in situ and use the remaining screw hole to stabilize the fracture. If the drill bit has broken off in the proximal femur, where there is only one screw hole, it must be removed. A bone trephine just larger than the bit may be useful in its removal.

Complications of femoral nailing

Femoral neck fracture

Christie and Court-Brown (1988) documented the problem of femoral neck fracture following femoral nailing. It is sometimes difficult to know if the femoral neck fracture was present at the time of nailing, but there is no doubt that in certain circumstances nailing can cause such a fracture. The approximate incidence of this complication may be as high as 1.5 per cent. An example of a femoral neck fracture is shown in Figure 23.14a. This was treated by the use of two AO screws placed behind the nail (Figure 23.14b). All iatrogenic femoral neck fractures in the author's centre have healed without problem.

Femoral neck fractures are associated with an incorrect choice of starting position. Too medial a starting point may weaken the femoral neck and cause a fracture. This complication however is so obvious that surgeons automatically guard against it. The femoral neck fractures that have occurred in the author's centre have in fact been associated with a lateral starting position in female patients with a narrow medullary canal. Another associated problem is the insertion of the proximal cross-screw above the lesser trochanter into the base of the femoral neck (Figure 23.15a and b). This also provides a stress riser in the base of the neck and may cause a fracture. The proximal location of the proximal cross-screw is caused by a failure to drive the nail fully home.

Proximal femoral comminution

A second consequence of incorrect placement of the intramedullary nail entry point is comminution of the proximal shaft of the femur (Figure 23.16). This occurs under three circumstances. If the proximal femur is inadequately reamed and the descending nail is wider than the medullary canal, a fracture of the proximal femur may occur. However, it is more common for proximal comminution to follow the incorrect initial placement of the nail. If the surgeon makes the initial bone defect too lateral in the greater trochanter, the nail may pass medially and impinge on the medial proximal femoral cortex, which causes a fracture. Alternatively, if the starting position is too anterior or posterior, comminution in the proximal femur may also occur. To avoid proximal comminution, careful attention should be paid to the initial placement of the nail and to correct reaming technique.

If proximal comminution occurs, a static lock is mandatory to prevent shortening or deformity. If this is done, there should be no problem following proximal comminution. The incidence of proximal comminution was 5 per cent over the first 3 years of femoral nailing in the author's centre, but with experience this figure has decreased considerably.

Pudendal nerve neuropraxia

When femoral fractures are reduced, countertraction is applied through the post on the orthopaedic table. A rare, but unpleasant, complication of excessive traction on the leg is a neuropraxia of the pudendal nerve. The most troublesome complication of this is anaesthesia of the scrotum and penis in the male and the labia majora and clitoris in the female. Fortunately, being a neuropraxia, the nerve damage is reversible and normal function usually returns after a few weeks. To avoid this complication, it is recommended that care be taken in positioning the patient on the orthopaedic table. Ideally the post should be placed so that it is in the groin opposite the side of the fracture. This ensures that the pudendal nerve on the side of the fracture is not being stretched excessively. The incidence of this complication in the author's centre is approximately 1.5 per cent but all cases have resolved spontaneously.

Gluteal pain

The most common reason for removal of a femoral nail is a persistent discomfort in the buttock during sitting. This is usually caused by deposition of bone around the proximal end of the nail and is relieved by removal of the bony deposit and the nail. Figure 23.17 shows a patient with bilateral gluteal discomfort on sitting.

If a nail is incorrectly inserted so that there is a considerable length of nail outside the bone, or if it migrates proximally after insertion, the bony deposition around the nail may be considerable. Figure 23.18a shows the bone laid down around a Küntscher nail that had migrated proximally but left in place for 10 years. The excised bony swelling is shown in Figure 23.18b. The patient was relieved of considerable buttock pain by its excision!

Complications of tibial nailing

Proximal comminution

The insertion of a straight tibial nail through an entry point on the anterior tibial cortex means that there are inevitably stresses on the anterior tibial cortex inferior to the entry point. As with femoral fractures, there may be comminution. The example in Figure 23.19 shows the upper tibia of a 64-year-old lady prior to the insertion of a tibial nail. Following nail insertion, a tongue of bone has been elevated from the anterior cortex. There was no significant instability and union occurred at 15 weeks.

Proximal comminution is more common and more important in proximal tibial fractures. If the entry point is close to the fracture there may be significant comminution which may be controlled by the insertion of the appropriate cross-screw, as shown in Figure 7.9a. The risk of proximal comminution is lessened by flexing the knee to at least 90 degrees during nailing. The straighter the knee, the greater the stresses on the anterior cortex of the tibia below the nail entry point and the higher the risk of proximal comminution. In nailing proximal fractures, the surgeon must always be aware of this potential problem and should be prepared to insert the lateral proximal cross-screw to control the fragments if necessary. A low entry point will also increase the risk of proximal comminution.

Neurological damage

Insertion of the distal cross-screws may cause damage to the sural or saphenous nerves, with numbness in the appropriate nerve distribution. This has occurred in about 2 per cent of patients in the author's centre and unfortunately has not responded to cross-screw removal.

Fracture site discoloration

As mobilization is easier and quicker than when using standard cast treatment, patients often regain mobility with virtually full weight bearing within a few weeks of surgery. Occasionally, full weight bearing is regained within 7–10 days and, when this occurs, a swollen discoloured area may appear on the skin overlying the fracture site (Figure 23.20). This is caused by an underlying subcutaneous haematoma which appears on the anteromedial border of the tibia. As it is warm to the touch, the question of infection may be raised, but the patient does not exhibit any other sequelae of infection and bone union is not delayed. The treatment is to restrict mobilization until the swelling and discoloration begin to settle. This usually takes 48 to 72 hours.

Knee pain

The most troublesome complication of closed tibial nailing is knee pain. This occurs in about 50 per cent of patients and is felt particularly on kneeling. The discomfort is such that in the author's centre, about 41 per cent of patients have had their tibial nails removed because of knee pain. If the nail is very prominent there may be actual restriction of knee extension, but this is unusual (Figure 23.21).

There does not appear to be a relationship between knee pain and damage to the patella tendon during insertion. The incidence of pain is the same if the nail is initially inserted to the medial side of the patella tendon or through the tendon. The nail should be hammered as far as possible into the tibia to minimize knee pain, but even if this is done, some patients will experience significant discomfort. The treatment is nail removal after fracture union, and in most cases this abolishes the discomfort.

Calcaneal pin insertion

Most surgeons rightly criticize the prolonged use of calcaneal traction. However, if the transfixion pin is only in place for an hour or so, there are virtually no complications, although care must be taken when positioning the pin to avoid neurovascular damage. One neuroma related to the transfixion pin has been encountered in Edinburgh.

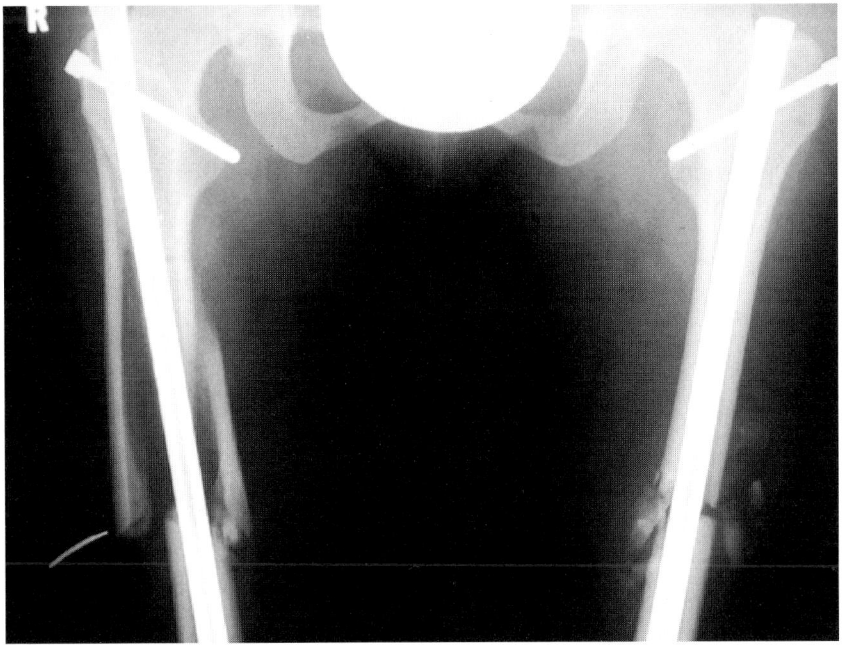

Figure 23.1

Bilateral closed femoral fractures in an 18-year-old female. The left femur was nailed in 40 degrees of external rotation. The mal-rotation is clearly seen by an examination of the width of the cortices above and below the fracture site. If the fracture is properly aligned, the cortical widths should be identical. If there is comminution, as in the right femur, it may be more difficult to rely on the cortical width to assess rotation.

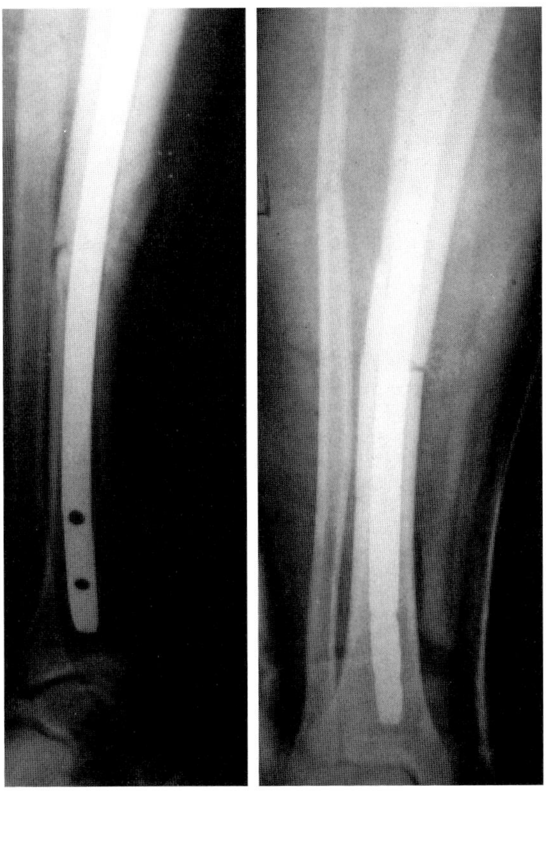

Figure 23.2

a A varus recurvatum deformity reproduced by incorrect placement of the guide wire and the surgeon leaning on the fracture site during nail insertion. Correct placement of the transfixion pins is very important when very distal femoral or tibial fractures are nailed.

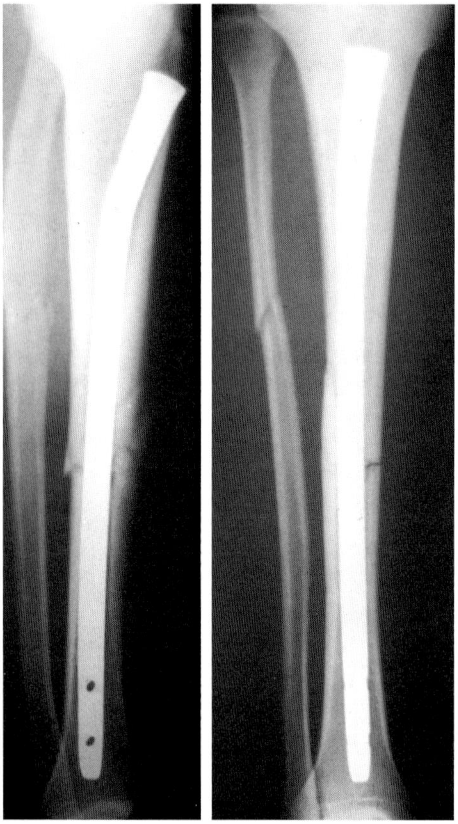

Figure 23.2 *continued*

b The patient was returned to the operating theatre and the original nail removed. After renailing, good alignment was achieved.

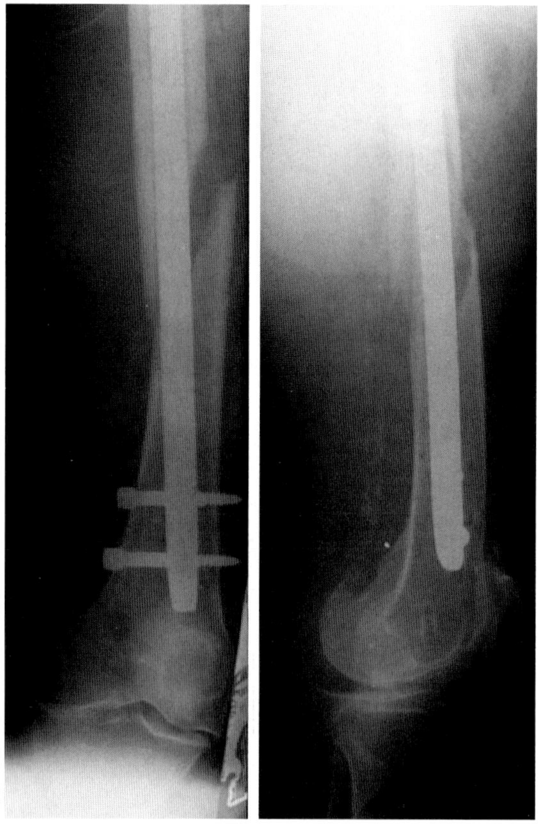

Figure 23.3

The surgeon should always remember that the nail will follow the guide wire. If the guide wire is incorrectly placed, then insertion of the nail may cause an angular deformity, as seen here. It is important, particularly in distal fractures, to centralize the guide wire in the distal fragment.

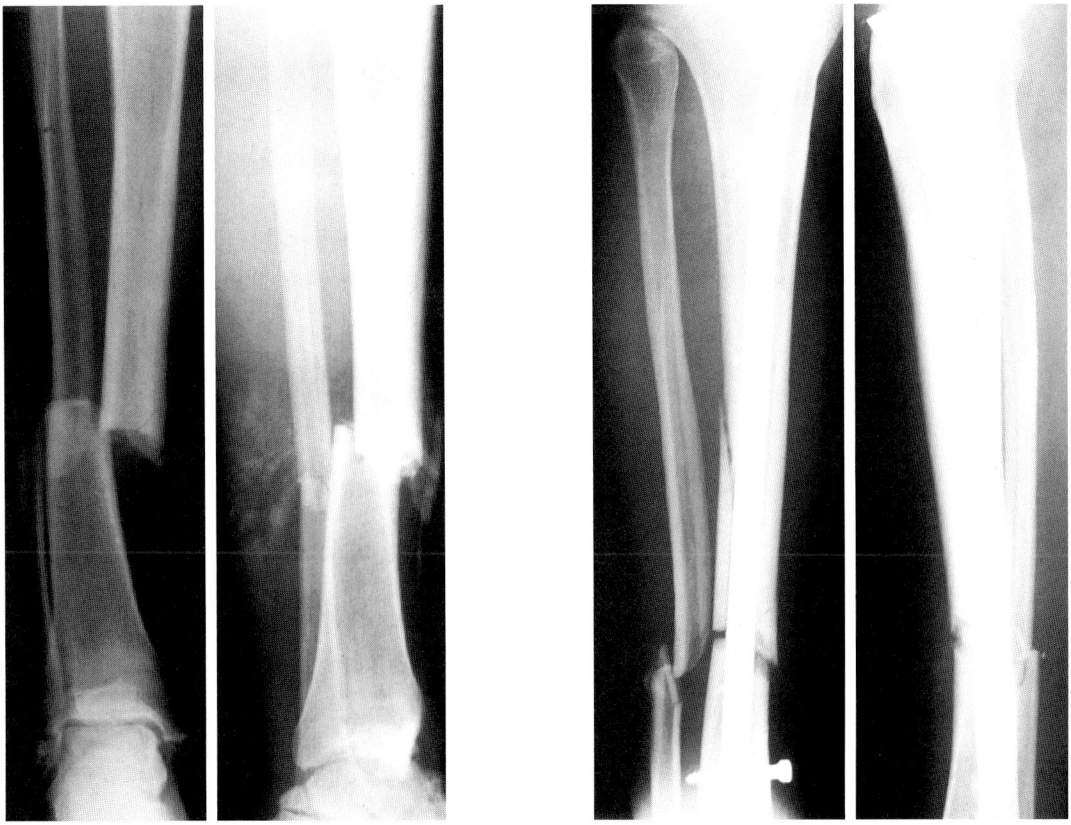

Figure 23.4

a A closed tibial fracture. Examination of the X-ray scan shows an undisplaced fracture on the medial side of the distal end of the proximal fragment. Even this degree of comminution is more safely treated with a statically locked nail as there may be other undisplaced fracture lines which will displace as the nail is passed down the diaphysis.

b In this case, the previously noted bone fragment has not displaced but a lateral bone fragment has. The surgeon has incorrectly treated this fracture with a distal dynamically locked nail. Had a proximal cross-screw been inserted at this stage, none of the subsequent problems would have occurred.

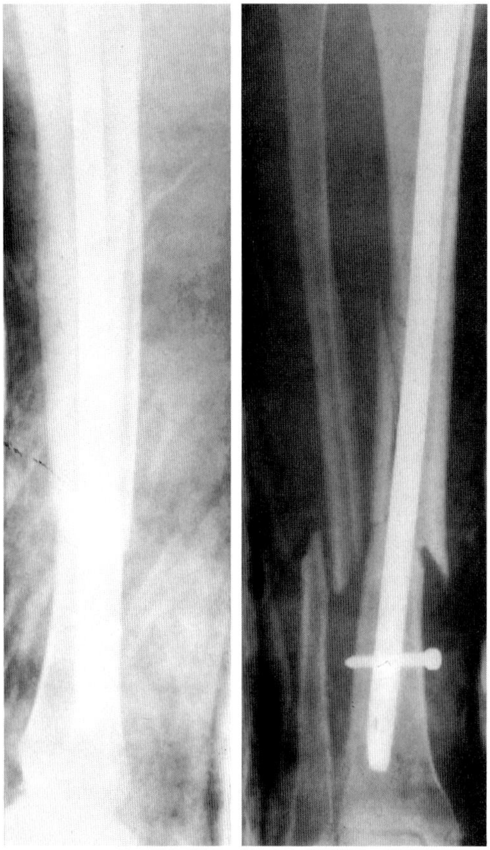

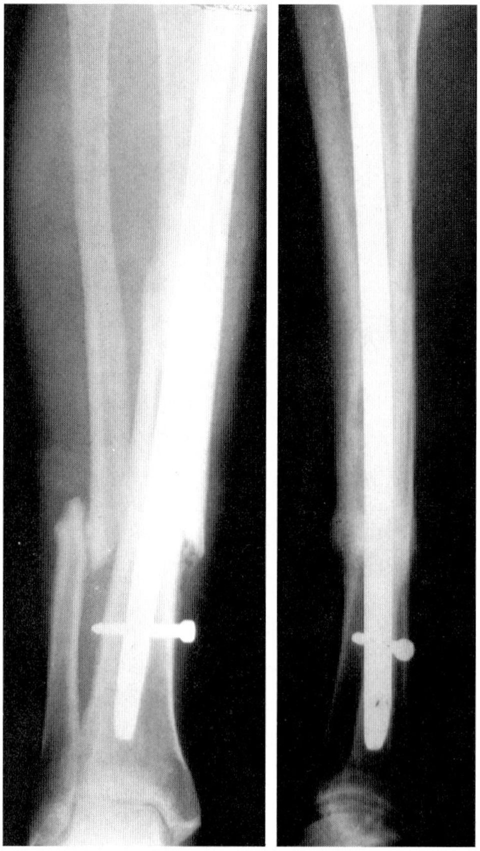

Figure 23.4 *continued*

c There has been displacement of the lateral bone fragment and shortening of the tibia. Even at this stage, a reasonable result could have been achieved if a proximal cross-screw had been inserted.

d Fracture union has occurred but there is marked shortening. This series of X-ray scans serves to highlight the requirement for a static lock if there is any doubt about the stability of the fracture.

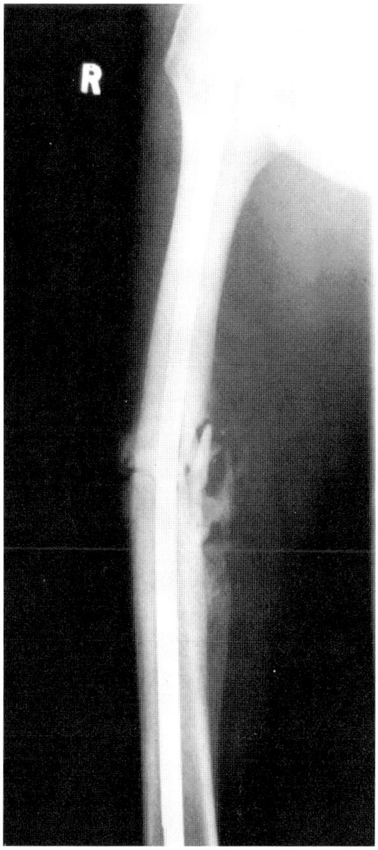

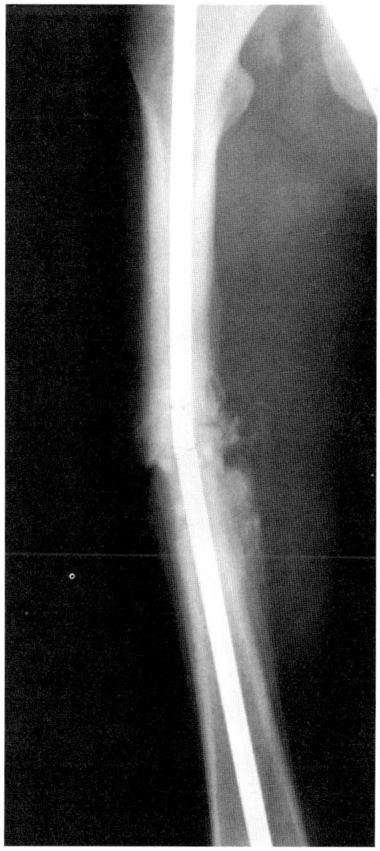

Figure 23.5

a A small diameter Küntscher nail used to stabilize a femoral diaphyseal fracture. The use of such nails is inappropriate as they frequently bend.

b Once the nail has bent, union of the fracture is unlikely and nail breakage is virtually inevitable. At this point, the two halves of the nail must be removed and an adequate intramedullary nail inserted.

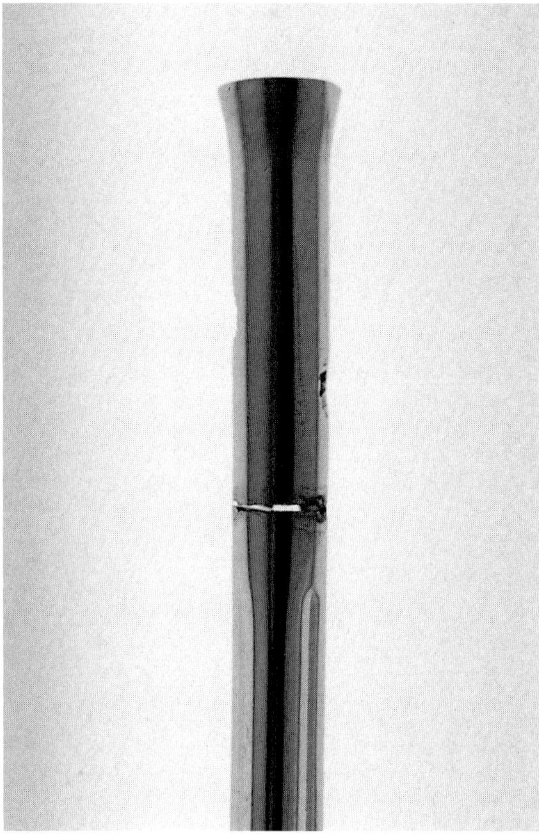

Figure 23.6

Failure of a Grosse-Kempf femoral nail at the junction of the solid and slotted portions of the nail. This problem is no longer seen as this area of the nail has been strengthened. However, surgeons may encounter old nails which have broken in this area. Removal of the proximal portion is easy, but removal of the distal part much more difficult.

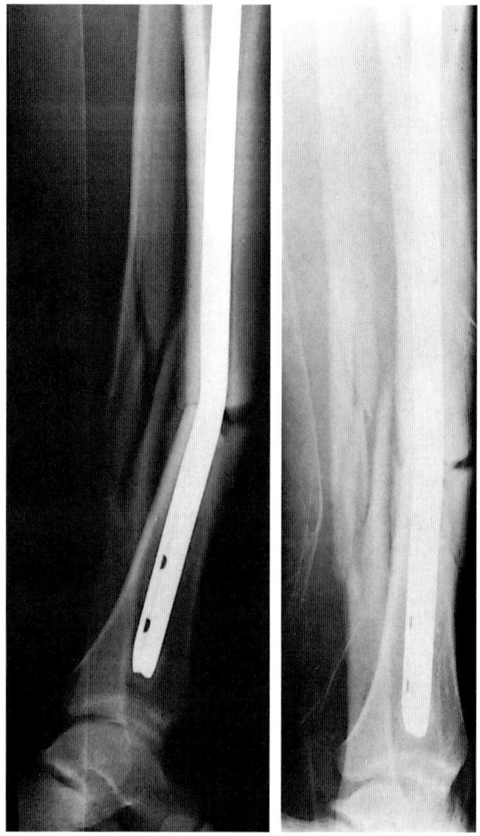

Figure 23.7

Bending of a Grosse-Kempf nail. The angle was reduced by approximately 50 per cent by the surgeon. This allowed the nail to be extracted in the usual manner and a new nail to be inserted.

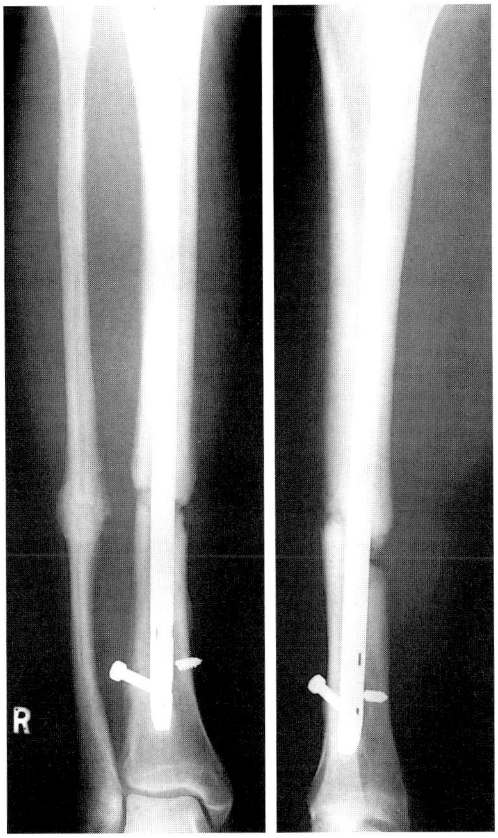

Figure 23.8

Cross-screw failure is rare. This distal cross-screw broke after 6 weeks. The two halves were removed and a new cross-screw inserted.

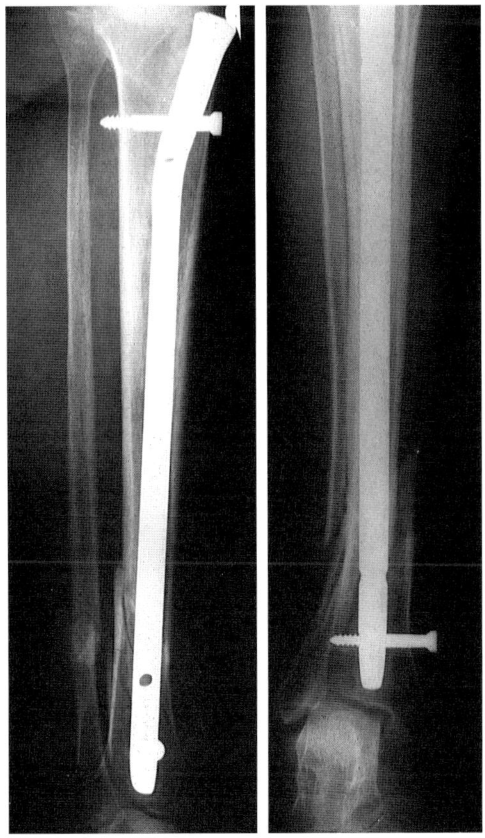

Figure 23.9

Despite the incomplete insertion of a number of cross-screws over the last 8-year period, failure of distal cross-screws to hold a distal fragment is extremely rare. In this case, however, the distal cross-screw did back out, allowing for displacement of the fracture. The bone was extremely osteoporotic. The distal cross-screws were removed and two more inserted. The fracture healed in correct alignment. Two distal screws should be used in osteoporotic bone.

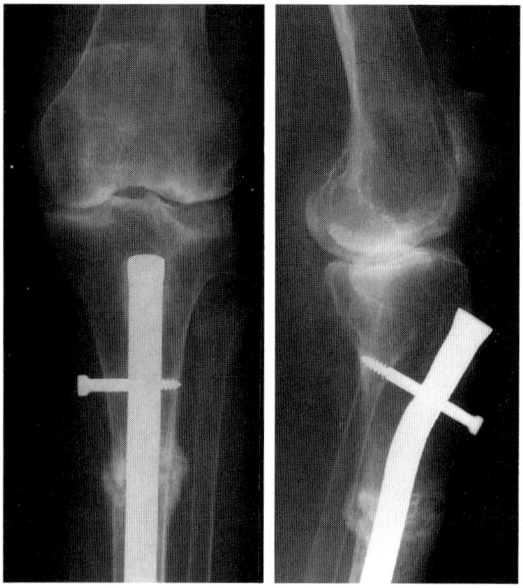

Figure 23.10

Cross-screws should be fully screwed home. If they are not, there may be irritation over the head of the screw. This is most common with the proximal antero-posterior screw of the tibial nail.

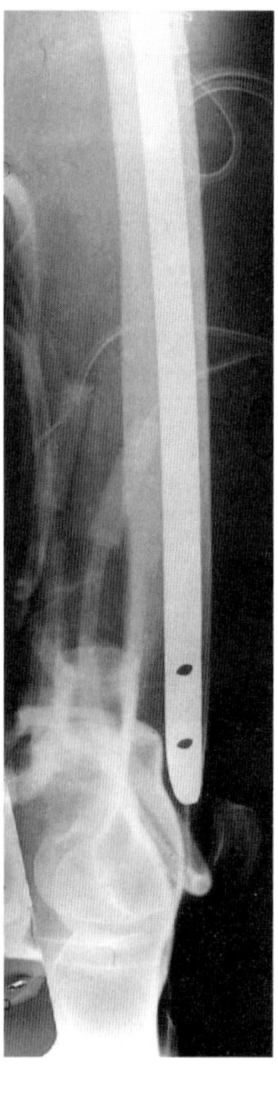

Figure 23.11

If osteoporotic or osteomalacic bone is being nailed, care must be taken not to breach the cortex. Here the guide wire was incorrectly placed and the distal end of the nail has breached the cortex anteriorly. Because of the danger of subsequent fracture, the patient was renailed.

Figure 23.12

There is frequently abundant callus formation associated with the use of intramedullary nails. Occasionally this can cause discomfort as in this case where normal quadriceps function was prevented. The callus mass was removed surgically.

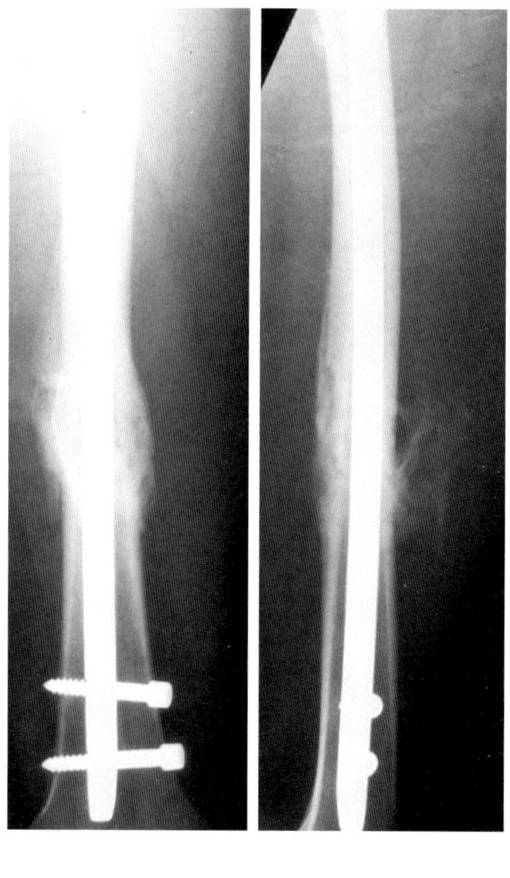

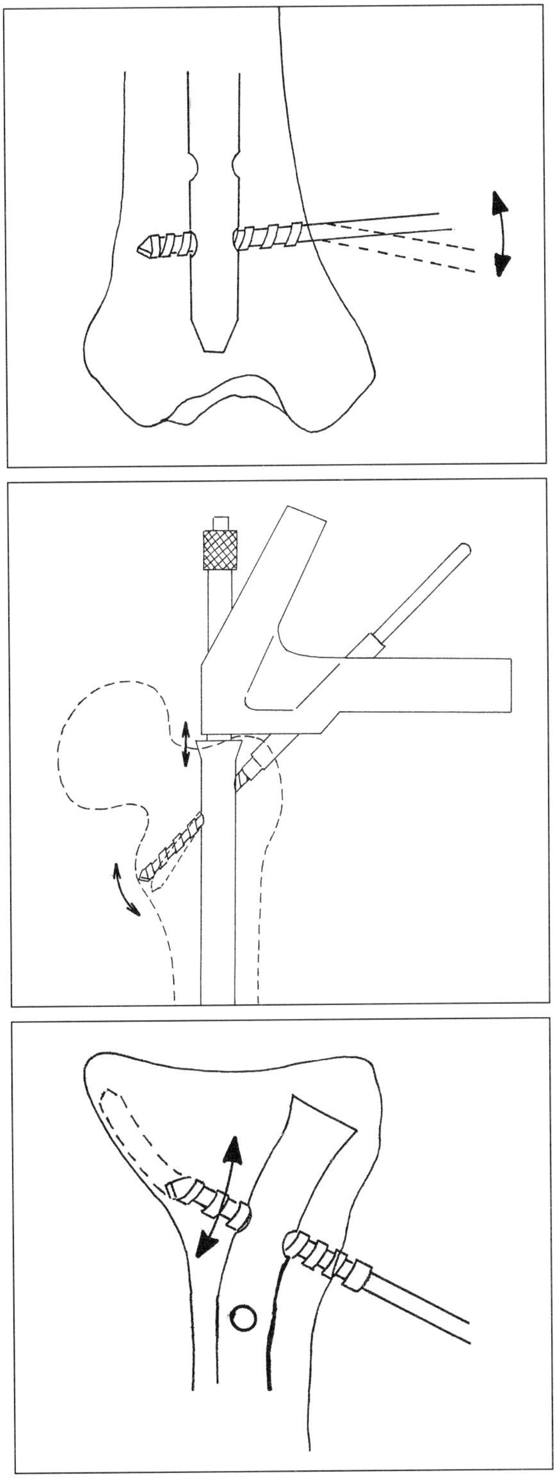

Figure 23.13

a A free-hand technique may be associated with breakage of drill bits during insertion of distal femoral and tibial cross-screws. This is shown diagrammatically here. The surgeon usually inserts the drill at an angle and, realizing this, attempts to straighten the drill bit after it has passed through the nail. This is clearly impossible and the result is a broken drill bit.

b If the proximal femoral or tibial jig is not tightly applied to the nail there is a tendency for the drill bit to bend as it passes through the proximal screw hole. Rotation of a bending drill causes breakage. It is important to make sure that the proximal jigs are tightly secured to the nail.

c If the antero-posterior proximal tibial screw is to be inserted, the drill bit may slide up the posterior cortex rather than pierce it. This happens if the drill bit is blunt.

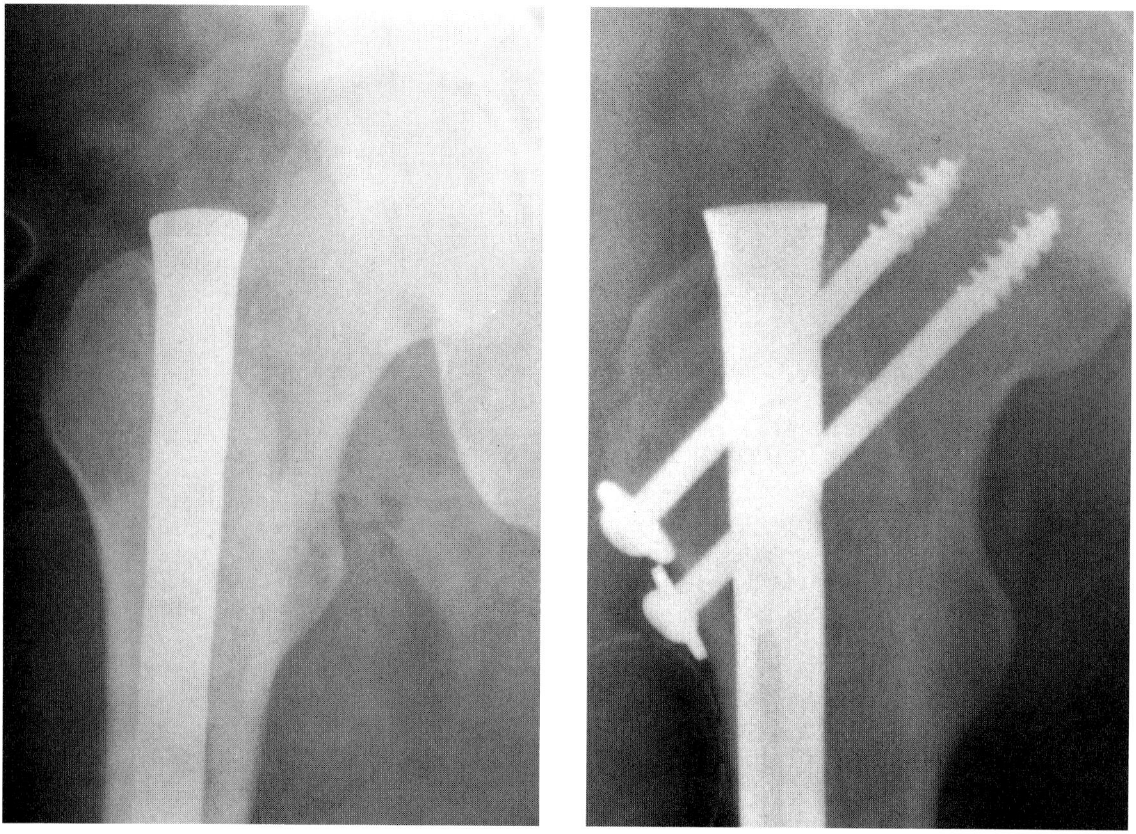

Figure 23.14

a A subcapital fracture associated with closed intramedullary nailing. Although subcapital fractures may occur in association with diaphyseal femoral fractures, pre-operative X-ray scans in this patient showed no evidence of fracture.

b These fractures are easily treated by the insertion of cancellous bone screws. They are inserted posterior to the intramedullary nail. Two screws adequately stabilize the fracture.

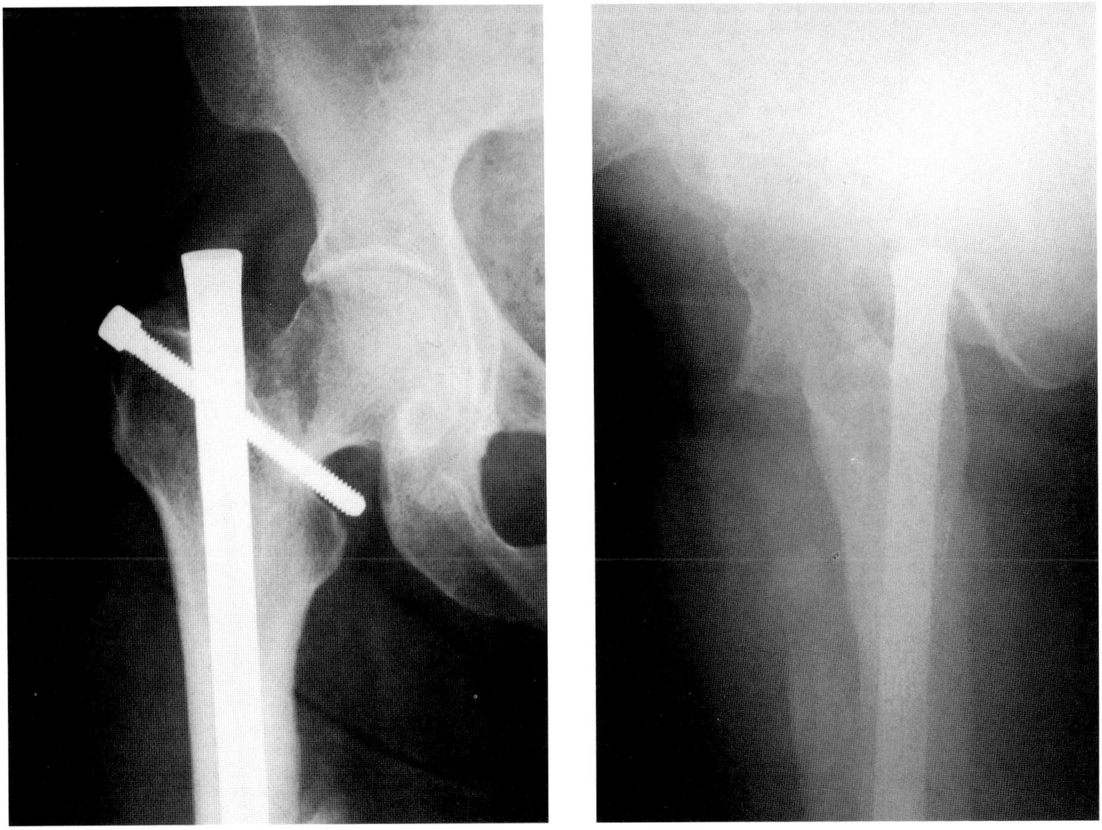

Figure 23.15

a If the femoral nail is not inserted fully into the femur, the proximal cross-screw may be inserted above the level of the lesser trochanter. Combined with an incorrect starting point, this may cause a femoral neck fracture.

b Examination of the lateral view suggests that, in this case, the starting point was somewhat anterior. The considerable displacement of the femoral neck fracture can be seen.

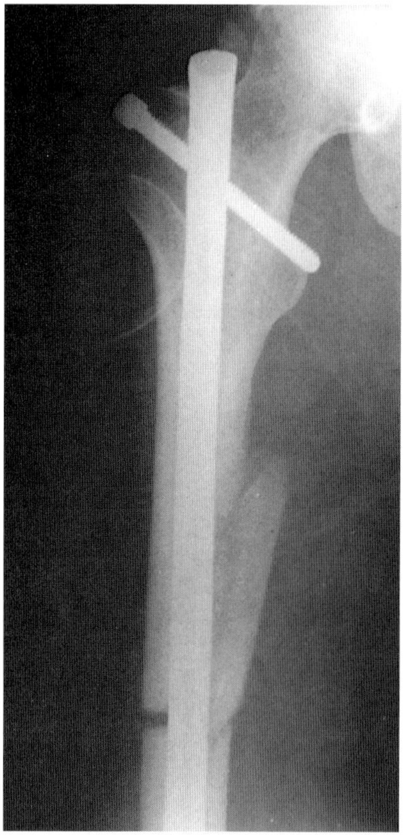

Figure 23.16

Incorrect placement of the starting point may also cause proximal comminution of the femur. This is rarely a problem provided the proximal comminution is located below the level of the lesser trochanter. A statically locked nail must be used.

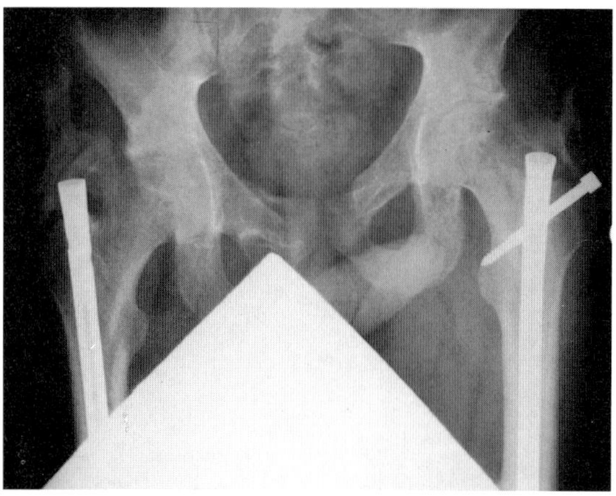

Figure 23.17

Calcification seen around the proximal ends of bilateral femoral nails. This is a common radiological appearance and may be associated with gluteal pain. The calcific deposits are usually excised at the time of nail removal.

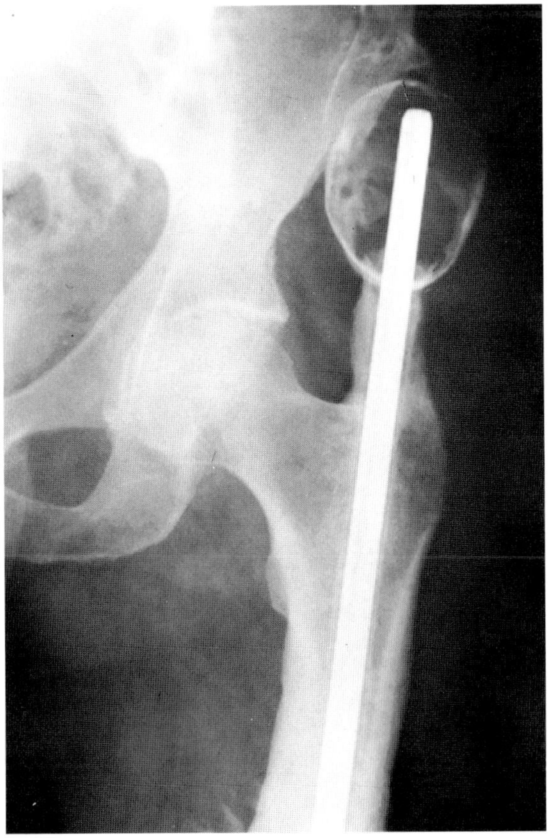

Figure 23.18

a A considerable quantity of bone may be laid down around the proximal end of the femoral nail. This Küntscher nail had been inserted 10 years earlier for a mid-diaphyseal femoral fracture but had migrated proximally.

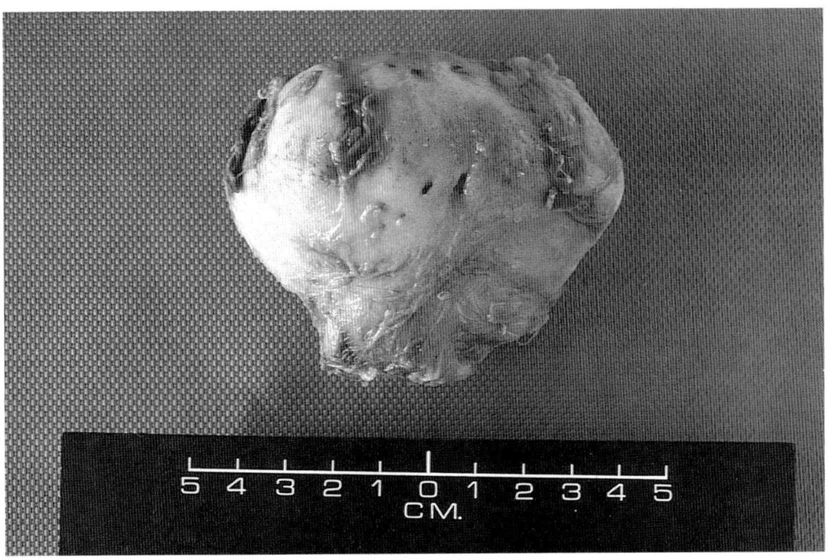

b The excised mass measured 9 cm by 6 cm.

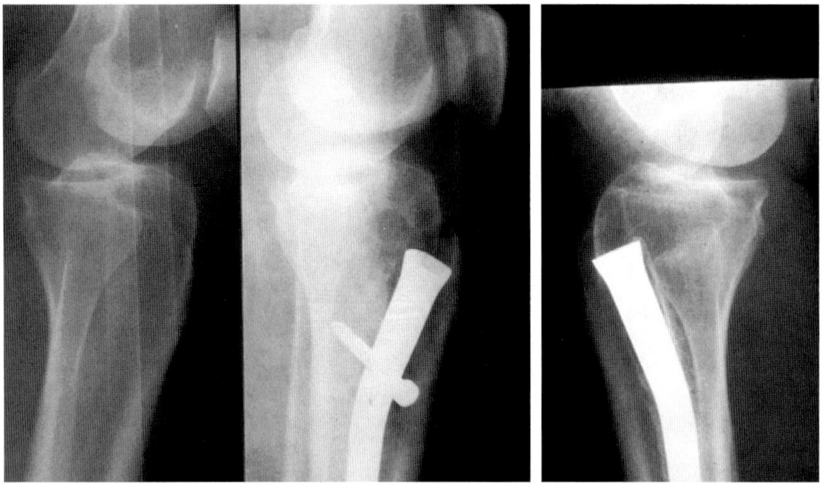

Figure 23.19

Proximal comminution of the tibia following nailing. A pre-operative lateral X-ray scan of the proximal tibia (left) shows no evidence of proximal fracture. Postoperatively (centre) there is a definite fracture but after healing of the tibial fracture, it is clear that the proximal comminution has also healed (right).

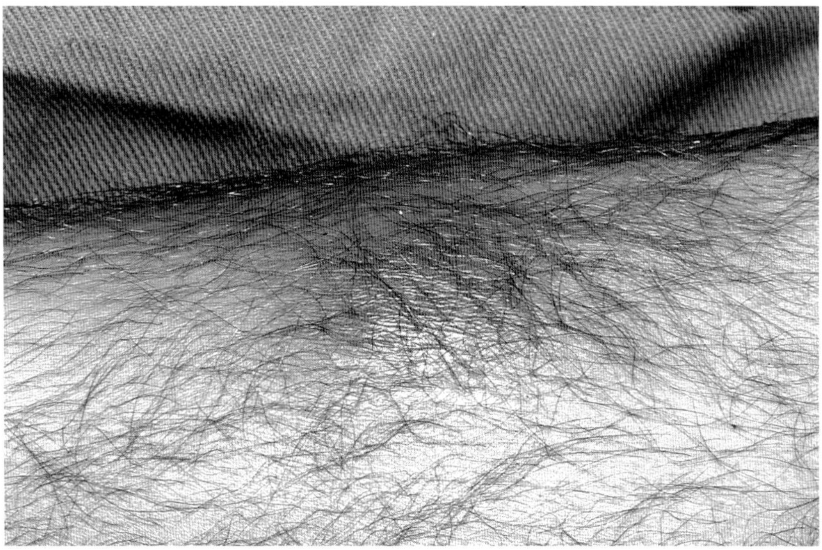

Figure 23.20

Swelling and redness adjacent to a tibial fracture. The clinical signs mimic those of infection but in fact represent a subcutaneous haematoma which resolves after a period of rest.

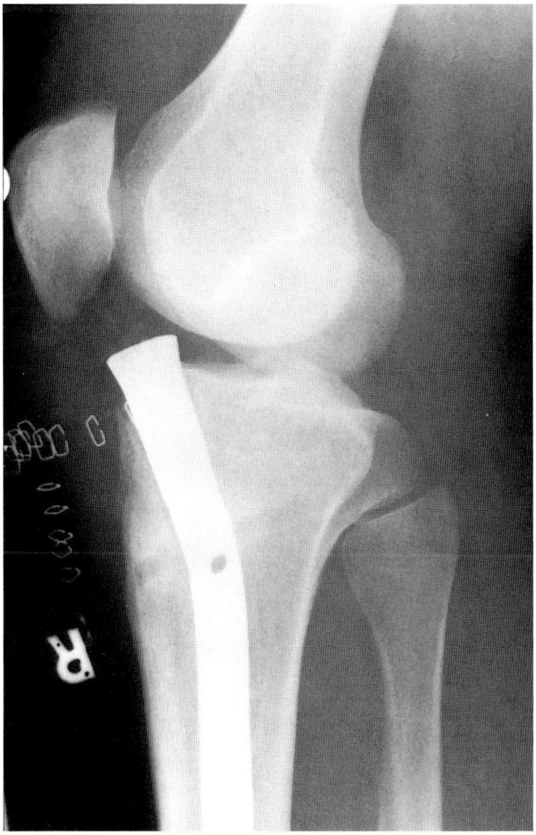

Figure 23.21

Knee pain may be associated with prominence of the tibial nail proximally. If the nail is very prominent there may be restriction of knee movement, as in this case. This degree of protrusion was produced by an unwise failure to replace the proximal cross-screw after exchange nailing of a Type IIIa fracture. The old screw track is clearly seen and is approximately 1 cm below the screw-hole. The patient was returned to the operating theatre and the nail position reduced by traction. A proximal cross-screw was then inserted.

SELECT READING

- Barron SE, Robb RA, Taylor WF et al, The effect of fixation with intramedullary rods and plates on fracture-site blood flow and bone remodelling in dogs, *J Bone Joint Surg* (1977) **59A**:376–85.
- Behr JT, Apel DM, Pinzur MS et al, Flexible intramedullary nails for ipsilateral femoral and tibial fractures, *J Trauma* (1987) **27**:1354–7.
- de Belder KRJ, Distal migration of the femoral intramedullary nail, *J Bone Joint Surg* (1968) **50B**:324–33.
- Böhler J, Percutaneous internal fixation utilizing the x-ray image amplifier, *J Trauma* (1965) **5**:150–61.
- Böhler J, Closed intramedullary nailing of the femur, *Clin Orthop* (1968) **60**:51–67.
- Bone LB, Johnson KD, Treatment of tibial fractures by reaming and intramedullary nailing, *J Bone Joint Surg* (1986) **68A**:877–87.
- Born CT, Delong WG, Shaikh KA, et al, Early use of the Brooker-Wills interlocking intramedullary nail (BWIIN) for femoral shaft fractures in acute trauma patients, *J Trauma* (1988) **28**:1515–22.
- Bostman O, Vainionpaa S, Saikku K, Infra-isthmal longitudinal fractures of the tibial diaphysis: results of treatment using closed intramedullary compression nailing, *J Trauma* (1984) **24**:964–9.
- Bostman A, Varjonen L, Vainionpaa S, et al, Incidence of local complications after intramedullary nailing and after plate fixation of femoral shaft fractures, *J Trauma* (1989) **29**:639–45.
- Brooker AF, Brumback RJ, Brooker-Wills nails in treatment of infra-isthmal injuries of the femur, *J Trauma* (1988) **28**:688–91.
- Browner BD, Pitfalls, errors, and complications in the use of locking Küntscher nails, *Clin Orthop* (1986) **212**:192–208.
- Browner, BD, Edwards CC, *The Science and Practice of Intramedullary Nailing* (Lea and Febiger: Philadelphia 1987).
- Brumback RJ, Reilly JP, Poka A, et al, Intramedullary nailing of femoral shaft fractures. Part I: Decision making errors with interlocking fixation, *J Bone Joint Surg* (1988) **70A**:1441–52.
- Brumback RJ, Uwagie-Ero S, Lakatos RP, et al, Intramedullary nailing of femoral shaft fractures. Part II. Fracture healing with static interlocking fixation, *J Bone Joint Surg* (1989) **71A**:1324–31.
- Chadwick CJ, Hayes AG, Treatment of femoral shortening after medullary nailing, *Injury* (1988) **19**:35–8.
- Chan K-M, Leung Y-K, Cheng J-C-Y, et al, The management of type III open tibial fractures, *Injury* (1984) **16**:157–65.
- Chan KM, Tse PYT, Chow YYN, et al, Closed medullary nailing for fractured shaft of the femur – a comparison between the Küntscher and the AO techniques, *Injury* (1984) **15**:381–7.
- Chapman MW, Closed intramedullary bone-grafting and nailing of segmental defects of the femur: a report on three cases, *J Bone Joint Surg* (1980) **62A**:1004–8.

- Chapman MW, The role of intramedullary fixation in open fractures, *Clin Orthop* (1986) **212**:26–34.
- Christie J, Court-Brown CM, Femoral neck fracture during closed medullary nailing: brief report, *J Bone Joint Surg* (1988) **70B**:670.
- Christie J, Court-Brown CM, Howie CR, et al, Intramedullary locking nails in the management of femoral shaft fractures, *J Bone Joint Surg* (1988) **70B**:206–10.
- Cierny G, Byrd HS, Jones RE, Primary versus delayed soft tissue coverage for severe open tibial fractures: a comparison of results, *Clin Orthop* (1983) **178**:54–63.
- Clancy EJ, Winquist RA, Hansen ST, Non-union of the tibia treated with Küntscher intramedullary nailing, *Clin Orthop* (1982) **167**:191–6.
- Clifford RP, Beauchamp CG, Kellam JF et al, Plate fixation of open fractures of the tibia, *J Bone Joint Surg* (1988) **70B**:644–8.
- Court-Brown CM, Christie J, McQueen MM, Closed intramedullary tibial nailing. Its use in closed and Type I open fractures, *J Bone Joint Surg* (1990) **72B**:605–11.
- Court-Brown CM, McQueen MM, Compartment syndrome delays clinical union, *Acta Orthop Scand* (1987) **58**:249–52.
- Court-Brown CM, Wheelwright EF, Christie J et al, External skeletal fixation in the management of type III open tibial fractures, *J Bone Joint Surg* (1990) **72B**:801–4.
- Denker, M, Technical problems of medullary nailing: a study of 435 nailed shaft fractures of the femur, *Acta Chir Scand* (1965) **130**:185–9.
- Donald G, Seligson D, Treatment of tibial shaft fractures by percutaneous Küntscher nailing: technical difficulties and a review of 50 consecutive cases, *Clin Orthop* (1983) **178**:64–73.
- Dugpace TW, Schutzer SF, Deafenbaugh MK, et al, Compartment syndrome complicating the use of the hemi-lithotomy position during femoral nailing. A report on two cases, *J Bone Joint Surg* (1989) **71A**:1556–7.
- Ekeland A, Thoreson BO, Alho A, et al, Interlocking intramedullary nailing in the treatment of tibial fractures: a report on 45 cases, *Clin Orthop* (1988) **231**:205–15.
- Franklin JL, Winquist RA, Benirschke SK, et al, Broken intramedullary nails, *J Bone Joint Surg* (1988) **70A**:1463–71.
- Gustilo RB, Anderson JT, Presentation of infection in the treatment of one thousand and twenty-five open fractures of long bones, *J Bone Joint Surg* (1976) **58A**:453–8.
- Gustilo RB, Mendoza RM, Williams DN, Problems in the management of Type III (severe) open fractures: a new classification of Type III open fractures, *J Trauma* (1984) **24**:742–6.
- Hæger K, *The Illustrated History of Surgery* (Starke: London 1988).
- Hanks GA, Foster WC, Cardea JA, Treatment of femoral shaft fractures with the Brooker-Wills interlocking intramedullary nail, *Clin Orthop* (1988) **226**:206–18.
- Hansen ST, Winquist RA, Closed intramedullary nailing of the femur. Küntscher technique with reaming, *Clin Orthop* (1979) **138**:56–61.
- Harper MC, Fractures of the femur treated by open and closed intramedullary nailing using the fluted rod, *J Bone Joint Surg* (1985) **67A**:659–708.
- Harper MC, Carson WL, Curvature of the femur and the proximal entry point for an intramedullary rod, *Clin Orthop* (1987) **220**:155–61.
- Harper MC, Henstorf J, Fractures of the femoral neck associated with technical errors in closed intramedullary nailing of the femur: report on two cases, *J Bone Joint Surg* (1986) **68A**:624–6.
- Henley MB, Intramedullary devices for tibial fracture stabilisation, *Clin Orthop* (1989) **240**:87–96.
- Hey Groves EW, Some clinical and experimental observations on the operative treatment of fractures, with especial reference to the use of intramedullary pegs, *Br Med J* (1912) **2**:1102–5.
- Hindley CJ, Closed medullary nailing for recent fractures of the tibia, *Injury* (1988) **19**:180–4.
- Hofmann A, Jones RE, Schoenvogel R, Pudendal nerve neuropraxis as a result of traction on the fracture table: a report on four cases, *J Bone Joint Surg* (1982) **64A**:136–8.
- Hooper GJ, Lyon DW, Closed unlocked nailing for comminuted femoral fractures, *J Bone Joint Surg* (1988) **70B**:619–21.
- Huckstep RL, The Huckstep intramedullary compression nail, *Clin Orthop* (1986) **212**:48–61.
- Huckstep RL, Stabilisation and prosthetic replacement in difficult fractures and bone tumours, *Clin Orthop* (1987) **224**:12–25.
- Hunter SG, Deformation of femoral intramedullary nails: a clinical study, *Clin Orthop* (1982) **171**:83–6.
- Incavo SJ, Kristiansen TK, Retrieval of a broken intramedullary nail, *Clin Orthop* (1986) **210**:201–2.

- Johnson KD, Johnston DWS, Parker B, Comminuted femoral shaft fractures: treatment by roller traction, cerclage wires and an intramedullary nail or an interlocking intramedullary nail, *J Bone Joint Surg* (1984) **66A**:1222–35.
- Johnston EE, Marder RA, Open intramedullary nailing and bone grafting for non-union of tibial diaphyseal fracture, *J Bone Joint Surg* (1987) **69A**:375–80.
- Kempf I, Grosse A, Abalo C, Locked intramedullary nailing: its application to femoral and tibial rotational, lengthening and shortening osteotomies, *Clin Orthop* (1986) **212**:165–73.
- Kempf I, Grosse A, Beck G, Closed locked intramedullary nailing: its application to comminuted fractures of the femur, *J Bone Joint Surg* (1985) **67A**:709–20.
- Kempf I, Grosse A, Rigaut P, The treatment of non-infected pseudarthrosis of the femur and tibia with locked intramedullary nailing, *Clin Orthop* (1986) **212**:142–54.
- Ker NB, Maempel FZ, Paton DF, Bone cement as an adjunct to medullary nailing in fractures of the distal third of the femur in elderly patients, *Injury* (1984) **16**:102–7.
- Klemm K, Die Stabilisierung infizierter Pseudarthrosen mit dem Verriegelungsnagel, *Langenbecks Arch Chir* (1973) **334**:595–666.
- Klemm KW, Treatment of infected pseudarthrosis of the femur and tibia with an interlocking nail, *Clin Orthop* (1986) **212**:174–81.
- Klemm KW, Borner M, Interlocking nailing of complex fractures of the femur and tibia, *Clin Orthop* (1986) **212**:89–100.
- Kovacs AJ, Richard LB, Miller J, Infection complicating intramedullary nailing of the fractured femur, *Clin Orthop* (1973) **96**:266–70.
- Kunex JR, Lewis RJ, Closed intramedullary rodding of pathological fractures with supplemental cement, *Clin Orthop* (1984) **188**:183–6.
- Küntscher G, Die Marknagelung von Knochenbruchen, *Langenbecks Arch Chir* (1940) **200**:443–55.
- Küntscher G, The Küntscher method of intramedullary fixation, *J Bone Joint Surg* (1958) **40A**:17–26.
- Küntscher G, *Practice of intramedullary nailing* (CC Thomas: Springfield 1967).
- Leighton RK, Waddell JP, Kellam JF, et al, Open versus closed intramedullary nailing of femoral shaft fractures, *J Trauma* (1986) **26**:923–6.
- Levin PE, Schoen RW, Browner BD, Radiation exposure to the surgeon during closed interlocking intramedullary nailing, *J Bone Joint Surg* (1987) **69A**:761–5.
- Lidgren L, Onnerfalt R, Infected non-union of the tibial shaft treated by Küntscher intramedullary reaming and nail fixation, *Acta Orthop Scand* (1982) **53**:669–74.
- Lidgren L, Torholm C, Intramedullary reaming in chronic diaphyseal osteomyelitis: a preliminary report, *Clin Orthop* (1980) **152**:215–21.
- Lindenbaum SD, Fleming LL, Smith, DW, Pudendal nerve palsies associated with closed intramedullary femoral fixation, *J Bone Joint Surg* (1982) **64A**:934–8.
- Lottes JO, Treatment of fractures of the femur with a heavy, large cored three-flanged medullary nail, *Surgery* (1951) **29**:868–84.
- Lottes JO, Medullary nailing of the tibia with the Triflange nail, *Clin Orthop* (1974) **105**:253–66.
- Maatz R, Lentz W, Arens W, et al, *Intramedullary Nailing and Other Intramedullary Osteosyntheses* (WB Saunders: Philadelphia 1986).
- Macausland WR, Medullary nailing of the fractures of the long bones, *Surg Gynecol Obstet* (1947) **84**:85–9.
- MacAusland WS, Eaton RG, The management of sepsis following intramedullary fixation for fractures of the femur, *J Bone Joint Surg* (1963) **45A**:1643–53.
- McGraw JM, Lim EVA, Treatment of open tibial shaft fractures. External fixation and secondary intramedullary nailing, *J Bone Joint Surg* (1988) **70A**:900–11.
- MacMillan M, Grosse RH, A simplified technique of distal femoral screw insertion for the Grosse-Kempf interlocking nail, *Clin Orthop* (1988) **226**:252–9.
- McQueen MM, Christie J, Court-Brown CM, Compartment pressures after intramedullary nailing of the tibia, *J Bone Joint Surg* (1990) **72B**:395–7.
- Marks PH, Paley D, Kellam JF, Heterotopic ossification around the hip with intramedullary nailing of the femur, *J Trauma* (1988) **28**:1207–13.
- Matsen FA, *Compartmental Syndromes* (Grune and Stratton: New York 1980).
- Matsen FA, Winquist RA, Krugmire RB, Diagnosis and management of compartmental syndromes, *J Bone Joint Surg* (1980) **62A**:286–91.
- Maurer DJ, Merkow RL, Gustilo RB, Infection after intramedullary nailing of severe open tibial fractures initially treated with external fixation, *J Bone Joint Surg* (1989) **71A**:835–8.

- Medinov®, *Charactéristiques et mode opératoire du clou centromédullaire pour femur et pour tibia* (Medinov®: Roanne 1990).
- Medoff RJ, Insertion of the distal screws in interlocking nail fixation of femoral shaft fractures: technical note, *J Bone Joint Surg* (1986) **68A**:1275–7.
- Melis GC, Sotgia F, Lepori M, et al, Intramedullary nailing in segmental tibial fractures, *J Bone Joint Surg* (1981) **63A**:1310–18.
- Merianos P, Cambouridis P, Smyrnis P, The treatment of 143 tibial shaft fractures by Ender nailing and early weight bearing, *J Bone Joint Surg* (1985) **67B**:576–80.
- Merle D'Aubigne R, Maurer P, Zucman J, et al, Blind intramedullary nailing for tibial fractures, *Clin Orthop* (1974) **105**:267–75.
- Miller ME, Ada JR, Webb LX, Treatment of infected non-union and delayed union of tibia fractures with locking intramedullary nails, *Clin Orthop* (1989) **245**:233–8.
- Miller ME, Davis ML, MacClean CR, et al, Radiation exposure and associated risks to operating-room personnel during the use of fluoroscopic guidance for selected orthopaedic surgical procedures, *J Bone Joint Surg* (1983) **65A**:1–4.
- Moran CG, Gibson MJ, Cross AT, Intramedullary locking nails for femoral shaft fractures in elderly patients, *J Bone Joint Surg* (1990) **72B**:19–22.
- Mubarak SJ, Hargens AR, *Compartment Syndromes and Volkmann's Contracture* (WB Saunders: Philadelphia 1981).
- Murphy CP, D'Ambrosia R, Dabezies EJ, et al, Complex femur fractures: treatment with the Wagner external fixation device of the Grosse-Kempf interlocking nail, *J Trauma* (1988) **28**:1553–62.
- Olerud S, Karlstrom G, The spectrum of intramedullary nailing of the tibia, *Clin Orthop* (1986) **212**:101–12.
- Owen R, Tsimboukis B, Ischaemia complicating closed tibial and fibular shaft fractures, *J Bone Joint Surg* (1967) **49B**:268–75.
- Pankovich AM, Adjunctive fixation in flexible intramedullary nailing of femoral fractures: a study of twenty-six cases, *Clin Orthop* (1981) **157**:301–9.
- Pankovich AM, Tarabishy IE, Yelda S, Flexible intramedullary nailing of tibial shaft fractures, *Clin Orthop* (1981) **160**:185–95.
- Papagiannopoulos G, Stewart HD, Lunn PG, Treatment of subtrochanteric fractures of the femur: a study of intramedullary compression nailing, *Injury* (1989) **20**: 106–10.
- Patzakis MJ, Wilkins J, Wise DA, Infection following intramedullary nailing of long bones, *Clin Orthop* (1986) **212**:182–91.
- Rand JA, An KN, Chao EYS et al, A comparison of the effect of open intramedullary nailing and compression-plate fixation on fracture-site blood flow and fracture union, *J Bone Joint Surg* (1981) **63A**:427–42.
- Rao JP, Allegra MP, Benevenia J, et al, Distal screw targeting of interlocking nails, *Clin Orthop* (1989) **238**:245–8.
- Rorabeck CH, The treatment of compartment syndromes of the leg, *J Bone Joint Surg* (1984) **66B**:93–7.
- Rorabeck CH, Castle GSP, Hardie R, et al, Compartmental pressure measurements: an experimental investigation using the slit catheter, *J Trauma* (1981) **21**:446–9.
- Rhinelander FW, Phillips RS, Steel WM, et al, Microangiography in bone healing. II: Displaced closed fractures, *J Bone Joint Surg* (1968) **50A**:643–62.
- Rush LV, *An Atlas of Rush Pin Techniques* (The Berivon Company: Meridian 1955).
- Rush LV, Rush HL, A technique for longitudinal pin fixation of certain fractures of the ulna and of the femur, *J Bone Joint Surg* (1939) **21**:619–26.
- Schwartz JT, Brumback RJ, Lakatos R, et al, Acute compartment syndrome of the thigh, *J Bone Joint Surg* (1989) **71A**:392–400.
- Seligson D, *Concepts in Intramedullary Nailing* (Grune and Stratton: Orlando, Florida 1985).
- Soeur R, Intramedullary pinning of diaphyseal fractures, *J Bone Joint Surg* (1946) **28A**:309–31.
- Søjberg JO, Eiskjaer S, Møller-Larsen F, Locked nailing of comminuted and unstable fractures of the femur, *J Bone Joint Surg* (1990) **72B**:23–5.
- Star AM, Whittaker RP, Schuster HM et al, Difficulties during removal of fluted femoral intramedullary rods, *J Bone Joint Surg* (1989) **71A**: 341–4.
- Stothard J, Sinha BMK, Maughan PA, Double fractures of AO intramedullary femoral nails, *Injury* (1989) **20**:119–21.
- Strachan RK, McCarthy I, Fleming R et al, The role of the tibial nutrient artery, *J Bone Joint Surg* (1990) **72B**:391–4.
- Sugarman ID, Adam I, Bunker ID, Radiation dosage during AO locking femoral nailing, *Injury* (1988) **19**:336–8.

- Thoreson BO, Alho A, Ekeland A, et al, Interlocking intramedullary nailing in femoral shaft fractures. A report of forty-eight cases, *J Bone Joint Surg* (1985) **67A**:1313–20.
- Trueta J, Cavidias AX, Vascular changes caused by the Küntscher type of nailing, *J Bone Joint Surg* (1955) **37B**:492–505.
- Tscherne H, Haas N, Krettek C, Intramedullary nailing combined with cerclage wiring in the treatment of fractures of the femoral shaft, *Clin Orthop* (1986) **212**:62–7.
- Velazco A, Whitesides TE, Fleming LL, Open fractures of the tibia treated with the Lottes nail, *J Bone Joint Surg* (1983) **65A**:879–85.
- Walters J, Shepherd-Wilson W, Lyons T, et al, Femoral shaft fractures treated by Ender nails using a trochanteric approach, *J Bone Joint Surg* (1990) **72B**:14–18.
- Watson-Jones R, Bonnin JG, King T, et al, Medullary nailing of fractures after fifty years with a review of the deficiencies and complications of the operation, *J Bone Joint Surg* (1950) **32B**:694–729.
- Webb LX, Winquist RA, Hansen ST, Intramedullary nailing and reaming for delayed or non-union of the femoral shaft, *Clin Orthop* (1986) **212**:133–41.
- Weinstein AM, Clemow AJT, Starkebaum W et al, Retrieval and analysis of intramedullary rods, *J Bone Joint Surg* (1981) **63A**:1443–8.
- Weller S, Kuner E, Schweikert CH, Medullary nailing according to Swiss study group principles, *Clin Orthop* (1979) **138**:45–55.
- White GM, Healy WL, Brumback RJ, et al, The treatment of fractures of the femoral shaft with the Brooker-Wills distal locking intramedullary nail, *J Bone Joint Surg* (1986) **68A**:865–76.
- Winquist RA, Closed intramedullary osteotomies of the femur, *Clin Orthop* (1986) **212**:155–64.
- Winquist RA, Hansen ST, Clawson DK, Closed intramedullary nailing of femoral fractures: a report of five hundred and twenty cases, *J Bone Joint Surg* (1984) **66A**:529–39.
- Wiss DA, Flexible medullary nailing of acute tibial shaft fractures, *Clin Orthop* (1986) **212**:122–32.
- Wiss DA, Fleming CH, Matta JM, et al, Comminuted and rotationally unstable fractures of the femur treated with an interlocking nail, *Clin Orthop* (1986) **212**:35–47.
- Yoslow W, Lamont JG, Alternative method for removing an impacted AO intramedullary nail, *Clin Orthop* (1986) **202**:237–8.
- Zimmerman KW, Klasen HJ, Mechanical failure of intramedullary nails after fracture union, *J Bone Joint Surg* (1983) **65B**:274–5.
- Zucman J, Maurer P, Primary medullary nailing of the tibia for fractures of the shaft in adults, *Injury* (1970) **2**:84–92.

Sources

The author wishes to acknowledge Howmedica Ltd for their kind permission to reproduce Figures 6.4 and 20.3.

INDEX

BOXN|+|+|+|+|+|+|+

BOOKS 27+32+29+32+32+14+